Advance Praise for *Sound Mind, Sound Body*

"*Sound Mind, Sound Body* is a profound exploration of the nature of health in its widest sense, and healing in its many dimensions. Beyond that, it is a guide to the well-lived life, a clarion call for meaning, purpose, and values as the centerpiece of true success and satisfaction. Kenneth Pelletier has rendered us all a service."

—DANIEL GOLEMAN, coeditor, *Mind/Body Medicine*

"For more than twenty years, Dr. Pelletier has pioneered the creation of the field of mind/body medicine and optimal health. In *Sound Mind, Sound Body,* he extends his groundbreaking research even further by providing us with living prototypes of prominent individuals and their lifestyle practices, pointing the way toward greater lifelong good health for everyone. This is truly a landmark book of the greatest importance."

—MICHAEL MURPHY, founder, Esalen Institute, author of *Future of the Body*

"Dr. Pelletier's research on highly successful people indicates that optimal health depends on much more than what you eat, how you exercise, and what vitamins you take. In particular, it involves how connected you are to other people, how you define purpose in your life, and how much you devote yourself to improving the welfare of others. *Sound Mind, Sound Body* is an excellent demonstration of the first principle of holistic medicine: We are more than just physical bodies."

—ANDREW T. WEIL, M.D., author of *Health and Healing* and *Natural Health, Natural Medicine*

"It is refreshing to hear a voice in our national health dialogue that speaks from clinical data in support of the premise that healthy folks are simultaneously anchored inwardly to spiritual roots, and outwardly to their community through compassion."

—RAM DASS, author of *Be Here Now*

"Dr. Pelletier goes beyond the familiar wellness guidelines to delve deeply into the essential inner lives. ill----- -- -'---'-- -----sonal challenges, and individualized he dozen highly prominent people. A fascinating and profoundly useful book."

"Dr. Pelletier's new book is by far his best and most important. He totally reframes our conceptions of what health is all about. When I turned the last page over, I was overcome with that rare epiphany: an understanding of health. And for someone approaching 70, that's seminal—and life-giving. Unless the Clinton administration takes Pelletier's book into account—seriously so—I'm afraid the only reforms we'll get will be cosmetic."

"*Sound Mind, Sound Body* is a lucid summary of the evidence that a sound mind not only inhabits but helps produce a sound body. Ken Pelletier makes it clear how mind and body can interact to foster good health. This book is an excellent overview of what is new and worth knowing in mind/body medicine."

"*Sound Mind, Sound Body* is a remarkable book—beautifully written, documented, and reasoned. The theme of 'broken bones heal strongest' offers a much-needed antidote to the cultural whine that traumatic or difficult periods of life need weaken the body and mind. The methods described for responding to and resolving traumatic incidents are extremely practical. And the interweaving of relevant and pithy comments from 53 exceptional individuals into a logical and nonrepetitive sequence is itself a tour de force."

"In this impressive examination of health in America, Ken Pelletier argues convincingly that to achieve optimal mental and physical health, we must devote fewer resources to strategies aimed at avoiding or treating disease and more toward creating a *health*-care system that fosters a deep and abiding sense of purpose and genuine caring about others. With its broad-ranging and

comprehensive review of mind-body research and fascinating stories of extraordinary people who have succeeded in this quest, this book will help many to do likewise. Pelletier's message, if heeded, will dramatically improve our individual and national robustness."
—REDFORD WILLIAMS, M.D., Director, Behavioral Medicine Research Center at Duke University; coauthor, *Anger Kills: Seventeen Strategies for Controlling the Hostility That Can Harm Your Health*

"Dr. Ken Pelletier describes the cutting edge of mind/body research while exploring the motivations, world views, and struggles of highly successful people to give an extremely interesting and human perspective on health and illness, reminding us that it's not the challenges we face as much as how we cope with them that ultimately influences our health and the quality of our lives. This book will truly inspire people to change their lives."
—JON KABAT-ZINN, Ph.D., Director, Stress Reduction and Relaxation Program, Associate Professor of Medicine, University of Massachusetts

"If you think the secrets to health, vitality, and longevity are to be found only in modern medicine, you are in desperate need of this book. Medical science, as magnificent as it may be, is helpless without *you*, for the key to lifelong health lies within each of us, as this book makes clear.

"Dr. Kenneth Pelletier has emerged over the past two decades as a veritable prophet of the future of health care. *Sound Mind, Sound Body* is an invaluable vision of what lies ahead."
—LARRY DOSSEY, M.D., author of *Healing Words, Meaning & Medicine*, and *Recovering the Soul*

"*Sound Mind, Sound Body* is a sane prescription for healthy living that is remarkably easy to follow. A diet of altruism and loving-kindness, spiced with a sense of purpose in life, moderately low in fat and high in fiber, can make our personal and collective world a better place to live. It is refreshing to read the personal stories and scientific studies that support an attainable and sustainable approach to health. This book will take its place alongside *Mind as Healer, Mind as Slayer* as one of the classics of the new medicine."
—JOAN BORYSENKO, Ph.D., President, Mind/Body Health Institute

"Most of what we know about health comes from a study of sick people, but *Sound Mind, Sound Body* corrects this incomplete picture of health with a refreshing account drawn from in-depth interviews with some of the healthiest high-achievers Dr. Pelletier could find. These are real people who manage to attain high levels of health despite disabilities, illnesses, and crises. Their success appears to be related to their drive toward a deeper purpose and meaning in life—rather than arduous personal health regimens of diet and exercise.

"*Sound Mind, Sound Body* is a highly readable, fascinating book that will inform and inspire those facing life-threatening illness or those just wishing to pursue the deeper meanings of health."
> —DAVID S. SOBEL, M.D., Director of Patient Education
> and Health Promotion, Kaiser Permanente,
> coauthor of *Healthy Pleasures* and *The Healing Brain*.

"Nothing is more common than the notion that health is not the same as the absence of disease. Nothing is less common than an understanding of the difference. Now *Sound Mind, Sound Body* promises to remedy this situation once and for all. Based on Ken Pelletier's extraordinary study of a fortunate few who have found health on their own, this ground-breaking book offers a unique gift—the wisdom of health. We, as individuals and as a society, cannot afford to turn this offer down. Simply put, this is required reading for all those who value the human experience."
> —DONALD M. VICKERY, M.D.,
> President and CEO, Health Decisions, Inc.

"An intriguing and thought-provoking treatment of an important subject: preventing illness and promoting health. Read it and be well!"
> —DIANA CHAPMAN WALSH,
> President, Wellesley College

SOUND MIND, SOUND BODY

A New Model for

Lifelong Health

.

DR. KENNETH R. PELLETIER

A FIRESIDE BOOK
Published by Simon & Schuster
NEW YORK   LONDON   TORONTO   SYDNEY   TOKYO   SINGAPORE

FIRESIDE
Rockefeller Center
1230 Avenue of the Americas
New York, New York 10020

First Fireside Edition 1995

FIRESIDE and colophon are registered trademarks of Simon & Schuster Inc.

Designed by Karolina Harris
Manufactured in the United States of America

10 9 8 7 6 5 4 3 2 1

Library of Congress Cataloging-in-Publication Data
Pelletier, Kenneth R.
Sound mind, sound body : a new model for lifelong health/
Kenneth R. Pelletier.
p.   cm.
1. Health. 2. Mental Health.
3. Mind and body. 4. Conduct of life. I. Title.
RA776.5.P39   1994
613—dc20   94-3181 CIP
ISBN: 0-671-77000-4
ISBN: 0-684-80251-1 (Pbk.)

The ideas, procedures and suggestions in this book are intended to supplement, not replace, the medical and psychological advice of trained professionals. In addition, all matters regarding your health require medical supervision. Consult your physician before adopting the medical suggestions in this book, as well as about any condition that may require diagnosis or medical attention. The authors and publishers disclaim any liability arising directly or indirectly from the use of this book.

To Shaughnessy, Sullivan, Kanaloa, Zoe and
Cherokee for illuminating the path of the heart.

Oh, Great Spirit, whose voice I hear in the winds,
And whose breath gives life to all the world—
Hear me.

I come before you, one of your many children.
I am small and weak,
I need your strength and wisdom.

Let me walk in beauty, and make my eyes ever behold
The red and purple sunset.
Make my hands respect the things you have made,
My ears sharp to hear your voice.
Make me wise so that I may know the things
You have taught my people,
The lesson you have hidden in every leaf and rock.

I seek strength
Not to be superior to my brother,
But to be able to master myself.

Make me ever ready to come to you
With clean hands and straight eyes,
So when life fades as a fading sunset,
My spirit may come to you without shame.

Chief Yellow Lark
Lakota Sioux

CONTENTS

CHAPTER ONE

If You Don't Know Where You're Going,

Any Road Will Get You There

On a crisp fall morning in 1977 I received a telephone call from the wife of a friend and former professor of mine, Gregory Bateson. Lois was calling to tell me that her seventy-two-year-old husband had been admitted to Moffitt Hospital at the University of California School of Medicine in San Francisco. Exploratory surgery had revealed an inoperable tumor in his right lung, and his doctor had suggested radiation and chemotherapy.

Gregory Bateson was a man who devoted his life to asking challenging questions. He was known for being both a hard scientist and a philosopher—one of the twentieth century's few generalists. His father had been a leading British biologist and pioneering geneticist, William Bateson, a member of the circle of academic nobility that included Aldous Huxley and Charles Darwin. A pioneer in his own right, Gregory conducted field research in anthropology, wrote numerous books, including the seminal *Steps toward an Ecology of Mind* (which remains a classic), and taught at literally every major international university. He was analytical, agnostic, and perpetually fascinated by the intricacies of patterns, processes, and paradoxes. At the time of his surgery he was serving on the Board of Regents of the University of California and was a mentor to then-Governor Jerry Brown.

Just before he was diagnosed with cancer, Gregory was immersed in writing a book with his daughter, Mary Catherine Bateson. They had been collaborating on the project for several years, and it represented the culmination of a lifetime of research and experimentation. When Dr. Michael Stulborg, Gregory's physician at UCSF, told him that the radiation and chemotherapy would affect him mentally, Gregory realized that such treatment would impair his ability to finish the book. He also realized, however, that he had to do something to fight the disease that was threatening his life.

During the course of Gregory's treatment Dr. Stulborg became very interested in his patient's books. He not only understood Gregory's desire to remain lucid but also, by removing administrative obstacles, supported his patient's wish to take an active role in his own care. This kind of collaborative effort, innovative in 1977, has since served as a prototype for many of the participants in my study. Navigating between an individual's need to fight a life-threatening illness and the desire to remain intellectually acute is one of medicine's greatest challenges.

When I got the call from Lois, it was nearly five years since I had been Gregory's student. At that time I was an assistant clinical professor of psychiatry and of medicine spending much of my clinical and research time using behavioral medicine and meditation therapy with my patients. "You know that Gregory's skeptical about mind-body interaction," Lois reminded me, "but he trusts you. I am calling you because you value this 'necessary unity' of mind-body interaction and use it in your clinical practice. Right now Gregory needs to decide whether to accept or reject chemotherapy and radiation, and we would like you to help him make that decision. He doesn't know it, but the doctor says he only has thirty days to live. Will you see him?"

That same afternoon, in the sterile atmosphere of the hospital, I sat down next to Gregory's bed and we began our work together. First we determined that there was something from Gregory's past—though we weren't sure what—that was driving him to finish the book. Consciously he was aware of his lifelong commitment to research and his firm commitment to seeing projects through to fruition, but something else was motivating him as well. Gregory eventually agreed with my idea that deep relaxation, and the subsequent elicitation of repressed memories and images, might benefit him in his quest to understand his subconscious motivation.

After learning some basic meditation techniques, Gregory began to experience vivid imagery and memories from his early life. It wasn't long, however, before his skepticism took over. He couldn't help intellectualizing about the value of doing these exercises and asking me what I expected he would get out of them. At first I tried to answer his questions, but my answers just encouraged him to challenge me more. Finally I asked him to take the approach of Coleridge and consider a "willing suspension of disbelief," and we proceeded with regular sessions over several weeks.

During our first few sessions Gregory would always fall asleep during the relaxation part of the exercise. At first I was sympathetic, assuming that this poor man was simply exhausted. But then I began to realize that he was falling asleep at precisely the same point each time. To keep him awake, I asked if I could put my fingernail on his hand and poke him gently when he started to doze off. We later realized that by falling asleep he had been avoiding a painful memory about his father and a task that they had never completed together. During the meditation he experienced a vivid image of an intense discussion between himself and his father in the family library. By reliving this encounter, Gregory realized why he had to finish writing his book: Radiation and chemotherapy were out of the question.

As I was leaving Gregory's room that day, in walked Ram Dass, in full beard and flowing white tunic and pants. Formerly known as Dr. Richard Alpert at Harvard University, Ram Dass left Harvard in the sixties to become one of the architects and spokesmen of the burgeoning counterculture. He wrote the influential *Be Here Now* and became a leading figure in introducing Eastern meditation practices into Western culture. He looked at me and said, "I'm here to help him die and you are here to help him live. Well, Ken, which of us do you think he'll choose?" With that he entered Gregory's room. A short time later Ram Dass emerged from the room, smiled, and said, "It's you, Ken."

Bedridden as he was, Gregory revealed a zest for life. He was compelled by something much deeper than the pursuit of the perfect physical condition, which many of us erroneously equate with health. He was operating out of courage and that indefatigable need to persevere to fulfill one's purpose, no matter what the challenge.

For more than two and a half years beyond the terminal prognosis of "thirty days to live," Gregory Bateson carried on with his remarkably productive life. During that time his book, *Mind and Nature: A Necessary Unity*, was completed. The memory of his father that we had unearthed made finishing the book a matter of honor to Gregory. Having accepted an advance on the project, he felt he had to uphold his end of the bargain despite his terminal illness. When Gregory died at the Green Gulch Zen Center north of San Francisco, he had inspired many people by living his life fully and vitally to the very end.

WHAT IS HEALTH?

My experience with Gregory, who was terminally ill but actually healthy, led me to conclude that health is not completely describable in traditional biological or psychological terms. Countless occasions over the next several years reminded me again and again that there is much more to health than cholesterol counts or blood pressure—that health is the psychological adjustment to the extraordinary experience of living life in its fullest expression. As the Greek philosopher Herophilu♦ put it approximately 300 B.C.: "When health is absent, wisdom cannot reveal itself, art cannot become manifest, strength cannot be exerted, wealth becomes useless, and reason is powerless." Again and again in my own experience it was becoming evident that health is not an end but a means to fulfill the purpose of life itself.

Those early stirrings of a fundamental concept began to take shape for me several years later over dinner with Norman Cousins. "One of my favorite cartoons," chuckled Norman with his characteristic impish grin and raised eyebrows, "was in the *New Yorker*: Two yogis are sitting cross-legged at the edge of a cave on top of a very high mountain in the Himalayas. They obviously had just been interrupted in their meditations by a seven forty-seven jet that had passed overhead. One of them looks over at the other and says, 'Ah, they have the know-*how*, but do they have the know-*why*?' " Norman continued: "For me the question of *why* we live is more important than how we live. And *why* we seek health is of greater significance than particular practices and potions. For several years now I have met with terminal cancer patients in their sixties and seventies at the Wellness Community [a cancer self-help program founded by the attorney and psychologist Dr. Harold H. Benjamin in Santa Monica, California] and found them to be more vital, more alive, and, yes, healthier than many of the students jogging through the UCLA campus on their way to a health food store! So how do we define this inner state of health in a way that includes people during periods of illness and crisis; those with disabilities; adults and children of all ages; individuals of all ethnic backgrounds; as well as those who are already committed to mind, body, and environmental health practices? What is health? And most importantly, why do we seek it?" In his inimitable way Norman had framed one of today's most formidable questions with simplicity and clarity.

During the past decade health was narrowly defined as "the absence of disease," and health practices focused on "preventing" heart attacks, "avoiding" cancer, or "coping" with stress. Today national surveys indicate that health is the number-one concern both in the

United States and internationally, as the over 77 million baby boomers enter middle age and look forward to a longer life expectancy than past generations. But if our striving for health mainly involves an endless succession of aerobic workouts, a boringly regimented diet, or an outrageous investment in cosmetic surgeries, then our misguided preoccupation with health is literally worse than disease. The narcissistic preoccupation with personal attractiveness and the outward appearance of vitality has replaced our cavalier disregard for the health consequences of our hazardous lifestyles.

So how can optimal health be achieved and sustained? With increasingly longer lives ahead of us, what lies beyond career, child rearing, and retirement? Questions raised in the name of health are synonymous with those eternal issues driving the world's great spiritual quests for meaning. For the vast majority of our population that has already attained a measure of material security, these are pressing and timely issues.

Sound Mind, Sound Body is based on the results of the first ongoing study to address the vital question: What is health? It explores how personal health practices and a sense of meaningful purpose play a major role in both inner fulfillment and professional success, and it offers practical, effective techniques for achieving physical, mental, and emotional equilibrium throughout the ebbs and flows of life. However, this is much less a how-to book than a testament to the human capacity to grow, face new challenges with conviction, and learn from any situation. Each individual discussed in this book demonstrates that health is an ever-evolving process, and that there is even a healthy way to be ill and a good way to die. By their example you will witness that health is not superficial or one-dimensional, but an integration of body, mind, spirit, and environment. Most importantly, their stories show that achieving optimal health is indeed possible.

Health is an attitude or orientation comprising our basic values and beliefs about ourselves and the world around us. It is an inner quality that gives rise to particular health practices but cannot in itself be reduced to those practices. There is no lifestyle—no matter how disciplined or hedonistic—that guarantees freedom from disease and disability or ensures longevity. Some people do everything right and die young, while others break all the rules and get away with it. Truly to grasp the deepest meaning of health, it is necessary to broaden its definition beyond the physical. Optimal health requires an integration of physical, mental, spiritual, and environmental well-being. For example, if we work harder to nurture community projects, philanthropic efforts, and our extended families, we might find ourselves less frightened by the specters of illness, disability, and old age, less preoccupied with individual survival, and our outlook on life would indeed be healthier.

Health needs to be recognized as an ongoing process of self-discovery, manifesting a positive influence on the world around us. It is a means to living a successful and satisfying life. In 300 B.C. the Greeks referred to health as the *physics*, or the "healing force within." Our current term *health* is derived from the Old English *hale*, meaning "whole." Where did our culture go wrong? How have we lost that fundamental essence of health—the concept of the body, mind, spirit, and nature as inextricably bound and functioning in concert as a whole? Only recently have we begun to rediscover the truth behind this perennial wisdom.

Good health allows us to enjoy our families, participate in our communities, and live to know our grandchildren, while providing us with the opportunity to contribute to our time in history. It allows us to find personal fulfillment, to enjoy our sexuality, to be creative and productive, but it does not confer these things upon us. While it permits us to seek a satisfying and complete life, it is not a substitute for one. We must be careful not to expect too much from diets, jogging, or the "right" cholesterol level, because we cannot control our genetic, predetermined propensity to disease or alter our biological destiny with a breakfast of bran or a weight-training regimen.

There seems to be a growing disillusionment and backlash against narcissism in the name of health. In his article entitled "Through a Glass, Darkly," published in *Newsweek* in December 1991, the playwright and bartender Jeff Morris gave some "bartenderly advice": "Jogging, Stairmasters, aerobics classes and diets are not the answer. They only relieve the symptoms: stress, anxiety, poor physical condition. They do nothing to effect change or to alleviate the causes of our problems. All the effort that goes into focusing on one's self can be detrimental in the long run. All the energy we exert in the name of health and the glorification of the self is diverting and sapping us of the energy we need to come to terms with what our real problems are: the economy, AIDS, human rights, the environment, education— these things can't be fixed unless people think more about other people and less about themselves." From a bar in New York to the pages of *Newsweek* to mainstream research, it is clear that new model of health must supersede the superficial outward appearance of health or fixation on any single influence such as cholesterol levels or minutes of exercise per week.

Individual efforts are necessary but insufficient for optimal health. We need to create approaches and systems in economics, environment, politics, and in the delivery of medical care, that elicit and sustain individual strategies. One major objective of the Sound Mind– Sound Body research was to lay the foundation for a model of health that would incorporate both individual and collective influences. As a first step I focused on individuals who have made major contributions to the world *beyond* their own personal success and security. From interviews with them I was able to learn a great deal about how people can achieve a balance between personal and professional fulfillment and attempt to achieve the ancient ideal of "a sound mind in a sound body." This sense of optimal health as a personal and societal responsibility is the focus of my research, my clinical practice, and this book.

MEDICAL CRISIS IN AMERICA

Medical care in this country reflects our cultural values of materialism. We throw money at problems, believe that external solutions can solve internal problems, prefer simplistic approaches to reality, and worship high technology. Furthermore, we believe that modern medicine can and should cure all ills, that medical care is a basic right, and that death is the enemy to be conquered at all cost. We reason that if some medical care is good, more of the same must be even better.

Underlying the nearly $3 billion in medical care expenditures each day are the personal choices and lifestyle decisions made by millions of individuals. Each day we choose health or illness simply by choosing how to live. In 1990 the United States Surgeon General released *Health 2000: Objectives for the Nation*, which elaborated the goals for health care in the coming decade. It also listed the twenty-one major causes of illness and death today; *nineteen* are entirely lifestyle related—the result of destructive lifestyle choices.

Such findings are a minuscule fraction of the dire facts reported every year in every mainstream professional journal and by every major professional society and government agency. Since the early 1980s, tax "reforms" have actually decreased the income of the poorest 20 percent of our nation and simultaneously withdrawn access to health care. At the 1990 meeting of the American Public Health Association, the president, Dr. Myron Allukian, stated unequivocally, "The United States has a health care system that does not promote health, that does not care, and is not a system, in spite of the dedication of thousands of caring health workers. It is a fragmented patchwork of procedure-oriented services enmeshed in a voluminous paper payment trail with little relevance to community-based needs. It provides more and more treatment, at higher and higher costs, to fewer and fewer of the have-nots in our society."

Perhaps in a system devoid of empathy or compassion, it would be conceivable to distance ourselves from the have-nots—the homeless children, warehoused elderly, and teenage girls having babies—but the negative impact of the misdirected disease management system reaches all of us, whether we are actually receiving medical care or not. Be it in the form of higher taxes or limited and increasingly expensive insurance coverage, the juggernaut runs over everyone. Considering the medical care system from a consumer's point of view, Allukian described the current system as one "where consumers are receiving an unknown product of unknown quality of an unknown but higher and higher cost. It's been estimated that some eighty-nine thousand Americans a year die or are permanently disabled due to medical negligence. Something is wrong with our nonsystem." More so than any other aspect of modern life, concerns about medical care touch every person, at every age. There are no innocent bystanders when children have easier access to guns and drugs than to immunizations and family planning. This fundamental problem can be solved not by spending more money, but rather by creating a true health care *system* that insists on appropriate, equitable levels of care for informed consumers.

What is the cause of this deplorable state of affairs, and how do we pull ourselves out of it? First it is essential to consider how so many well-intentioned individuals and institutions have become mired in such a calamity. Perhaps the key is a lack of direction. Medical care no longer has a well-defined goal. Without a clear destination, wandering is inevitable. If we are to transform the present disease management industry into a *health care system*, then health—not the for-profit management of disease—needs to be restored as its bottom-line goal. A true health care system is one that encourages preventive techniques and practices to enhance and sustain the health of the vast majority of people and makes appropriate disease management technologies available and affordable to those who really need them.

In the now-classic 1960 *Harvard Business Review* article entitled "Marketing Myopia," Harvard business professor Theodore Levitt focused on the railroad industry at the turn of the century as an archetype for all enterprises that lose sight of their purpose and direction. According to Levitt, "Railroads did not stop growing because the need for passenger and freight transportation declined. That grew. . . . They let others take customers away from them because they assumed themselves to be in the railroad business rather than in the transportation business." As such alternative modes of transportation as automobiles, airplanes, and even telephones evolved, the railroads failed to advance and diversify. By defining themselves too narrowly, they failed to ascertain or act upon their customers' needs and desires. As a result they served fewer people less well at higher, noncompetitive prices, with less consumer satisfaction. Sound familiar?

Applying this analysis to the automobile manufacturing and oil production businesses, Levitt concluded that "there is no such thing as a growth industry. . . . The history of every dead and dying 'growth' industry shows a self-deceiving cycle of bountiful expansion and undetected decay. There are four conditions which usually guarantee this cycle: 1) the belief that growth is assured by an expanding and more affluent population; 2) the belief that there is no competitive substitute for the industry's major product; 3) too much faith in mass production . . .; and 4) preoccupation with a product that lends itself to carefully controlled scientific experimentation, improvement, and manufacturing cost reduction." While no analogy is ever perfect, it is increasingly evident that the disease management industry does adhere to these fatal precepts. Fortunately its demise will give rise to a true health care system, one that will not lose sight of its purpose by becoming preoccupied with self-perpetuation.

Words like *purpose*, *mission*, and *values* may seem inappropriate relative to the Goliath of the medical-industrial complex, but they nonetheless identify very real—and very critical—issues. Most health care professionals abhor the idea that they are in business, but this denial is precisely what produces professional myopia. Market forces—consumer preferences, changing social values, customer dissatisfaction, and so on—are repugnant to health care professionals because such elements are associated with selling, while in fact, selling and marketing—at least in this situation—are fundamentally different. Selling involves using tricks and techniques to get people to exchange cash for your product. Marketing is concerned with the values underlying the exchange; it views the entire business process as a tightly integrated effort to discover, create, arouse, and satisfy customer needs, to borrow Levitt's definition. Clearly the purpose of health care should not be to create or arouse needs, but its job certainly is to discover and satisfy needs. Up until a few years ago the disease management industry occupied a unique status among businesses: it controlled both the demand and supply of its product. Fortunately that era is over—and not a day too soon.

Within such a closed system, Levitt observes, "What gets short-changed are the realities of the market. Consumers are [viewed as] unpredictable, varied, fickle, stupid, shortsighted, stubborn, and generally bothersome. This is not what the engineer-managers say, but deep down in their consciousness it is what they believe." At the root of the dissatisfaction expressed with the disease management industry is the fact that all too many patients have been and still are treated in a demeaning manner. Dr. Tom Ferguson, physician, author, and founder of *Medical Self-Care* magazine, reflects on this unfortunate state of affairs: "The best way to get doctors off of their pedestals is for patients to get up off their knees." As overstated as that may seem, we at least need to restore an equality, dignity, and renewed sense of purpose between patients and doctors even to hope for a true health care system.

Faced with the magnitude and complexity of such daunting problems, how can we as individuals begin to address these formidable challenges involving millions of lives, billions of dollars, and decades of well-meaning but misguided efforts? The Chinese poet Lao-tzu said that "the journey of a thousand miles begins with one step," and that is precisely where we must begin. Each person is directly and indirectly affected, both personally and financially, when he or a family member receives medical care of any kind, from a simple throat culture to major hospitalization.

We as individuals need to examine the factors that are driving up costs. We should all become more actively involved, by talking with our doctors, questioning our medical bills, and challenging the assumptions on which present care is based. We need to become informed consumers, knowing what to expect and demanding what we want. Above all, we need to realize that there is no magic third party guaranteeing our rights as patients and paying our medical bills.

More and more large companies today are either self-insured or paying directly for their own medical costs and assuming the responsibility of processing claims. But small businesses are unable to self-insure. They are forced to pay excessively high rates to insurers who seek to make up for the relatively small profit margins on policies negotiated with large companies, or more often than not, small businesses are forced to drop coverage. Given that more than 80 percent of all companies in the United States employ fewer than fifty workers, their collective decisions have enormous repercussions. Fortunately some major insurance companies, such as Blue

Shield, Healthnet–Qual Med, Prudential, Blue Cross/Blue Shield, and Aetna, are creating innovative coverages for large and small businesses, which include health promotion programs to contain costs. Major corporations like Johnson & Johnson, Du Pont, AT&T, and General Motors have redirected a large portion of their corporate medical expenditures toward health promotion and disease prevention programs.

Much of my own work over the last ten years has focused on the development and evaluation of such innovative health and medical programs in the work site. As director of the Stanford Corporate Health Program at the Stanford University School of Medicine, I work with such corporations as American Airlines, IBM, Bank of America, AT&T, Apple, and Levi-Strauss to create these types of programs, and every one of the more than fifty published evaluations of these programs has shown objective, quantifiable proof of increased health and decreased cost. These efforts are also a practical demonstration that individual strategies are a necessary but not entirely sufficient condition for optimal health. For example, an individual's decision to quit smoking must be elicited and sustained by a program that assists him or her in quitting and provides incentives to remain smoke-free. Work site "clean air" policies, which prohibit smoking completely, and a national policy to eliminate glamorous advertising of an addictive and lethal product, working in synergy with individual efforts, result in the precondition of optimal health for individuals and institutions alike.

Why are such synergistic policies so slow in coming? Perhaps the most pernicious characteristic of our outmoded biomedical model is that it defines health in terms of biological measures such as blood pressure, weight, and the absence of disease. It separates the mind from the body and relies on the "doctor knows best" belief that the means to health lie outside ourselves in medication, high-tech surgery, or the latest breakthrough in genetic engineering. To a significant extent this orientation was formalized in the writings of the highly influential seventeenth-century philosopher René Descartes. His treatises characterized the body as essentially a complex machine and illness as the manifestation of a breakdown in one of the machine's parts. The role of medicine—and ultimately the physician—was to identify and repair the broken part. Within this model disorders of the mind and spirit and their corresponding influence on health and disease were seen as separate and distinct from the functioning of the physical machine. With Leeuwenhoek's invention of the microscope and the identification of microbes and bacteria, along with the historical impact of research by Dr. Louis Pasteur and Dr. Robert Koch, the dominance of Descartes's model was assured. Illness was explained as an attack upon the machine by external bacteria or as the consequence of a nutrient deficiency. Medicine was logical, predictable, and wholly physical. Practical applications of these discoveries resulted in vaccines and antibiotics, both of which have for centuries prevented and cured various diseases without regard to the intangible domains of the mind or spirit.

More recently an increasing number of geneticists are challenging the inordinate amount of funding dedicated to the Human Genome Project, which is focused on the mapping of the entire human DNA. While this is surely an important scientific undertaking, it is the logical extension of a reductionist, mechanistic, and limited approach to science. One of the project's most articulate critics is geneticist Dr. Richard C. Strohman of the University of California at Berkeley, who observes, "The wide acceptance of the concept of genetic diseases, and the confusion of rare monogenic (single cause) disease with the more common polygenic (multiple cause) human disease, is seen as the single most important historical development underlying the widespread belief in the paradigm question. . . . 98 percent of disease is not single-gene determined. . . . A new biomedical research outlook would shift to a focus on the organism-environment interface." Surely research on single-gene disease and subsequent gene replacement therapy is important, but its focus compared to the whole spectrum of human health issues is extremely narrow.

Lost in the shadow of Descartes's diehard rationalism is the fact that the mind's influence on health had been recognized by medicine since its very beginning, however underestimated or poorly understood. Early in the fourth century B.C. Hippocrates, the founder of Western medicine and of the Hippocratic Oath, equated health with a harmonious balance of mind, body, and the environment. By contrast he concluded that disease was due to a disharmony of these elements. In the second century A.D. the Greek physician Galen observed that "melancholic" women appeared to be especially susceptible to breast cancer.

During the Renaissance, Dr. Thomas Sydenham extended Hippocrates' observations about the "healing power of nature," proposing that a person's internal adaptation to external forces was a major factor in disease and health. Writing in 1725, Dr. George Cheyne noted in *An Essay of Health and Long Life* that "it is most certain that 'tis easier to preserve Health than to recover it, and to prevent Diseases than to cure them." In the mid-nineteenth century, the eminent

French physician Dr. Claude Bernard, who defined the role of the pancreas in digestion, also emphasized the role of the *"milieu interieur,"* or inner state, as essential to understanding health and disease. At the beginning of this century that idea was given a scientific basis by Harvard physiologist Dr. Walter B. Cannon, who first described the "fight-or-flight response," the internal adaptive response of the body to a threat.

This fight-or-flight response was essential to survival when humans faced frequent physical threats and dangers, such as wild animals searching for food. By contrast the stresses we face today are much more likely to be psychological and interpersonal—ones that cannot be handled by fighting or fleeing. The late Dr. Hans Selye, a pioneering stress researcher at McGill University, demonstrated in the 1950s that the body reacts to modern stresses as though it were facing a real physical threat. Today research indicates that the way people cope with incipient illness may be at least as important as the biological pathogens themselves in determining health or illness. A variety of psychological factors including mood, personality characteristics, social support, coping techniques, suppressed anger, a sense of hopelessness or a sense of purpose, psychological vulnerability, and defensiveness can each affect the way a person handles and overcomes potential illness and disease. It is also increasingly evident that what goes on in the mind of the individual is at least as important as what goes on inside the body. As the eminent physician Sir William Osler once observed, "It is as important to know what patient has the disease as it is what disease the patient has."

Until we restore the whole *individual*—body and mind—to the center of our health care system, we will continue to spend billions of dollars on excessive surgeries and unwarranted medications, while relegating the individual to a passive role devoid of responsibility or authority. Bear in mind that individual responsibility should not be equated with "victim blaming" or the idea that a person's thoughts or actions bring on cancer or any other disease. Instead, restoring individual responsibility recognizes that there are critical lifestyle choices we can all make to increase the likelihood of sustained health. It encourages us to become as active as possible in our own treatment. Such an approach does not imply blame or assign guilt. It simply recognizes the fact that conscious, individual choices underlie many of the major causes of death and disability in the United States today.

Individuals can have a profound impact on their own health as well as on the shaping of a true health care system. Surely the first step is to set a goal or objective. If that objective is health, rather than just the absence of disease, then a new model of health must be defined with specific strategies to achieve and sustain it. This new model of health can set the fundamental direction for individuals and the nation as a whole and lead us toward a true health care system by providing a basis for our day-to-day decisions. The new orientation will involve and empower all of us—individuals and institutions alike—to be integral and responsible participants in our own health, as well as that of others less fortunate, across the nation and throughout the world. It has major implications for how we structure the future of medical care, how we provide access to basic services for the 37 million uninsured Americans, and how we care for the exploding number of elderly. Most important, this new direction is realistic, achievable, and vitally relevant to the health issues and challenges of the twenty-first century.

THE SOUND MIND–SOUND BODY STUDY

Countless volumes have been written describing every conceivable disease of body and mind, but there is a virtual vacuum of data and information on health itself. Dr. Evan G. Pattishall of Pennsylvania State University wrote in the November 1989 issue of the *Annals of Behavioral Medicine*:

> We have been so indoctrinated in the methodology of the biomedical model that we still think too much in terms of the disease model: how disease develops, how it can be cured, or how it can be prevented. If we study 25 people who are exposed to, say, an influenza virus and five develop the illness, we tend to study the five who developed influenza, when we should be exerting even more effort studying the twenty who didn't become ill. This is more than just another way of saying, as the World Health Organization did a couple of generations ago, that health is more than the absence of disease. We are slowly learning that there are tremendous biological, social, and behavioral variabilities within and between the normal. Understanding stress and learning to cope with individual, group, and environmental variabilities, and using their potentials to promote health, has become an exciting area for research and practice.

Certainly as a first step toward a health model it is necessary to begin developing a body of knowledge about those twenty people who did not succumb to influenza, about individuals who cope extremely well with chronic diseases such as arthritis and heart disease, as well as those individuals who rarely if ever experience illness until the very last few months of their lives.

Surprisingly, one area where this approach to a model of health rather than disease has been developed most fully is in the supposedly inevitable process of aging. Among the most insightful and influential articles in the last decade was "Human Aging: Usual and Successful," published in the July 10, 1987, issue of *Science* magazine. According to the authors, Dr. John W. Rowe of the Harvard Medical School and Dr. Robert L. Kahn of the University of Michigan, "successful aging" is actually healthy aging, as manifested by individuals who live unusually long lives while remaining in excellent physical and psychological health. "Usual aging" simply describes a statistical average, and given the high incidence of premature disease in our population, is a rather dismal yardstick.

Rowe and Kahn also examined the biological markers or indicators by which researchers commonly measure the aging process. Among these indices are carbohydrate metabolism or the increasing impairment of the ability to metabolize blood glucose; osteoporosis or the tendency for the bones to decline in density, leading to more fractures late in life; supposedly normal increases in blood pressure and cholesterol; and declines in intellectual functions such as memory and verbal ability. Although the standard textbooks using a disease model indicate that such declines are normal, inevitable, and irreversible, the evidence from a health model indicates just the opposite is true in a healthy or successful aging model. Every one of these supposedly inevitable declines can be slowed, halted, and even reversed, according to a growing body of both animal and human research. There is abundant research that diet and exercise can remedy impaired carbohydrate metabolism and insulin intolerance as well as osteoporosis. In fact, research indicates that physically active older men actually have an ability to metabolize blood sugar identical to that of young athletes. Likewise, programs that work with people to improve memory, recall, and intellectual skills such as reading have been shown to reverse mental deterioration in as few as five sessions.

Such outcomes are not the result of improved pharmacology or surgery. They are the result of an increased sense of control over one's own health and environment; the provision of social support during periods of death and bereavement; assistance at critical transition points in one's life, such as retirement or relocation to a new home; and an enhanced sense of autonomy and purpose. Rowe and Kahn concluded, "These recommendations have in common a thrust to-

ward health promotion and disease prevention in the elderly. A revolutionary increase in life span has already occurred. A corresponding increase in health span, the maintenance of full function as nearly
as possible to the end of life, should be the next gerontological goal.
The focus on successful aging urges that goal for researchers, practitioners, and for older men and women themselves." If this approach
is applicable to aging, which is certainly considered one of life's im-
mutable events, then certainly such an approach should be applicable to every chronic disease as well as to the study of personal
strategies for optimal health.

Drawing upon such insights and new directions, my research has
focused upon the best, rather than the worst, we can anticipate of both
individuals and the institutions which help us elicit and sustain optimal health. The Sound Mind–Sound Body study is an inquiry into the
nature of health based upon a series of extensive interviews with fifty-
three prominent individuals who represent prototypes of optimal
health. Beginning in 1978, Laurance S. Rockefeller funded this five-
year research project as well as several others that made similar inquiries into different populations, including individuals who gave up
lucrative careers to enter public service, women who became altruists, and other people who sought to transcend the limitations of personal, material achievement. Periodic meetings have been held with
the researchers who conducted these related studies, and their findings are discussed throughout this book.

In any new field of inquiry some boundaries need to be established. For example, in a study of coronary heart disease, individuals may be selected for research based on specific criteria including
family history, blood pressure, cholesterol levels, and other relevant
risk factors and characteristics. The Sound Mind–Sound Body project focused on individuals who met a three-tiered set of criteria: 1)
All of the participants are "prominent" in the sense that they are acknowledged by their peers as accomplished in their chosen profes-
sions or businesses. Attainment of wealth per se was not a criterion.
2) All the individuals selected had publicly indicated prior to selection that they adhered to personal health practices that enabled them
to sustain the demands of their careers; and 3) Either explicitly or im-
plicitly, each participant conveyed the personal conviction that he or
she was acting out of a deep sense of purpose and higher or spiritual
values.

One of the most striking findings of the study is that material abundance, the alleviation of narcissism with the onslaught of old age, and
an exercise/diet regimen simply are not enough to make people

healthy and fulfilled. The key factor seems to be a moving beyond purely materialistic and competitive concerns to the discovery of a deeper meaning. The subtle but critical dimensions of psychological and spiritual growth seemingly play a more important role in a healthy life than has previously been estimated.

Altruistic or self-transcending behavior derived from an individual's sense of higher purpose or spiritual values is receiving renewed attention from many different quarters of inquiry, ranging from medicine to evolution. From an evolutionary perspective, altruistic behavior may actually sacrifice the individual for the greater good. Dr. Herbert A. Simon of Carnegie Mellon University notes in an article published in *Science* that altruism is not inconsistent with the strictest Darwinian assumptions. In fact, he concludes, "Altruism, either defined socially or as defined genetically, is wholly compatible with natural selection and is an important determinant of human behavior." Rather than seeing altruism as inherently self-sacrificing, Simon observes that "altruists are fitter than selfish individuals. . . . altruism will not only survive, but will gradually permeate the entire population. . . . one might even rename the accompanying altruism 'enlightened selfishness.' "

Adherence to "enlightened selfishness" turned out to be one of the most striking similarities among the individuals I interviewed. Every participant consistently cited a deep sense of altruism as the primary motivation infusing his or her larger service to humankind. And it seems the participants are not alone. According to Allan Luks, executive director of Big Brothers/Big Sisters of New York City and author of *The Healing Power of Doing Good*, over 90 million Americans are engaged in altruistic volunteer work. In his book, he cited the classic ten-year study of over twenty-seven hundred people living in Tecumseh, Michigan, indicating that men who did not engage in volunteer work were two and a half times more likely to die from various causes than their peers who did volunteer work. Of course it may be argued that people who volunteer are happier and healthier to begin with, but most researchers believe that providing helpful services to others provides a strong antidote to stress and depression. Individuals with emotional problems often find that helping others with similar difficulties is particularly beneficial and satisfying, which may account for the success of such support groups as Alcoholics Anonymous, Narcotics Anonymous, and Gamblers Anonymous. More and more retired and elderly individuals are devoting their spare time to helping others. One popular activity is the Foster Grandparents Program, in which volunteers over sixty are teamed with children who are emotionally or physically handicapped, abused, or neglected. From this growing body of research, and from every interview in my study, it is clearly evident that altruism is good for both the self and others. Surely it ought to be a mainstay for any future model of health.

With the 1980s came a distorted approach to health—that of neurotic self-absorption in the latest fad diet, exercise, or relaxation method. While the narcissism that motivates this approach is not the focus of this book, we must understand why it still runs rampant and how it contradicts the model of health we seek to establish. In *Worried Sick* Dr. Arthur J. Barsky of Harvard University noted that Americans have become "prisoners of health, a society plagued by a sense of dis-ease and malaise and a seemingly constant need for medical care." Attaining a state of health is thought tantamount to achieving not only freedom from disease, but longevity and moral virtue. Yet good health is not valued as a means to accomplishing other fundamental personal goals, such as raising a family; rather it has become a substitute for them. We have replaced the religious quest to save our souls with the secular quest to preserve our bodies. Attaining a state of wellness is like attaining a state of grace, but for many the highest purpose of human activity is not to purify the soul, but to purify the body, and the appearance of perfect health is now the object of conscious, sustained, and deliberate endeavor.

Our pursuit of the youthful, beautiful body fuels an enormous cosmetics industry, a stampede on plastic surgeons' offices, and a mass convergence on the weight rooms and whirlpool baths of health clubs devoted entirely to the care and worship of the body. With the combination of vigorous exercise, restricted diets, and modern biomedical technology, we believe we have the power to control our biological destiny, to avoid disease, and to drink from a genetically engineered fountain of youth. We have come to the facile conclusion that if health-promoting behavior is moral and virtuous, then illness must be the result of a moral failure or lapse. With physical conditioning we attempt to fortify ourselves against an increasingly menacing environment filled with health hazards, violence, and the potential for large-scale man-made as well as natural disasters.

In an essay in the *Harvard Medical Journal*, entitled "The Body as Our Temple," Barsky observes that "daily life is a mine field through which we must thread our way. We are in danger of being struck by a drunk driver, engulfed in warfare, or murdered with a handgun; there are poisoned Halloween candies and Tylenol capsules laced with cyanide; we read about ticks with Lyme disease, mosquitos with AIDS, and killer bees." Confronted with a hazardous world, we try to assert control in the one sphere of influence that remains ours—our bodies and our personal habits. In a world where dangers seem out of our control, we retreat to shore up our own physical integrity, to attempt to ensure survival by building resistance and stretching endurance. Again Barsky notes that, "powerless to stem the seepage of toxic wastes into our drinking water, unable to avoid carcinogens in our vegetables, at the mercy of a psychopath who would assault us on the street, we check our blood pressure, fortify our diet, and carry weights with us as we jog." Faced with such a threatening external macroenvironment, we seek control over our internal microenvironment in the name of health.

But the current prescriptions for how to achieve "health" are a bewildering barrage of instant diets, panacea exercises, and stress management nostrums. In short, our program for achieving health parallels the disease model in that we seek something *outside* of ourselves as a solution.

But what life direction do we really seek in the name of health, beyond the superficial paradigm of the eighties? What inspires some people to make extraordinary decisions requiring great courage at a time of a personal health crisis? Somehow a crisis puts some people in touch with a deep inner resource, which in turn empowers them to do more with their lives than just strive for the perfect physique. But is a crisis always necessary? What can *we* learn from those who have embarked on such personal odysseys?

Throughout this book questions such as these will explore true optimal health as an ongoing process in which we exercise individual choice throughout every stage of our lives. The answers will come from hundreds of hours of background searches and structured interviews with specially selected individuals, their families, and associates, and from a wealth of insights, anecdotes, and data on their personal histories, perspectives, and lifestyle practices. Some of these people are prominent in the public eye; others are not necessarily well known outside of their professional circles. All are, however, representative of their peers and colleagues in that they share the same pressures and hassles of daily life. And although their personal strategies for health and success may not be unique, they are men and women from whom there is a great deal to be learned simply because they defy the current conventional approach to health.

Case studies provide a level of detail and entry into a person's life that few works of fiction can match. Freud himself was a master of individual studies. His classic accounts of Dora and the Rat Man stand as both literary and clinical masterpieces. Despite an increasing concern about confidentiality and malpractice suits, the recent popularity of the neurologist Dr. Oliver Sacks's book *The Man Who Mistook His Wife for a Hat* and the hit movie *Awakenings* demonstrate the compelling depth of and growing interest in individual life stories. In 1987 Dr. Richard Green of Yale University reported the results of his fifteen-year study of a group of apparently "feminine" young boys and "nonfeminine" controls using a case study method to speculate on the development of male homosexuality. Although such a study could have been reduced to statistics, he chose the case study format to develop his compelling and insightful book *The "Sissy Boy Syndrome" and the Development of Homosexuality.* Another book that influenced my choice of research method is *Love's Executioner and Other Tales of Psychotherapy* by noted psychiatrist Dr. Irving P. Yalom. His book is an extraordinarily brilliant and compassionate account of ten patients suffering from such conditions as promiscuity, obsession, obesity, and severe depression. In it the case study approach allows for each individual to speak out on his or her own behalf and provide a personal perspective on illness and treatment.

Inherent in case studies are some acknowledged and necessary limitations, such as a certain degree of generalization, potential bias in selecting any relatively small number of cases, and a lack of certain statistical analyses. Yet the use of intensive case studies is often the only method available in the early stages of a new area of study, be it astronomy or medicine. This case study approach has led to the discovery of new diagnostic categories, for instance multiple personalities in psychiatry; the development and refinement of surgical procedures, including coronary bypass, beginning with Dr. Christian Barnard's pioneering surgeries; discoveries involving the separate and distinct functions of the left and right hemispheres of the brain; and currently, evidence that advanced heart disease can be reversed through behavioral interventions only. There is no control group in case studies, but as Dr. Abraham Maslow explained, "I have not deliberately worked with an ad hoc control group, i.e., non-self-actualizing people. I could say that most of humanity is a control group, which is certainly true. . . . It is my strong impression that there is not a sharp line between my subjects chosen as self-actualizing and other people." This is the approach I took with the Sound Mind–Sound Body research project. Had I chosen a more rigorous reductionistic approach and statistical methodology, my research might have yielded harder data and more refined hypotheses, but the impact and complexity of the individuals, their lives, and their development would be lost. By allowing the human beings to speak for themselves, it is possible to capture the rich multidimensional quality of their lives and obtain their own opinions on why they have developed in the ways they have.

For the Sound Mind–Sound Body study a total of fifty-three individuals were interviewed. Each session lasted two to three hours, and each person was given a complete transcript to review for accuracy after the interview was over. After reading the transcripts, twenty participants requested that their information be used anonymously because of the revealing nature of the discussions, and two asked to withdraw from the study completely. Of the fifty-one active participants, there were twenty-one women and thirty men between the ages of twenty-eight and ninety-six, who resided in various regions throughout the United States. Forty-eight of the fifty-one active participants also completed a standardized Health Risk Appraisal donated by Johnson & Johnson to compare their attitudes, health practices, and medical conditions to national norms.

Data garnered from the interviewees were analyzed to identify similarities in the lives of the participants that would explain how they achieved a healthy balance of mind, body, and environment. After identifying more than two dozen elements common to the participants, the researchers, consultants, and I worked together to pare the thousands of pages of information down to the most crucial, most significant findings. Each of the following chapters will discuss one of these important themes, which, along with the research data, form the foundation of a model of health that will require many years or even decades of further research and refinement.

When Abraham Maslow undertook his pioneering case studies of "self-actualizing" people, he explained that he sought to "study the extraordinary to understand the ordinary." That is my approach as well. These people, however successful in whatever field, are far from perfect by their own standards, and they too have many of the same qualities and experiences that you and I do. They were born and reared under vastly different social and economic circumstances, ranging from inherited wealth to a few dollars and a vision. They have suffered setbacks, disappointments, and life-threatening illnesses, and have experienced the joys, triumphs, and sense of awe that inspire all of us. They struggle through the same daily woes of living as we all do, but do so with more awareness and wisdom than most. They are remarkable—not because of a special genetic endowment, but by virtue of living life to its full expression.

It is easy to distance ourselves from these same challenges by reasoning that these individuals are somehow exceptional and therefore unlike us. But these are real stories about real people who have struggled with and triumphed over life's travails. Despite adversity they listened to their inner voices and developed the skills to turn their visions into realities. There is no attempt in this book to portray these individuals as representing unattainable ideals. Everyone interviewed emphasized that they had *learned* their skills and that others could do the same. Although the successful people profiled here are prototypes, their personal strategies are replicable by anyone, and their diversity can provide thought-provoking insights for any individual seeking to attain the same degree of personal and professional fulfillment. The answers lie not in simplistic techniques and glib nostrums. The lifestyle change that many of these individuals have undertaken has been as subtle as a shift in perspective from seeing a glass as half-empty to seeing it as half-full.

Since many of the interviewees are notoriously reclusive, I started with a few long-standing friends—Norman Cousins, Saul Zaentz, Laurel Burch, and Michael S. Currier—and branched out by referral and recommendation. So in a sense this *is* a random sample, and certainly representative of the health lifestyles and attitudes that are possible for all of us. Coincidentally, several of the people interviewed were independently selected by my friend and colleague Dr. Warren Bennis, Distinguished Professor of Business Administration at the University of Southern California, to be included in his excellent book *On Becoming a Leader*. Among those who overlapped in the two studies are television producer Norman Lear, John Sculley of Apple Computer, and James Burke of Johnson & Johnson. Bennis selected these people as leaders, defining that term as "people who are able to express themselves fully. By this I mean that they know who they are, what their strengths and weaknesses are, and how to fully deploy their strengths and compensate for their weaknesses. They also know what they want, and how to communicate what they want to others, in order to gain their cooperation and support. Finally, they know how to achieve their goals." Those characteristics hold true for all of the people interviewed in my study, not so much as leaders in business, but as leaders in *living*.

Despite the prominence of the individuals chosen for my research, this is *not* a *Lifestyles of the Rich and Famous* approach with an emphasis on materialism, narcissism, and superficial excess. Interviewing fifty or even five hundred randomly selected men and women would perhaps constitute a more objective survey but would render a study of what is average and mediocre rather than what is possible and inspiring. In studying concert pianists, you would learn little or nothing from a scientifically rigorous study of hundreds of novices performing five-finger exercises. For too long and in too many aspects of research, we have focused on averages and overlooked the vast range of excellence in human performance. Beyond their individual credentials and anecdotes, the participants in this study all share an absolute vigor in pursuing all that life has to offer. There is a passion in their humor, commitments, insights, careers, and relationships.

Why would a successful actor like Dennis Weaver take time away from lucrative movie and advertising offers to start the LIFE (Love Is Feeding Everyone) program with actress Valerie Harper? What is it that compels John Sculley, chairman of Apple Computer, to move beyond his professional position to fulfill a "mission" of peace and understanding between the United States and Soviet Union? How did the assassination of John F. Kennedy profoundly alter both the personal and professional direction of Norman Cousins, who emerged from a major depression with a new vision of the "greater purpose" in his life? These individuals and the others I interviewed describe in the following pages how they developed their ability to rise to these challenges, as well as the personal strategies they use to maintain optimal health under the most trying circumstances.

Throughout the book, a participant's title at the time of the interview is noted, but over the course of the four-year study, some job positions have changed and two remarkable individuals, Norman Cousins and John E. Fetzer, have died, but the essence of the interviews remains intact. Below is a selected listing of the individuals who agreed to be identified by name among those who were interviewed for the study:

James A. Autry, vice president of Meredith Corporation
Zane E. Barnes, chairman and CEO of Southwestern Bell Corporation
Laurel Burch, founder and president of Laurel Burch Associates
James E. Burke, chairman of the board, Johnson & Johnson
Norman Cousins, author and founder of *Saturday Review*
Michael S. Currier, president of the New Cycle Foundation
John E. Fetzer, founder and president of the John E. Fetzer Foundation
Dr. Murray Gell-Mann, Nobel Prize laureate in physics
Gordon Getty, composer and philanthropist
Eileen Rockefeller Growald, founder of the Institute for the

Advancement of Health

T. George Harris, editor-in-chief of *American Health* and
　Psychology Today

Paul Hawken, founder, chairman, and CEO of Smith & Hawken,
　Incorporated

Dr. Dorothea R. Johnson, AT&T corporate vice president

Joan Konner, dean, Columbia University School of Journalism

Walter Landor, founder and president of Landor Associates

Norman Lear, producer, chairman, and CEO of Act III
　Communications, Incorporated

Joshua Mailman, founder and president of the Threshold
　Foundation

United States Senator Claiborne Pell

David Rockefeller, banker and philanthropist

United States Congresswoman Claudine Schneider

Robert Schwartz, founder of the Tarrytown Conference Center

John Sculley, chairman and CEO of Apple Computer

Wayne Silby, founder and president of the Calvert Fund for
　Social Responsibility

Brandon Stoddard, president of ABC Entertainment

Anthony S. Tiano, president of KQED-TV

John L. Tishman, founder and president of Tishman
　Construction

Lindsay Wagner, actress and health spokeswoman

Dennis Weaver, actor and founder of LIFE (Love Is Feeding
　Everyone)

Saul Zaentz, coproducer of *One Flew over the Cuckoo's Nest* and
　producer of *Amadeus*

All of the participants told me that they found the interview questions challenging and fun, since they were finally being asked about issues important to them. After I finished interviewing the actor Dennis Weaver, for example, he remarked that he was surprised by how quickly the time had passed. With a broad smile and a sigh he quipped, "It is certainly a pleasure to have a three-hour interview which feels like three minutes, rather than a three-minute interview which feels like three hours."

Each chapter contains excerpts from interviews that most vividly illustrate the chapter theme. While these interviews are, in fact, scientific case studies, I have attempted to preserve the candid, often dramatic tone of the actual conversations, which were often filled with deeply personal stories, insights, and psychological strategies.

Additional scientific findings further support the conclusions drawn from the interviews and lead to the concluding element in each chapter: specific recommendations that you can adopt to enhance your own personal health and performance. These "action steps" focus on basic stress management techniques, visualization and mental imagery practices, psychological strategies, dietary practices, coping skills, and other practical guidelines to help you achieve optimal health in your daily life.

Each chapter also progresses naturally from the preceding one, from the inner formative experiences of early childhood to the adult development of personal convictions and outer practices in their lives and careers. Most important, the concluding chapter addresses the role of optimal health as a mainstay in the development of a true health care system.

A SOUND MIND IN A SOUND BODY . . . IN A SOUND WORLD

Individuals interviewed in the Sound Mind–Sound Body study play important roles on the world stage—not only directly through their professional offices, financial involvement, or public visibility, but with their bold and visionary attempts to inspire and help us lead healthier lives. All of us are living together in historical, social, and environmental turbulence as we approach the twenty-first century. These challenging times call for new insight into lifestyles and attitudes that promote health and give us the freedom to live satisfying and successful lives. There are signs of unprecedented ferment, both positive and negative, all around us: Unexpectedly, the Berlin Wall dividing East and West Germany came crumbling down amid wild celebration, with joblessness and ethnic violence rising from the rubble. Over forty years of Cold War ended, as Gorbachev's *glasnost* took off without him and the Communist leader and his Soviet Union collapsed together, leaving a Commonwealth of Independent States with no idea of how to survive in their newfound independence. International television has shown us thousands of Chinese students and workers demonstrating in Beijing's Tiananmen Square in the name of democracy, then being slaughtered. Deforestation of Brazil's rain forest is directly affecting the skin cancer incidence of farmers exposed to more ultraviolet radiation in Kansas. Houses on the seashore of the East and West coasts of the United States are washing out to sea as graphic testimony to the unequivocal fact that the levels of the world's oceans are rising as a result of the greenhouse effect, with serious health consequences to follow. Personal physicians to the Dalai Lama have pronounced that AIDS may be only the first of a series of modern plagues prophesied in Tibetan medical texts of thousands of years ago. According to the firm of Arthur D. Little, medical costs are so out of control in the United States that by the year 2000 all of the profits of all of the Fortune 500 companies will be equal to their medical expenditures!

Delays in both understanding and action are perhaps inevitable, as are anachronistic views of ourselves and the world around us. After all, it took the Catholic Church more than 350 years to offer a formal apology to Galileo! On October 31, 1992, Pope John Paul II finally announced that the Church had wrongly accused the Italian astronomer for his heretical views of astronomy. Even with this gesture, the pontiff still criticized Galileo, insisting that the Copernican model placing the sun at the center of the solar system should have been stated as a "hypothesis" rather than an absolute truth: after all, no one had adequate proof of the Copernican model in the seventeenth century. Hopefully, it will not take three hundred years for us to redress the limitations, misconceptions, and misdirection of the present disease management industry.

It is increasingly evident that our hospitals, intensive care units, and morgues are the repositories of a collective social pathology. Medicine itself is symptomatic of a greater societal ill for which resources are limited and choices need to be made. These choices extend far beyond medicine into the realms of ethics, social responsibility, and morality, where answers are not amenable to the scientific method. Finding solutions will require that we be both creative and iconoclastic. Every individual and society pays dearly when social and economic problems become medical cases. Breakdown of the family, alcohol and chemical abuse, high-risk sexual behavior, violence, chronic unemployment, and environmental destruction lead directly to growing demands on an already overwhelmed health care system. Jogging, cosmetic surgery, and low-fat diets are not the answer; they only relieve the symptoms of a far deeper malaise. Energy spent in a misplaced narcissistic preoccupation with a narrow definition of health distracts individuals and organizations from coming to terms with our real sickness. To find a cure we need to go far beyond the medical sphere and into the timeless realms of ethics and morals, life and death. These are issues that require us all to become involved, no matter how limited or far-reaching that involvement may be.

CHAPTER TWO

Broken Bones Heal Strongest

Beyond his many literary and political achievements, the late Norman Cousins became internationally recognized for his moving personal accounts of how he overcame arthritis and coped with a life-threatening heart condition for many years. When his *Anatomy of an Illness as Perceived by the Patient* was published in 1979, he was already well-known, but his name had not yet become a household word, nor had he been embroiled in the controversy that *Anatomy* would incite.

Two years earlier, after the publication of my book *Mind as Healer, Mind as Slayer*, Norman wrote me, telling me that it had inspired and helped him to focus his reflections on his recovery from ankylosing spondylitis, a degenerative arthritis of the spine. For many years we worked together—from his writing the introduction to my book *Holistic Medicine* in 1979 to our giving joint lectures in which Norman presented the personal aspects of recovery from major illness and I provided the scientific documentation.

Despite our long friendship I was surprised to hear Norman describe, during our interview for this book, a connection between his ability to cope with illness as an adult and an early childhood trauma. At the age of nine he had contracted tuberculosis and was confined to a sanitarium. "My life became entirely different," he reflected as we talked in his home in the hills above the UCLA campus, where he was a senior lecturer at the School of Medicine, "because I had been sheltered up to that point. I was put into a public sanitarium because my parents were of modest circumstances. I discovered that there was a hierarchy—that the kids seemed to be divided into two categories. There was a larger category of those who believed they would never get out of that place alive. They had seen kids carried out dead or dying and accepted that as the expected outcome. Then there was the other group of kids who would not accept that outcome as inevitable. They were determined to rise above it and get out of there alive. In short, I think we followed the paths of our expectations.

"Kids can be pretty brutal, but I learned a great deal about the importance of a belief system. One of the unfortunate aspects of life in the TB sanitarium was that if you began with a mild case, it actually got worse from being there [as a result of being with other sick children]. When and if you did overcome it, you not only triumphed over the original problem but the compounded one. . . . We learned a lot about survival during that time, and it has affected my entire life. It helped me, in Dewey's phrase, to come to full possession of my powers. From that time on, with each of my illnesses, the sting was gone from the crisis because I knew I was going to make it. My doctors didn't always share that sentiment, but what *I* knew was what made the difference in my recovery."

Today Norman Cousins, who died of a heart attack in 1990, remains an inspiring example of how illness can lead to liberation and self-discovery, rather than to inevitable breakdown and despair. He successfully demonstrated that it is possible to strike a vital balance between the best biomedical technology and a deeper, inner sense of conviction.

CHILDHOOD TRAUMA—DISASTER OR DISCOVERY?

Surely, the intensity of Norman Cousins's childhood trauma left him with an indelible sense of self-efficacy, a confidence that he could determine his life's direction and successfully overcome challenges as an adult. This sense of certainty, which grew out of a potentially life-threatening childhood trauma, was shared by almost every participant in the Sound Mind–Sound Body study. Most had experienced a major health or life crisis prior to age ten, and virtually everyone had undergone a traumatic event by age eighteen. Whether incest, the death of both parents, or a near-fatal automobile accident, these early life traumas significantly affected the character and life direction of these individuals. But it was the ways in which they coped with these potentially devastating events that formed the core of the inner strength they would call upon as adults. Interestingly, each individual's relationship with his or her father was a significant early life memory that came up frequently in the interviews. Positively or negatively, this relationship played a critical and formative role in both the men's and women's development, in that all of the participants exhibited a clear and profound desire to meet the expectations and demands of their strikingly strong fathers. This theme, the focus of the present chapter, will reoccur throughout the book.

Such experiences as Norman Cousins's tuberculosis, especially when suffered at an early age, are thought to predispose individuals to later adult impairments, including alcoholism, depression, and an array of psychological as well as physical disorders. Psychotherapy, oriented toward uncovering the early antecedent traumas of adult disorders, is predicated on the hypothesis that early life experiences determine the development of an individual throughout adulthood. Most often the effect is found to be negative. In 1991 Dr. Naomi Breslau of the Department of Psychiatry at the Henry Ford Hospital in Detroit, Michigan, published an insightful article in the *Archives of General Psychiatry*. She studied a random sample of 1,007 young adults in Detroit for evidence and antecedents of posttraumatic stress disorders. She concluded that the young adults most likely to actually suffer posttraumatic stress disorders were those who experienced early separation from parents, exhibited early symptoms of neurosis and depression, and had a family history of anxiety. Out of the 1,007 people interviewed, 394 reported experiencing early life trauma and about 9 percent of those 394 developed posttraumatic stress disorders. Nine percent sounds relatively small but in fact indicates that these disorders are one of the most common problems affecting our general population.

Dr. Lawrence Kohlberg, a prominent developmental psychologist, reviewed the research on the predictability of adult adaptation and health based on childhood experiences. He and his colleagues concentrated on the key longitudinal studies (in which the same subjects were observed repeatedly over a period of time) in the three areas of emotional development, sexual development, and social behavior. They concluded that the pervasive belief that early life experience determines adult behavior is generally a myth, the two major exceptions being schizophrenia and sociopathic disorders, both of which appear to be determined by a combination of genetic and early environmental forces.

Consistent with Kohlberg's findings, research on stress has indicated that an individual's *reaction* to a traumatic event is usually more significant than the event itself. My study further confirms this research, demonstrating that traumatic events in childhood often serve as catalysts for the later development of such positive adult characteristics as altruism, compassion, commitment, and resistance to psychological and physical illness. In spite of this accumulating evidence the myth of "unhealthy child, unhealthy adult" continues to be promulgated, and people are made to fear that early life trauma spells the absence of health, achievement, and happiness in adulthood.

But what about those who have moved beyond illness and mediocrity into the domain of true success and optimal health? The participants in my study who suffered early childhood trauma apparently became self-reliant by necessity and thereby discovered their own inner strengths. Although at the time they did not consciously acknowledge these newfound assets, they experienced a sense of their ability to "control" or exert a profound influence over the course and direction of their lives, setting their journey toward personal and professional success in motion.

Psychologist Dr. Victor Goertzel and his wife, Mildred, also studied prominent individuals, and their research provides some of the few quantitative results in this area. In *Cradles of Eminence*, they researched the biographies of four hundred historical figures. Later they focused on contemporary success stories in *Three Hundred Prominent Personalities: A Psychosocial Analysis of the Famous*. Among their extensive findings the most relevant to the Sound Mind–Sound Body study is that more than one-fourth of these people lost one or both parents early in their lives. The Goertzels also found that those who had failure-prone fathers (Carl Jung, Thomas Edison, Charles Dickens, and Upton Sinclair) seemed to be motivated by their fathers' failure, recognizing at an early age that failure need not be a dead-end if one is willing to take risks. Approximately sixty-four of the three hundred prominent people were delinquent as children (Al Jolson, Muhammad Ali, Bob Dylan, Ingmar Bergman, and Babe Ruth). Another 25, suffered serious or chronic illnesses in childhood, were isolated from their peers, and spent a great deal of time alone (Leonard Bernstein, T. S. Eliot, Pope John Paul II, and Louis Leakey). Additionally, twenty-four showed signs of mental illness and ten had a mentally ill parent. Reflecting on these findings, the Goertzels noted, "There is reason to believe that a child needs some experience with frustration to be able to cope effectively with disappointment and disillusionment as a young adult . . . creativity and contentment are not compatible." Although my study indicates that professional creativity and success are remarkably compatible with personal contentment, it is also consistent with the findings that early childhood trauma can have a significantly positive outcome. However, it is important to remember that trauma is not a prerequisite to creativity, and that even in the presence of early life trauma the participants in my study have in fact achieved a sense of contentment in both their personal and professional lives while also being creative.

Among the most insightful research and writing on the phenomenon of positive adaptation to childhood trauma is the work of Dr. Emmy E. Werner, professor of human development and research at the University of California at Davis. From her own research and that of others, Dr. Werner has identified four common characteristics among "resilient children": 1) an active, evocative approach to solving life's problems and challenges; 2) a tendency to perceive their experiences constructively despite their pain and suffering; 3) an ability, from infancy, to gain other people's positive attention; and 4) a strong faith or set of spiritual values as the basis for a vision of a meaningful life. Dr. Werner elaborates on this inner sense of spiritual values: "Resilient children seem to have been imbued by their families with a sense of coherence. They manage to believe that life makes sense, that they have some control over their fate, and that God helps those who help themselves. . . . It enables them to love despite hate, and to maintain the ability to behave compassionately toward other people." In effect the trauma can serve as a precondition for the adult development of empathy and compassion.

Empathy is the ability to put oneself emotionally in another's situation—that is, to imagine and perhaps actually to experience the pain of another human being. There is a growing body of evidence that empathy is a predictor of adult optimal health, that it can be learned, and that it may even be genetically inherent. In February 1993 the American Association for the Advancement of Science at its annual meeting focused on "what it means to be human." According to the Harvard Medical School neurobiologist Dr. Terrence W. Deacon, the fact that chimpanzees and dolphins perform complex language tasks makes it increasingly difficult to determine what really makes us humans unique. Based on his research, he asserts that empathy may hold the key as the trait that forms the essence of human, moral reasoning. He theorizes that the human brain has evolved in a way that allows humans to uniquely "represent to ourselves what goes on in other people's minds." While both the genetic basis of empathy and the nature of our uniqueness are currently being debated, there is compelling research that empathy is both essential to health and can be learned even under the most adverse circumstances. Research in 1993 by a University of Helsinki psychologist, Dr. Mirja Kalliopuska, with four thousand young people between ages fourteen and twenty revealed that the individuals found to be more empathetic were also more confident and more sensitive, while also being assertive. She also developed methods to increase empathy based upon a four-month study involving six- and seven-year-old children. Reflecting on her research to date, Dr. Kalliopuska concludes that "empathy can be trained in babies and grandparents alike"; she herself has successfully trained children, teachers, nurses, doctors, and retired people. It seems that development and enhancement of empathy and compassion can grow out of both traumatic and positive childhood experiences and can also be elicited throughout life.

Results of my own research concur with both Werner's and Kalliopuska's conclusions. The ability early in life to discover and adhere to inner values amidst chaos or trauma appears to serve as a major formative influence on adult personal and professional endeavors. Perhaps the most significant data in this area is presented in Harvard psychiatrist Dr. Robert Coles's *The Spiritual Life of Children*, the eighth and last of his series on children, two volumes of which won the Pulitzer Prize in 1983. Coles relates that children ponder complex issues of morality and ultimate meaning and debunks the long-held view that children are emotionally fragile and will fall apart under the slightest stress. He finds that whether children are raised in religious or atheistic families, they place a remarkable emphasis on the spiritual side of their lives. Yet although such higher concerns are universally present, their spiritual advisers take many unorthodox forms, whether "a friend or potential enemy, an admirer or critic."

Critics of Coles argue that he uses insufficient scientific method and relies too heavily on case studies rather than data analysis. To this he has responded, "We have such an appetite in America for labeling people. We want fast, inclusive, easily remembered categories. Psychology, psychoanalysis, and psychiatry are secular religions, and people want the priests of these religions to just give them the stages, the cycles, the phases. I've spent a lifetime resisting that." Despite Coles's caveat, the spiritual dimension of early life trauma does appear to be possibly the single most important influence on individual conduct throughout adulthood. Personal and career choices, as well as involvement in philanthropic activities and public service, grow out of a search for a deeper meaning and purpose in life. Whether researchers label types of children as "stress resistant," "invulnerable," "resilient," or even "superkids," the well-documented phenomenon is a key foundation in building a model of health.

In the now-classic research on concentration camp survivors, psychiatrist Dr. Victor Frankl used case studies and anecdotes to build his argument that daunting circumstances can be overcome. More recent research by the renowned Dr. Aaron Antonovsky, an Israeli medical sociologist, underscores Frankl's insights. In his book *Health, Stress, and Coping*, Dr. Antonovksy examines how women from different ethnic backgrounds adapt to menopause. Among them is a group of women who survived Nazi concentration camps. Overall these women were in worse mental and physical health than others were who were not interred. However, he also found a smaller subset of survivors who were healthy in all physical, psychological, and social measures. Noting this unusual group, Antonovsky observes, "Despite having lived through the most inconceivably inhuman experience, some women were reasonably healthy and happy, had raised families, worked, had friends, and were involved in community activities." To account for this success, he proposed that certain individuals can draw upon resistance resources and support systems, including friends, education, mentors, family, money, or a worldview that he termed a "sense of coherence." This sense of coherence builds confidence that things will work out as well as can reasonably be expected and contributes to an individual's belief that he or she can in fact influence this outcome positively.

Even poverty is not inherently damaging to all who experience it. Although it surely affects an individual's health negatively, there are a small number of individuals who thrive despite or because of it. The futurist John Naisbitt, author of *Megatrends*, writes, "I grew up in real poverty. We didn't have any money. My father, bless his heart, refused to join the WPA [Work Projects Administration]. I have images of all the WPA guys building the curbs and the streets in Salt Lake. My father had too much pride for that. He would go around and knock on doors to see if he could shovel snow or do odd jobs. I remember as a kid we sometimes lived for days on just flour and water. I remember being teased by my schoolmates for the shabbiness of my clothes. Somewhere along the line I decided I had to get through. I vowed at the time that I would never be that poor again." That precocious tenacity, sense of coherence, and certainty that he could and would control his own destiny is consistently evident in every one of the Sound Mind–Sound Body interviews. Surely there are many well-known instances of people who endured great poverty as children, vowed never to be poor as adults, and grew up to be ruthless robber barons, amassing great wealth without a shred of compassion for those they exploited. While this scenario does happen, it is not inevitable. The few longitudinal studies that have tracked children from infancy or preschool years through adolescence and into adulthood indicate that some minority children did well in school despite chronic poverty and discrimination, that children of psychotic parents can grow up intact, and that divorce is not inevitably disruptive.

FROM CHILDHOOD TRAUMA TO ADULT TRANSCENDENCE

A recent study by Dr. Peter Ebersole and Dr. Joan Flores of the California State University at Fullerton contributes additional insights on the issue of coping with trauma. Reports were gathered from ninety-six volunteers on the amount of positive growth they may have experienced from what they judged to be their most difficult life crisis. Most often the traumas involved other people who were close to them. For twenty-seven of the participants the trauma was the illness or death of a family member; for twenty-six, the breakup of a meaningful relationship; and for ten, the divorce of their parents. Among the other traumas were their own injury or sickness, sexual abuse or incest, or failure at school or work. Most significantly, the participants emphasized the ability to "transcend" the experience or rise above the crushing short-term trauma by developing a positive attitude about the experience or its long-term consequences. For the majority of the individuals in the Ebersole and Flores study, as in my own research, the long-term impact was positive. Particularly striking is the fact that while gaining this new perception of a single event, the subjects also underwent a profound change in their outlook on life. Instead of the experience causing a breakdown, it brought forth a breakthrough to a new and deeper appreciation of themselves and others. A traumatic experience, therefore, is not inherently destructive and may be one means by which a person continues to evolve and come to a more meaningful understanding and appreciation of life itself.

Certainly one individual who transcended trauma and now embodies true health is T. George Harris. At the time of our interview, Harris was editor-in-chief of both *Psychology Today* and *American Health* magazines, roles that epitomized his personal and professional commitment to both the mind and the body. One colleague described

Harris as a "gold card member of the New York aristocracy" with his undergraduate education as a Phi Beta Kappa from Yale University, followed by Oxford, and his 1979 marriage to Ann Roberts, the daughter of the late Nelson Rockefeller. Harris, however, was certainly not born into privilege, or even into good health.

Harris describes himself as a "seventh-generation Kentucky hillbilly, a descendant of Daniel Boone, and a farm boy who suffered from most of the deprivation diseases including rickets and infantile paralysis." Through hard work, diligence, an astute intellect, and a drive to achieve, he became an Eagle Scout, a 4-H conservation champion, and his high school's valedictorian. When he was seventeen, he moved away from his rural upbringing and volunteered to fight in World War II. He recounted to me with present-time vividness his experience of more than 116 missions behind German lines, his award of a Bronze Star for gallantry and of a field commission in Bastogne during the Battle of the Bulge for "leadership under fire." That accolade might aptly be applied to every aspect of his life, from his childhood to the present day.

Returning from World War II, Harris enrolled at the University of Kentucky as a history major but became fascinated by the newly emerging field of social psychology. Yale University was the bastion of this new field, so he transferred there, graduated in only three years, then won a scholarship to study at Oxford University. While at Yale he returned to Tennessee to work for the daily *Clarksville Leaf Chronicle* every summer. "Working on the paper made me a better student. I probed harder and wrote with a touch of clarity, while Yale's faculty helped me build a theory of social change that I've spent my whole life testing and revising through magazine reporting. You see, I'm still between the street and the tower!" When Harris graduated from Yale in 1949, T. S. Matthews, the managing editor of *Time* magazine, was just about to launch his college recruiting experiment. After over twenty-two hundred candidates were narrowed down to five, Harris was hired. For more than thirteen years, he worked under "*Time*'s catholic definition of news," writing cover stories on people including Billy Graham, David Riesman, and Adlai Stevenson. Following his own heart and inclinations, he was drawn to the early populist protests by blacks, reported on the newly emerging Black Muslims, examined the John Birch Society, and was one of the first to detect and champion a fledgling women's movement.

Always a man to strike out on his own, he made use of his psychological background—"not to mention my combat training"—to take over *Psychology Today* in 1969. At the time it was a tiny, near-death magazine with an unimpressive number of subscribers, but he skillfully managed to raise the circulation to more than one million. When the magazine moved from California to its Manhattan office in 1975, Harris was fired for his freewheeling management style. (For example, he had installed a Ping-Pong table in the editorial offices.) Not one to stand still, he teamed up with the prominent publisher Owen Lipstein in 1981 to form the ground-breaking and successful magazine *American Health*. Seven years later he and Lipstein bought out *Psychology Today* and, among other things, reinstalled the Ping-Pong table.

Despite the enormous responsibility of being the editor-in-chief of two magazines, T. George Harris comes across as a dreamer with exuberant energy and an ever-present mischievous smile. Given his lifelong dedication to advocating a healthy body and mind, he was an ideal person to ask to define optimal health. After a moment of reflection, he proposed that "Health is functioning at your best, whatever it is that you do. There is so much evidence from research and data from our Gallup polls that the public understands health as being able to perform at your best in whatever you care about. . . . But there is also a lot of confusion about health. Wonderful confusions in some cases. A health crisis is probably one of the few times that people take the opportunity to reexamine what is generally an unexamined life. It is the conquest of that disease which becomes the conversion experience. There is a born-again self that comes out of crisis or disease, but that experience of renewal can also be self-generated by a decision to transform your life. More than fifty percent of the people who decide to get into exercise say they experience a form of total make-over. So the transformative experience of health does not have to be in the form of a present or past crisis."

Consistent with the observation that broken bones heal strongest, Harris believes that his childhood and adolescent traumas prepared him for the tribulations of adulthood. He remembers having grown up amidst great affection despite his difficulties: "I had rickets when I was born and must have been one of the last people in this country to have had that disease. That was partly due to my overprotective mother. She was determined to nurse but didn't have enough milk. She starved me to death—unknowingly, of course—until the doctor made her use Pet milk, which was the only formula available then. At the age of five I almost died of pneumonia. Then at eight I was paralyzed for over a year with infantile paralysis. Because of these afflictions, I was terribly small—too small to make the basketball team until I was a high school sophomore. Even then I was always the sixth man on a five-man team. I got more bench splinters than anybody I know.

"Just before I finished high school, I joined the Boy Scouts and went to camp. To be a Scout I needed to get the physical fitness merit badge, a camping merit badge, and a whole range of other badges. First I resisted because of my size, but then I got into push-ups and workouts so I could build up my scrawny little body. Since I was admittedly self-conscious, I would go down by the creek to be all by myself while I worked out. That went on for about thirty days, maybe more. I spent most of that summer living alone in the woods to strengthen my body. By seventeen, when I volunteered into the Army, I was lean enough and tough enough to score among the top three out of more than two thousand GIs on the standard fitness test." Looking at T. George Harris, now in his mid sixties, one sees a muscular, five-foot ten-inch man with more energy than the Hoover Dam. It is almost impossible to imagine that he was once a small, malnourished, sickly farm boy who managed to live through three life-threatening illnesses and went on to brave uncountable perils in combat in World War II. Today he is one of the most vital, optimally healthy individuals alive.

Harris's view of health is a combination of "healthy skepticism" and "a matter of heart and soul": "I'll eat fish and salads, but I'll also eat a really depraved dessert. Some people think it's awful that others jog just to look better, but let's face it, vanity has encouraged more healthy behavior than the desire for a long life has.

"Today our concept of health includes, if not centers on, something far more spiritual than diet and exercise. Health is a way for people to live and achieve and succeed with higher values." These values were instilled by Harris's mother from day one. "My mother was a visionary who lived by her ideals. Her spiritual values governed her life, and she was a confirmed conscientious objector. She read the Bible avidly and taught me to look to it for guidance. There is some fairly unequivocal language in the Bible—for example, 'Thou shalt not kill.' Being in the war, I had a tough time with this until I saw a movie about Sergeant York in World War I. He was a religious man who captured a whole company of German soldiers while quoting the Epistle to the Romans on the necessity of combating evil. From that point on I entered the battle with the avowed purpose of ending the war and stopping the killing as soon as possible. I became a relentless warrior."

Throughout T. George Harris's life is that seemingly paradoxical fusion: he's the relentless warrior dedicated to preserving life, the social altruist embracing the wealthy elite, and the spokesman for the fixation on the healthy body advocating the necessity of a spiritual core in optimal health. One close friend of his observed that "T. George has no pretensions of being a purist; in fact, he has no pretensions at all." Perhaps it is that remaining trace of his Kentucky heritage as a descendant of Daniel Boone that infuses his life with such refreshing irreverence for both his own personal shortcomings and any view of optimal health that does not include personal commitment and behavior governed by deeper spiritual yearnings.

TWO SIDES TO EVERY COIN

Many of the individuals in my study currently enjoy substantial financial security, but the vast majority were born into modest means. In addition they did not first become wealthy and *then* espouse altruistic values. Rather it was quite the opposite. When faced with each new crossroads or crisis, they consistently based their decisions on their inner values and commitments. Often the choices they made seemed wrong financially, but in retrospect they were profitable, both personally and monetarily.

Even for the five individuals born into great inherited wealth, including Gordon Getty and David Rockefeller, their childhood and adolescent crises were by no means cushioned and may, in fact, have even been exacerbated by their affluence. This observation is consistent with a five-year study by John Levy, the San Francisco founder of Inherited Wealth Consultants, who researched how parents of wealthy families might pass on the advantages of affluence to their heirs while minimizing the disadvantages. Because this was such a novel area of inquiry, Levy made significant discoveries through his interviews with approximately thirty wealthy parents and inheritors. He found, for instance, that children of inherited wealth often have "inadequate self-esteem," are "delayed in their emotional development," "lack adequate motivation," have "difficulty with self-discipline," are "bored with their lives," "suffer from extreme guilt," tend to be "suspicious, alienated, and isolated," and have "difficulty in the use of power."

However, Levy's pioneering work illuminates a key point relevant both to people who inherit wealth and to those who independently acquire it. According to Levy, "Psychological and spiritual growth are essential to the good life for everyone, but particularly for the affluent, because of their need to find meaning in their lives beyond the materialistic and competitive realms. Also, they are likely to have more leisure time to ponder, to be concerned about, and perhaps to do something about these aspects of their lives. For some this means more or less conventional church-oriented religion; for others a more individual way. We all find life more fulfilling if we have at least some sense of reality and significance beyond that which is just physical and rational, and this is particularly true for the rich, who end up realizing that material abundance just isn't enough for a satisfying life." Although those participants who inherited great wealth may have discovered this fact sooner, it was acknowledged by every individual in my study. Money is neither a panacea nor a plague; nor does it ensure that people will move beyond the narcissism of purely material pursuits. Many people have inherited equal or greater fortunes than have the few individuals in my study and have not turned to altruistic, philanthropic, or public service endeavors. Perhaps there is a subtle chemistry born of successful adaptation to early childhood trauma and challenge that remains an imponderable influence upon adult altruism.

Individuals can transcend pain and adversity, and even transform trauma, by shifting their perception of a crisis or event. There does not appear to be any secret or special technique to achieving this shift in perception, but it seems to involve a mental aikido or ability to accept constructively life's obstacles and learn from the experience. Those of us who did not acquire that strategy in early childhood must recognize that it is never too late to learn.

Consider the well-known designer Laurel Burch. Laurel is a highly influential jewelry, clothing, and graphic designer and president of Laurel Burch Incorporated, a $25-million-a-year business. Her designs are featured in over five thousand stores in ten countries. Since childhood Laurel, who suffers from a rare, congenital osteopetrosis, has endured over fifty fractures, numerous operations, and frequent pain. This type of osteopetrosis, not to be confused with the more common loss of bone calcium as one ages, is a genetic disease that creates abnormal patterns of bone density. The condition makes bones as fragile as glass and leaves the entire skeletal system susceptible to a fracture from the slightest impact or strain. In 1988 Laurel's dog innocently ran into her as she opened the door for their usual walk. As a result both her legs were fractured, she was confined to a hospital bed for weeks following surgery, and when she left the hospital, she was in a lower-body cast requiring months of immobility. Depressed, isolated, and removed from the creativity of her business, Laurel was distraught.

She plagued herself with questions—"Why does this have to happen to me?" "What have I done to deserve this?"—which only exacerbated her depression and caused her to withdraw further. Then something remarkable happened. "While immobile," Laurel remembers, "I found it so hard to move around, my body felt like a leaden weight and my spirits felt even worse. . . . Since I couldn't concentrate on my work, I hated my studio. Because of the damn cast I really wasn't sleeping well, and I stopped eating because I couldn't afford to gain any weight as it would aggravate the stress on my bones. Finally the only room I could stand to be in was my living room, so I had my mattress brought in and spent days lying there. My only relief was the fire I stared into at night. . . . All of my drawings and pottery turned deep brown, purples, and black as I just lay on the floor. My work up until that time was full of vibrant colors, exotic birds from my travels in Malaysia, soaring wild horses with Pegasus wings which reflected my feeling that I was flying too. Now I was crawling, without legs, close to the earth like some kind of lizard, like a salamander—all the lowly, stunted, and repulsive little creatures. It was when I felt like one of these creatures that I saw that they had a beauty too, just like the strange beauty I discovered in myself when there were no distractions and no way to take flight. . . . So I began drawing and painting frantically—lizards, salamanders, frogs, and newts. After I convinced my designers I had not gone crazy, we began the 'Celebration of the Earth' series, and it has proven to be one of the most successful and profitable lines we have ever developed."

Laurel's breakdown was clearly a precursor of her creative breakthrough. By having had to cope with fractures and pain since childhood, she was able to transcend a potentially devastating adult trauma and actually enter a period of intense insight. Her ability to empathize with lowly creatures allowed her to explore the rich landscape residing within her own creativity.

Empathy, that ability to experience vicariously another person's emotional state, is one of the most notable qualities to emerge from early personal trauma. As early as the first week of life, infants have been found to exhibit distress and cry in response to another infant's cry. Yet despite the presumed importance of empathy toward other people, there is relatively little research on the subject and even less on the factors that influence its development.

In 1990 Dr. Mark A. Barnett and Dr. Sandra J. McCoy of Kansas State University published a ground-breaking article indicating that an intense, distressful event early in life, such as a serious illness or injury, is directly related to the development of adult empathy, the capacity to experience the emotional response of another person. An adult can transform that early crisis into personal and professional creativity that touches the inner beings of others. Crisis has served as the creative wellspring of authors, artists, and scientists, since it inspires or even compels individuals to communicate their experience to others. As might be expected, the researchers also found that the women participants in their study were more empathetic than their male counterparts.

Drs. Barnett and McCoy interviewed fifty-six men and fifty-five women students who were led to believe that they were actually volunteering for two different projects. First the students completed the Distress Experiences in Childhood questionnaire. Then the same students watched a highly emotional therapy session acted out by a professional actress. Both the men and women who rated their early childhood experiences as the most stressful exhibited greater empathy toward the woman in the taped therapy session than did the other subjects.

Other research into the phenomena of empathy and spiritual orientation and my own study have illuminated specific commonalities among both children and adults. Research by Dr. C. Margaret Hall of Georgetown University has explored the function of family crisis in potentially precipitating empathy and spiritual values. Dr. Hall analyzed life history data from two hundred families that did not report familiar disruption and found that family members who successfully coped with crises appeared to live life more productively and experience greater satisfaction than people in families that reported few if any major problems. Her research indicated that successfully coping with a crisis had "far-reaching constructive effects on the quality of life" for every family member. Very often the crisis, ranging from physical abuse to a debilitating illness or death, prompted both the afflicted individual and the entire family to examine their fundamental values and life orientation. Although crisis is not a necessary prerequisite for the development of empathy, it clearly precipitates a "more dramatic rate of spiritual growth" among families in crisis. Dr. Hall also discovered that very often a single family member changes or deepens his or her values and beliefs and that it is that person who has the most impact on other family members. A supportive family environment or one positive adult role model appeared to be another significant factor, as was the influence of a parent or parents who taught their children to empathize.

Even beyond childhood, the degree to which parents give affection to their children and the degree to which they encourage independence are among the two most accurate predictors of adult happiness and social adaptability. During 1988 Dr. Judith Richman and Dr. Joseph Flaherty of the Department of Psychiatry at the University of Illinois interviewed one hundred randomly selected medical students to determine if there was a link between their views of how they were reared and their adult mental health. According to the study, depression and adult personality problems were associated with the father's coldness or emotional distance and with overprotection by either parent. Overprotective parents constrict and control their children rather than provide them with a supportive environment in which they can experience the seemingly inevitable crises of growing up. Adult states resulting from overprotection are quite the opposite of empathy and compassion. Overprotected students also reported low self-esteem, dependency, and rigidity, although it could not be determined from this study if these qualities led to or were caused by their reported depressions. Furthermore, their negative moods had an adverse effect on certain personality characteristics, particularly their sense of being in control of their lives. The students who grew up in rigid and emotionally limited homes felt that they could not influence the course of their lives. The distinction between feeling in control over the course and direction of one's life versus feeling helpless or hopeless to orchestrate it is a critical element found in my research. It is also a powerful indicator of adult mental and physical health or illness.

On the other hand, those students who said their parents had supported them emotionally and had encouraged them to be independent showed high self-esteem and intellectual flexibility. This important finding is consistent with Dr. Mark Barnett's conclusions as presented in 1987 in his definitive collection of monographs entitled *Empathy and Its Development*. After an extensive review of the empathy research, he determined that "children who are encouraged to feel good about themselves may be more inclined to empathize with others than children who are preoccupied with personal inadequacies and other concerns about the self. . . . Development of empathy would appear to thrive in an environment that encourages the child to experience a broad range of emotions and provides numerous opportunities for the child . . . to [develop] emotional sensitivity and responsibleness to others." In summary, early childhood trauma within a supportive family environment can become an important core experience for the development of highly positive adult coping skills and emotional maturity.

Today there is a growing consensus among child development specialists, educators, and public policy makers that the best time to lay the foundation for constructive adaptation and the acquisition of positive emotions is during childhood. Late in 1990 Dr. Emory Cowen, professor of psychology and psychiatry at the University of Rochester, received the Award for Distinguished Contributions to Psychology in the Public Interest for his work in emphasizing the importance of health promotion for children. Delivering his acceptance speech to the American Psychological Association, Cowen urged the nurturing of children's skills in "competency" and "resilience," especially for children from high-risk poor families of the inner city, where there is a high incidence of drug use, violence, and teenage pregnancies. Resilience is the ability to withstand trauma and emerge stronger. Cowen emphasized that society must "promote politics and conditions that enable people to gain control over their lives, on the assumption that doing so will reduce problems in living and enhance wellness."

Studying people who, like the participants in my research, have learned to persevere through—if not thrive upon—adversity can reveal helpful strategies for others living under chronically disabling conditions, children or adults. Apparently because of their own confrontations with hardship, these individuals have developed a strong empathy and compassion for people in circumstances similar to or even more tragic than what they have experienced themselves.

AN UNFORGETTABLE FATHER

Among the subjects of my study it was most often one or both parents who had influenced the outcome of childhood trauma. Dr. Michael Goldstein at UCLA has found that a child may be able to transcend a troubled home if a parent or any other supportive, stable adult is an influence. My own research uncovered two further nuances. First, for both the men and women, the father was cited far more frequently in the interviews than the mother, at least in terms of the influence each had upon the child's career as an adult. Secondly, the influence of the father persisted even when the traumatic incident itself had been caused by the father or when the child experienced his death.

This paternal influence was articulated by Robert Schwartz, founder of the Tarrytown Conference Center in New York and described by his peers as the "entrepreneur of entrepreneurs." Reflecting on his personal childhood experience and his later work with the founders of new business ventures, Bob observed, "The principal motivation of people who want to do something different, to be entrepreneurial, is primarily influenced by their father. The relationship of men or women in this kind of pursuit is always toward the father, often an absent one. My father died of stomach cancer when I was ten. He had been a powerful man, and as his condition grew increasingly worse, he remained strong. My father's death had a much more profound impact on me than I realized at the time. Every single entrepreneur has some aspect of that; their father was too powerful, too absent, too demanding, too this, or too that. Although they love their mother, the father is the premier figure."

Looking back at his childhood in Germany during the rise of the Nazis, designer and entrepreneur Walter Landor reflected upon his father's influence on his life. Although renowned as one of the world's most gifted designers, Landor acknowledges that "my ambition and achievement grew out of a situation where my childhood security was disturbed by political upheaval. If it hadn't been for that, I do not think I would have developed in the same manner. I was affected by such a combination of influences including, of course, my father and mother. I was born in Munich, raised there, and I observed my father as someone who possessed tremendous talent and perfectionism. But he did not receive the degree of professional recognition or compensation he deserved. . . . Knowing the injustice my father suffered, I felt I had to do better than he did. Somehow I learned to compensate for my father's shortcomings through my mother. She had a flair for putting things in order, and from her I learned the importance of organizational skills, which were lacking in my father. I have always managed to find someone to handle the details of business so I could focus on my artistic and intuitive abilities. My mother taught me the importance of business and how to delegate responsibility, but it was my father's sad plight which taught me it *must* be done."

Like Walter Landor, Nobel Prize laureate Murray Gell-Mann perceived his father's deficiencies. Dr. Gell-Mann remembers that "he would lock himself in a little room and work out mathematical equations and try to understand physics and astronomy theories. But he never became a serious physicist or astronomer and he never succeeded in understanding Einstein's general theory of relativity or Einsteinian gravitation, but he liked to think about them. He actually did succeed in understanding a certain branch of mathematics which was exceedingly obscure at that time but became important later. All of his work could have been quite usefully applied, but he wasn't very good at dealing with the world in general.

"A few years ago I read an article about great achievers. There seemed to be a general rule that they had all been given confidence by their upbringing. They were taught to feel good about themselves in some way or another. At the Academy Awards ceremony this year I saw Jodie Foster accept her award for best actress. She said she wanted to thank all her family, her mother, fathers, uncles, aunts, brothers, and sisters and so on for making her feel so good about herself and telling her that all her finger paintings were Picassos. Suddenly it struck me that I never felt that way. I have always doubted myself and felt insecure.

"It's been very hard for me to accomplish anything because I've been fighting a childhood obstacle of self-doubt. Somehow I never understood what was expected of me. People expected me to have good manners, but they never told me what that meant. They assumed that I would know. Because I was fairly bright, they assumed that I knew all these things, but how can you know facts without being exposed to them? I was always embarrassed because I was a perfectionist and yet I always found myself saying or doing something wrong because I didn't know what the rules were. Even now when I do research, I always delay a year and a half or two years before publishing results. By that time somebody else is usually doing it too. Fortunately I was doing things sufficiently in advance that even the delay did not completely cripple the research. But that's just one example. In so many different ways I just don't have enough faith in myself. At the root of my self-doubt is the way my family was structured. There was so much criticism and perfectionism. I mean, we didn't ever do finger painting. It was too sloppy. Anything I did was always held up to some very high standard. My father's criticisms were probably correct, but they did not affect me positively."

Throughout the interviews the vast majority of participants made similar statements. Not only did they cite the significance of their father's influence—positive or negative—but they also conveyed the need they felt to create their own, internal version of who he was. This self-induced, reconstructed role model built partially from memory and partially from fantasy was important because it invited the subjects to project their own values onto memory. The ability to reflect upon and consciously reconstruct an early life experience and thereby more fully comprehend it marks one of the most striking personal strategies in attaining optimal health. By this strategy we are able to contact the part of ourselves that some schools of psychotherapy refer to as the "inner child." It is that aspect of our person that remains emotionally immature, in both the negative and positive aspects of immaturity, despite the fact that the body grows taller, ages, and becomes an adult. As adults the participants in my study imagine their father, in effect, conversing with their inner child. Through this confrontation they are able to come to a more balanced resolution of their father's inordinate influence, positive and negative.

These findings are somewhat unusual since the majority of research in the area of empathy and prosocial behavior by Dr. Seymour Feshbach and other noted psychologists has indicated that the mother may play a particularly important role in her child's development of these qualities. This conclusion appears to be especially accurate with regard to African-, Asian-, and Mexican-American girls reared in poverty by mothers who are employed. However, in his extensive review of the scientific literature through 1987 Dr. Mark Barnett had anticipated my finding. He states that "fathers (as well as other important caregivers) have not always been included, or included as extensively as mothers, in studies of the child's social-emotional development. With many fathers becoming more actively involved in all aspects of child rearing, their contribution to their sons' and daughters' evolving capacities to empathize merits greater attention in the future." Although all my research participants were raised before any recent change in child-rearing practices, the influence of their fathers is unmistakable.

This finding has been confirmed independently in another ongoing study of the development of altruistic behavior by my colleague and friend Dr. Christie W. Kiefer of the Human Development and Aging Program at the University of California School of Medicine. His research was also independently funded by Laurance S. Rockefeller through the Institute of Noetic Sciences in Sausalito, California. During the course of a meeting convened by the Institute, Dr. Kiefer and I discovered the commonalities in our research regarding the dominant role of the father. In interviews with twenty individuals identified as "altruists," he found that "five of the altruists and two of the 'pocket altruists,' or not publicly active individuals, had fathers who either died or suffered debilitating illnesses or injuries early, or who were perceived by their child as ineffectual. Apparently, no father at all, or a reduced one, is better for producing altruism than a domineering father. . . . Children of warm fathers in my samples, even when they were not altruists, were more generous and had a more relaxed, playful attitude toward life. The altruists in particular were unusually curious about the world, and they all had a well-developed sense of humor." Kiefer also concluded that most fathers, while they mean well, have been raised in a competitive model emphasizing individualism. The model is of the self-reliant warrior in a world of similarly driven warriors.

In *Scripts People Live* Claude Steiner succinctly captured the resulting impact: "Individualism goes hand in hand with competitiveness. Since we stand or fall strictly on our individual efforts, it follows that we must think of everyone around us as individuals equally interested in succeeding and, in the mad scramble to the top, also necessarily invested in achieving superiority, or one-up status, to us. Being one-down is intolerable; the only alternative in our society is to try to stay one-up. Equality is not comprehended by us and often not even considered. Competitiveness is trained into human beings from early life in our culture." Two choices result. One is to adopt the model and become the fiercely competitive warrior, seeking domination over all and coping with the resulting isolation, separation, incessant insecurity, and fear of losing. The alternative is to create a larger whole so that the individual needs of many can be satisfied by shares of the larger pie. That choice appears to be a fundamental building block for the entrepreneur who is motivated to satisfy his or her own needs while creating new programs, products, and services that meet the needs of others as well. Competitive drive is not inherently negative or destructive; its value depends on how it is managed, directed, and manifested in the world.

Virtually all of the individuals in my research triumphed over circumstances that others might have found crushing. It is possible to identify the inner resources and outer circumstances that enabled them to prevail, with the hope that the knowledge can be useful to parents, children, and even traumatized adults who may not yet have been able to rise above their misfortunes. The participants in my research are "transcenders," to borrow a term coined by Katherine Northcraft, a psychiatric social worker from Indiana. According to Northcraft, transcenders have self-confidence and learn to think for themselves early on. They distance themselves emotionally from their parents and choose their own actions rather than do what would be expected of them in their environment. "In the worst of times, transcenders envision themselves elsewhere, imagining that they can do great things despite their surroundings." The ability to detach oneself from trauma, as opposed to denying it, and to envision a future goal beyond the immediate circumstances is an extremely important coping mechanism confirmed by my research. Certain children seem to be able to draw upon inner strength in the face of adversity, even when the trauma involves their parents, especially the father, and there is no evident source of external adult support.

Writer, producer, and director Norman Lear went through a painful boyhood trauma that was brought on by his father's poor judgment.

Although devastating at the time, the experience has had a long-term positive impact on his life and has been a pervasive motivating factor throughout his extensive television and film career. Norman has received innumerable accolades and distinguished awards, but to the public he is best known as the developer of television shows, including *All in the Family, Sanford and Son, The Jeffersons, Mary Hartman, Mary Hartman*, and *One Day at a Time*. Having started out as a comedy writer at the inception of network television, Norman has incorporated a comedic element into virtually all of his productions. He commented that comedy was essential because "I'm so passionate about the issues in my sitcoms that if I really stated how I feel without the comedy, people would be bored to tears with my preaching!" His personal philosophy might be summed up by his words, "People laugh hardest when they care the most."

Roots of these passionate convictions were established in Norman's early childhood. When he was nine years old, his father, whom he admired and loved, was sent to prison. There was a great deal of publicity at the time of the arrest and Norman's humiliation was only exceeded by his sense of loss and betrayal. Norman reflected, "My father was a great character, a rascal! If there was a little screw in his head that could have been adjusted a sixteenth of an inch in one direction or other, he might have known right from wrong. That got him into a bunch of trouble. . . . He always billed himself as a great salesman, but he was conned by a couple of other salesmen. He sold some bad stocks for them. Everyone told him that there was something wrong with these guys, but he refused to believe it.

"One day when I was nine, he flew to Oklahoma. Having a father who flew to Oklahoma was a big thing in Revere, Massachusetts, where we lived. He was going to bring me back a ten-gallon hat. . . . I will never forget that he was going to bring me back that hat. He never did come home from that trip. The police picked him up at the airport, and the next thing I knew there he was on the front page of the local paper . . . and my mother was selling all of our furniture and breaking up our home. One effect it had on me, I know, was to put a particularly high premium on honesty—in myself and others. Also, I think I can trace the fact that I love to wear the 'white hat' in all my work to the longing I felt for that ten-gallon hat that he had promised me."

It was not until he was twelve years old that Norman reunited with his father on a railway platform in New Haven, Connecticut, on their way to New York to begin life again. Out of the trauma of his father's arrest, and the religious convictions of his maternal grandfather, Norman developed a deep sense of honesty and integrity, which continues to pervade his prolific writing and passionate political activism.

A MIND-BODY CONNECTION

Practically every individual interviewed for the Sound Mind–Sound Body study fulfilled the medical truism that broken bones heal strongest. Having coped successfully with early life trauma, nearly all have carried with them the ability to triumph over crises that arose in their adult lives. Particularly in the case of those who overcame life-threatening disease as adults, such as Norman Cousins, Norman Lear, and Congresswoman Claudine Schneider, it is clear that both a psychological and a physical dimension characterized their remarkable recoveries.

There is growing evidence that unexamined psychological and physical traumas can lead to adult conditions of otherwise unexplained origin. Case studies have linked sexual abuse, psychological trauma, physical injury, and other repressed earlier experiences to adult physical disorders that do not have an organic basis. The phenomenon is a form of somatization disorder, in which the body expresses an injury that the mind cannot acknowledge. Since several individuals in my research experienced physical and sexual abuse in childhood, a study published in late 1990 is particularly relevant. Writing in *Annals of Internal Medicine*, a group of clinicians at a university-based gastroenterology clinic in North Carolina gave a confidential questionnaire to a group of women who entered the clinic. Approximately seventy-five women presented a history of functional gastrointestinal problems, that is, conditions with no evident physical cause, such as irritable bowel, spastic colon, nonspecific abdominal pain, and nonulcer indigestion. Among these women 31 percent reported at least one lifetime incident of rape or incest and 13 percent reported frequent physical abuse.

By contrast, of the patients with organic gastrointestinal symptoms, that is, those traceable to biological and lifestyle risk factors, only 2 percent reported sexual or physical abuse. Only 35 percent of the abused women had ever discussed their experiences with a professional therapist, and in only 17 percent of these cases were the clinic gastroenterologists aware of their own patient's history of abuse. This study adds to a growing body of medical literature indicating that patients with unexplained physical symptoms, ranging from intestinal tract problems to various forms of heart disease, may have a history of physical, sexual, or psychological trauma and abuse. The recognition of this possibility and the adoption of new clinical interventions to address it broaden the dimensions of the mind-body approach to true health care.

These findings, their implications, and ideas on how they can be applied will be more fully elaborated throughout this book. Effects of childhood trauma are evident in both mind and body. A growing number of studies have correlated early familial trauma or chronic instability with negative effects upon the immune system and greater susceptibility to disease. One study followed sixteen families for one year to determine why some people became ill with streptococcal infection resulting in strep throat while others did not. After accounting for all the medical factors, such as age, season, antibiotic use, and transmission, the best predictor was acute and chronic family stress. Another study followed the entire class of cadets at West Point for four years. Out of all the cadets who evidenced the presence of the Epstein-Barr virus, only 25 percent actually developed mononucleosis in the four years. Those cadets who developed mono, the study found, had fathers who were overachievers, had an unusually high level of drive toward a military career, and scored poorly in academic performance.

Further studies detailed later in this book which indicate that early life trauma may predispose adults to disorders ranging from psychosis to cancer, although there is a small but important subset of less vulnerable individuals and families who suffer the same or greater degree of trauma and do not become ill as children or adults. Although unexplored childhood traumas have a dramatic and often negative impact on adult mental and physical health, the interviews in my research and increasing evidence from other sources show that the long-term effect of such trauma is not inevitably negative; painful early experience can be transformed into a positive force in an individual's life.

By speaking out publicly, First Lady Rosalyn Carter raised women's awareness of breast cancer after her own surgery, Betty Ford made alcoholism recovery an occasion for celebration rather than shame, Dick Cavett and Rod Steiger made inspiring recoveries from severe depression, and Michael Landon created an indelible image of dying with dignity. Their heartfelt honesty, together with their positions of prominence, helped lift the stigma from conditions that affect the lives of millions. Likewise, the subjects of my research project, all prominent people, here reveal the depth and meaning of their early life traumas. Lessons they have learned are included in these pages to help you, the reader, make working with such personal crises more acceptable, and to show that it can result in lifelong benefits.

In effect these individuals learned at an early age to engage in a form of self-directed psychotherapy. Although evidence continues to show that early crises predispose people to adult disorders, it is becoming increasingly established that psychological and behavioral strategies can reduce the incidence of a wide range of health problems. Underlying the general model of mind-body interaction is the working assumption that inhibiting a person's thoughts, feelings, and behavior in response to a life crisis is associated with increased long-term stress and ultimately disease. Furthermore, a basic tenet of behavioral treatment for the entire range of lifestyle disorders, from depression to coronary heart disease, is that actively confronting the crises or difficulties actually reduces or eliminates the negative effects of the trauma. It is now well documented that the need for medical care in treating the full spectrum of acute and chronic diseases, including everything from surgical recovery to arthritis management, drops following psychotherapy and behavioral interventions. Individuals in my research appear to have learned, albeit not necessarily consciously as children or young adults, how to adopt personal coping strategies when confronted with crisis. Even more importantly, their coping skills increased throughout their lives, suggesting that anyone at any age can develop similar personal strategies for optimal health and performance.

One of the most memorable and striking of all the interviews is one that appeared *not* to fit the findings regarding early childhood trauma. Joan Konner's life, while unique in many ways, is nevertheless one of the best illustrations of how successfully to transform trauma, no matter at what age, into a positive experience.

Joan Konner is currently dean of the Graduate School of Journalism at Columbia University, where she also serves as a professor of broadcast journalism and publisher of the *Columbia Journalism Review*. Before her position at Columbia Dean Konner was president and executive producer of Public Affairs Television, an independent production company, in partnership with Bill Moyers. Their company produced Moyers's programs for public television, among them *Moyers: In Search of the Constitution; God and Politics; The Secret Government: The Constitution in Crisis*; and *Joseph Campbell and the Power of Myth*. In her work for public television and NBC News, Ms. Konner wrote and produced more than fifty documentaries and served as executive producer of several major public affairs series. She has won every major award in her field, including twelve Emmys from the National Academy of Television Arts and Sciences, the George Foster Peabody Award, two Ohio State Awards, and the Alfred I. du Pont–Columbia University Award.

I first met Joan Konner over twenty years ago when she filmed a documentary on my research. Little did I know how remarkable her personal odyssey had been. Unlike the others in my study, Ms. Konner described her life a "pretty uneventful up until thirty-nine. . . . I came to regard my upbringing as the trauma. It was traumatic to not have been exposed to many things. We were, in the social definition of the times, little girls who should be pretty and brush their teeth, look nice, be attractive to boys, to date and find a husband. No theater, not much reading, but education was extremely important. My parents were very conventional. . . . Then in 1969 my entire family passed away. It was not a massive accident; each death was unrelated. My mother suffered with a brain tumor for nine months. It was horrible. She was in the hospital for two weeks before she died. That day I came home from work to a message on my machine. 'Your mother passed away today. Come down to the hospital as soon as you can.' When I got to the hospital, the whole family was there, all dressed and walking around. So I asked, 'How come we're not home? We should be planning the funeral. Why are we in the hospital?' My father responded, 'Oh, I'm a patient.' I said, 'You're a patient?' He said, 'Yeah. Something went wrong in here,' pointing to his chest, 'and I don't know what it is. They are doing some tests on me.' That was the most horrible two weeks of my life. My father had always been vigorous, healthy, supportive, and totally, totally committed and involved with our family. He suffered a severely ruptured aorta just ten minutes after my mother died.

"They couldn't diagnose it for a week because some anomaly in his body prevented them. They knew the blood count was off, but they could not identify the problem. Throughout that week he suffered excruciating pain and hallucinations. I was absolutely convinced it was psychological: after all, he was experiencing the same symptoms my mother had. At the end of five days the doctor said, 'We don't know what this is. But his condition is getting worse, and the pain is killing him.' We rushed him to Mount Sinai, where even the doctors there couldn't figure out what was wrong with him. They decided to give him an angiogram and discovered that the situation was life-threatening: he had a ruptured aorta. They flew him by private plane down to Texas, where they operated, and then two or three days later he died. My sister died five months later from an undiscovered brain hemorrhage.

"She just couldn't stand the grief. Everything happened in such a bizarre fashion. As we were sitting in my father's hospital room, he was hallucinating, and I told her I thought it was psychological. He was calling to the grave, to our mom. When I told her that, she looked up at me and said, 'I feel it too!' I said, 'Oh, come on, you know Mom wouldn't want you to do anything other than live your life well and to the fullest.' 'No,' she insisted, 'I feel it too.'

"Compounding all of that was the fact that my marriage had been in trouble for a couple of years. Although I wanted to get divorced, I didn't see how I could do it. My husband was a nice guy, but we just didn't belong together. We were off the rail for a variety of reasons; it was just not working. Just before my mother got sick, I had spoken to my father about the divorce because I thought I'd need financial support with the kids. Then my mother dies, my father dies, my sister dies. At the time I was in therapy because of my marriage and because I was trying to handle losing my family. Then three weeks later my analyst died suddenly of a heart attack.

"To say that this was transformational is an understatement. I finally decided I had had enough unhappiness. This is it, I thought; the marriage has been miserable. I am just going to start over again right now. My husband and I separated gradually for the kids. That piece of life up to age thirty-nine was over. There are very few people that I am in touch with now that even know about that part of my life."

Joan Konner literally regenerated herself to reach unprecedented achievement in a male-dominated media empire. She had always been creative, and her extraordinary writing skill had actually manifested itself early in her life, but it flowered after the loss of her family and marriage. "When the kids were young—I think they were one and three—I got mononucleosis, and I was confined to bed for three weeks. So I started to write. At first I wrote poetry. Then I took some courses at the New School. I vowed that when the kids went to school full-time, I was going to work. Suddenly there it was upon me. I applied to journalism school at Columbia and received a letter that said the class was already accepted but to apply for next year. That was a fortunate delay, because you had to know how to type and I didn't. Since it was a requirement, I bought myself a book, and I did nothing but type, type, type for three weeks. Two weeks later I got a letter from Columbia saying that a space had been made available. It turned out that a woman from Bergen County had gotten pregnant and dropped out, so I was accepted. Divine intervention—do you believe it? For me it can be summed up as 'invisible hands.' "

Through her own hands and her "invisible hands," Joan Konner created a second life for herself after experiencing as an adult a series of major traumas. For a different individual, any one of those tragedies could have accounted for a later adult life of dysfunction and disease, but for Konner, as for every individual in my research, such trauma offered not a breakdown but a breakthrough.

One more crucial study of the mind-body connection merits mention. One of the most recent research findings indicates that writing about emotional trauma can have a clear, positive effect upon the human immune system. The study is in the field of psychoneuroimmunology, which links the mind (*psycho*), the brain and nervous system (*neuro*), and the body's cellular defenses against disease (*immunology*). Two of the most prominent researchers in this innovative field, Dr. Janice K. Kiecolt-Glaser and Dr. Ronald Glaser of the Ohio State University College of Medicine, and their colleague, Dr. James W. Pennebaker of Southern Methodist University, asked fifty undergraduate students to participate in a writing exercise for four consecutive days. Half were asked to write about one or more traumatic events in their lives, while the other twenty-five were allowed to choose a superficial topic. The research team measured the responses of the students' immune systems over the four days and kept track of their student health center visits both before and after the experiment. Analysis of blood samples collected each day indicated that the students who wrote about their traumatic experiences had an overall stronger immune system response. The experiment took place during the first week in February, immediately prior to midterm exams, a time marked by the highest illness rate of the entire school year. The students' health center use was monitored for four months prior to the experiment and for six weeks following. For the students who wrote about their traumas, the number of visits went significantly down, while visits for the students writing superficial stories went markedly up during the peak cold and flu season. These results suggest that exploring personal crises can have a positive effect on the immune system and reduce the need to seek medical attention.

In addition several students who wrote about the same trauma for each of the four days actually changed their attitude toward the life-troubling traumatic event in that short time. One woman, who had been molested at the age of nine by a boy three years older, initially emphasized her feelings of embarrassment and guilt. By the third day of writing, she expressed anger at the boy who had victimized her. By the last day, she had begun to put it in perspective. On the follow-up survey six weeks after the experiment, she reported, "Before, when I thought about it, I'd lie to myself. . . . Now I don't feel like I even have to think about it because I got it off my chest. I finally admitted that it happened. . . . I really know the truth and won't have to lie to myself anymore." Students who reexamined a personal trauma learned to see it as a positive growth experience, demonstrating the same ability that was common among the prominent individuals of my project. Based upon the data, the team of researchers concluded, "An important predictor of illness is the way in which individuals cope with traumatic experiences. It has been well documented that individuals who have suffered a major upheaval are more vulnerable to a variety of major and minor illnesses. However, the adverse effects of stress can be buffered by such things as a social support network and by a predisposition toward hardiness. . . . individuals tend to deal with trauma most effectively if they can understand and assimilate it." What is most significant about the study is that it provides a direct causal mechanism that links the confronting of personal traumas with an improvement in immunity as well as in subsequent health status. For now the key point is that what the individuals in my study learned to do unconsciously at an early age can be consciously undertaken by anyone at any age with profoundly positive consequences for both their mental and physical health.

French painter Georges Braque once mused, "The only thing that matters in art can't be explained." At the heart of optimal health there is always something inexplicable. Some people do everything right and die young, while others break all the rules and live to a ripe old age. One of the major dangers in our present attempts to define health within a model based on disease is the tendency to explain hastily everything we observe, preferably in biological or genetic terms, even if it means blaming the victim. Heart disease is the major chronic illness and cause of death in our society, and we currently believe that medical science has provided a scientific explanation for heart disease developed from the leading risk factors of cholesterol, high blood pressure, and smoking. That conclusion, however, is premature.

In *Healthy Pleasures* Dr. David Sobel, regional director of preventive medicine for the Kaiser Permanente Health Maintenance Organization in Oakland, California, has noted, "With one risk factor, you are twice as likely to develop coronary heart disease; with two, you are more than three times as likely; and if you had all three, the risk of heart attack increases sixfold. However, more than eight out of ten people with all three risk factors won't suffer a heart attack in the next ten years, and the vast majority who have heart attacks will not have all three risk factors." Even with a disease believed to be so inherently organic as coronary heart disease, with reliable biological and lifestyle risk factors, there remains an enigma regarding who will or will not suffer its consequences.

Problems of heart disease and other major chronic diseases may not find their solution in medical technology or even lifestyle; they may instead be rooted in the most fundamental elements of life itself. Increasingly, such psychosocial factors as hostility, discussed by Duke University cardiologist Dr. Redford Williams in *The Trusting Heart*, and social isolation, noted by University of California researcher Dr. Dean Ornish, are found to play a major, causative role in the development, treatment, and even the behavioral reversal of advanced coronary heart disease. Isolation, loneliness, and anger are often the emotional consequences of childhood trauma. Interviews with the participants in this research project indicated that they had experienced these emotions as deeply as anyone, yet they learned to emerge unscathed. Through these interviews it became clear that the presence or absence of successful adaptation to early childhood challenges is a critical determinant of adult psychological and physical health.

What insight have we gained so far into the foundations of optimal health? Summing up the personal histories and research presented in this chapter, it is increasingly evident that

• Early childhood and adolescent traumatic events are not inherently negative and can actually be a source of profoundly positive influence in adult years. Empathy is a positive and socially adaptive response that can and should be nurtured in children and young adults. What appears to be a breakdown may in fact become a breakthrough.

• For both men and women traumatic events involving the father appear to be most significant. They occur regardless of whether the father serves as a supportive role model or he is actually the cause of the traumatic event.

• When neither parent is a positive influence or both are absent, the presence of an older mentor such as a relative, counselor, friend, teacher, or clergyperson appears to be an effective surrogate for a supportive parent. Those who care for children in any capacity can help by decreasing the child's exposure to trauma and by increasing the protective influences of counsel, love, and support.

• Virtually every individual in this study was required to carry out a socially responsible task at a level appropriate to a young person, such as helping a grandparent or caring for a younger sibling. Such tasks of required helpfulness appear to lead to enduring and positive traits as adults in the form of empathy, altruism, and forms of philanthropy. Children can be encouraged at an early age to reach out beyond their nuclear family to care for animals, help a friend or relative, or become involved in a community project such as a school play or sport.

• Even in the absence of any supportive people or social conditions, some individuals are able to draw upon a precocious inner strength or self-efficacy that enables them not only to survive, but actually to thrive in the midst of isolating traumas. Whether support comes from another person or from inner strength, the positive response to trauma forms the basis for an enhanced ability to cope as an adult and for an altruism expressed through their professional work, philanthropy, or public service.

• Whether in trauma or not, children need to have instilled in them a sense of confidence that they can control and influence their lives to a marked degree and a sense of coherence, a feeling that events will work out as well as can be reasonably expected and that seemingly overwhelming odds can be surmounted. Evidence from research and my interviews clearly indicates that such an attitude can be taught and learned even under the most adverse circumstances. Adults can convey optimism as well as pessimism to children and serve as powerful role models of how to cope well or poorly with life's inevitable adversities. Talking directly with children about such an orientation to life, counseling them during their crises both large and small, encouraging them to have a hobby in which they can experience mastery and control as well as praise, and demonstrating these traits in everyday behavior are all practical means of instilling a sense of personal control and realistic optimism.

• Unexamined and unresolved traumatic events, especially in early childhood and adolescence, appear to have a negative impact on both psychological and physical health in later years. Preliminary evidence is beginning to develop causal links, at least in the instance of disorders related to the immune system.

• Confronting and successfully coping with traumatic events can be learned unconsciously at an early age and also consciously developed as an adult. Underlying the transformation appears to be a perceptual shift from seeing the glass as half-empty to seeing it as half-full. Viewing the traumatic event from an adult perspective enables individuals to see its long-term positive impact and let go of the inhibiting emotions, thoughts, and behaviors associated with increased stress and manifested as chronic disease.

• Transforming crises into a positive influence, either during childhood or adulthood, is not achieved through a naive conception of the "power of positive thinking" or by denial. Crises need to be acknowledged and accepted as normal. Positive meaning and understanding can be derived from these experiences, if they are not repressed. It is possible to achieve a positive outcome even without professional help, self-help groups, or an extended family.

• Childhood trauma is not a prerequisite for optimal health, nor, on the other hand, is such an occurrence inherently destructive. There is an ongoing cycle of and shifting balance between major and minor challenges and periods of serenity and content. This pattern changes throughout the life cycle and varies with the sex of the child. Most importantly, a balance needs to be struck between major, disruptive trauma and character-building challenge.

• Finally and arguably most importantly, these findings begin to provide a basis for the inclusion of the positive emotions in any comprehensive model of health. According to Norman Cousins, these include "the positive forces—love, hope, faith, will to live, determination, purpose, festivity, laughter—which are powerful antagonists of depression and help to create an environment that makes medical care more effective." Giving these positive emotions their rightful place in both research and clinical practice constitutes a major step in restoring the individual to the center of a true health care system. Individual efforts are a necessary but insufficient condition for optimal health. Families, schools, health providers, business, and government have an imperative to elicit and sustain those individual practices.

We can no longer cling to the simplistic model of health that views early life trauma as inherently causing adult mental or physical disorders. For the most part when a person is unhappy or disturbed, there is a tendency to scan the past and fixate on some early crisis as the source of the present problem. This is but one example of the re-

ductionistic, simplified, cause-and-effect view of reality that underlies much of our zeal to lay blame for every conceivable illness on
personal daily habits, conditions of modern life, or the latest discoveries from the "black box" of inherited traits announced by the Human Genome Project. Both the public and health professionals seem
to believe that anyone who has had a heart attack or cancer must have
lived a life of gluttony, sloth, and indulgence, unless they are excused
by reason of diabetic complications or genetically inherited hyper-
cholesterolemia. Writing in the *American Journal of Public Health*,
the epidemiologist Dr. Paul R. Marantz of Montefiore Medical Center in New York quipped, "We seem to view raising a cheeseburger
to one's lips as the moral equivalent of holding a gun to one's head."
Such oversimplified reasoning is the basis for the limited, guilt-in-
ducing, and anachronistic nature of our present model of health.

Medical science has supplanted religion as the main source of man-
dates about right living. Standards of good and evil are often replaced
by judgments of what is healthy or unhealthy. Data on what is hazardous to our health is ubiquitous in both the popular media and professional journals. Certainly it is helpful for us to try to explain what
we observe about general patterns of illness, because such explanations can lead to new prevention and treatment strategies. However,
taking broad, epidemiological data and applying them simplistically
to the individual may lead to grossly inaccurate conclusions. When
the victim is blamed, a person's already debilitating anxiety, pain, and
fear of death from an illness are compounded by feelings of guilt, re-
morse, and a naive sense of responsibility. General health-oriented
guidelines—cholesterol reduction, smoking cessation, physical activity, reduction of environmental carcinogens, and the entire host of
public health measures—are necessary and nobly conceived. However, doing everything "right" is not a guarantee of optimal health or
longevity.

Broken bones do heal strongest. Illness, limitation, suffering, and
isolation—all the initial and transient aspects of trauma—may awak-
en us to a deeper meaning that was previously buried within. This
new understanding in turn can move us to reassess our values, to sort
out what matters and what does not, to consider the meaning not just
of the trauma but of life itself. In such experiences can be found the
roots of empathy and compassion, as well as the foundation for the
adult attainment of optimal health.

CHAPTER THREE

Directing the Play of Life: Personal

Control and Optimal Health

Issues of personal control emerged as a major theme during the sixties and are continuing to intensify today. Following the guidelines of Dr. Benjamin Spock, parents of the postwar baby boom encouraged their children to choose the time and place for sleeping, eating, and even toilet training. Personal control became an ingrained value, which the children came to exercise as adolescents protesting a dehumanizing war, as young adults advocating environmental responsibility, and now as middle-aged, prominent figures taking charge in their own right.

Fueling this drive toward personal control is the unlimited array of choices available. Multitudes of competing brands of automobiles, running shoes, personal computers, foods, religions, political causes, and even types of cosmetic surgeries offer us choices from the sublime to the ridiculous. By contrast, anonymous violence, terrorist bombings, assassins who change the course of history, and environmental contamination all seem to suggest that people have no control at all. Our personal choices and opportunities for control range from total to virtually nil.

Control is such a pervasive issue that the World Health Organization (WHO) has incorporated it into its current definition of health: "A process of enabling individuals and communities to increase control over the determinants of health." This definition of health is a central theme throughout this book. It translates into changing individual lifestyle practices, creating a healthier environment, and becoming politically active.

For every individual in my study, the childhood and adolescent necessity of exerting personal control was a key influence in their lives. "Control" here is not meant in the sense of manipulating yourself or others; that is clearly a negative form of control all too familiar in everyday circumstances as well as an aspect of a particular kind of hostility demonstrated to be a major risk factor in heart disease. Manipulative, hostile control betrays a need of an individual to dominate himself and others while competing with them at every opportunity. Such a strategy ultimately fails, leading to frustration and increased hostility and fueling more of the same destructive, heart attack—inducing behavior. By marked contrast the participants in my study have confirmed the findings from extensive research that individuals can possess a healthy kind of control: an abiding certainty based on past experience that they can influence the course of their lives to a major degree. Actress Lindsay Wagner said, "I feel more like the director of the film than an actor in it. Actors are given lines, told where to stand, how to feel, what to say, but the director oversees, orchestrates, and exerts control over every part of the production. . . . That feels like what I experience now." Such a sense of personal control has profound consequences beyond individual choices. Collectively the impact of these aggregated choices dictates election outcomes, the foods available in supermarkets, and even the national economy.

By one interpretation the notion of personal control allows society to blame the victim by attributing his or her condition to helplessness or incompetence, while supposedly lending reassurance that control is possible for anyone. This naive egalitarianism overlooks the fact that people may be passive and despondent because their environment is overwhelmingly negative. Political conservatives have argued that minority children fail in school because they are helpless, an explanation that ignores the very real problems of economic inequality and the dire health consequences of poverty and homelessness.

A more balanced interpretation of control, on the other hand, does not lead to blaming the victim. Control is the conviction that we as individuals can affect the course and destiny of our lives. It is a healthy belief that one can effectively manage challenging situations. With this orientation people rarely feel helpless, hopeless, or isolated. From this perspective control refers not only to the person, but to his or her interaction with the environment. While control is usually a characteristic assigned to individuals, it is also a quality of the world that surrounds them. Given this model, it is possible to develop personal strategies and interventions that can be directed to both the individual and the environment.

Once an individual voluntarily or involuntarily experiences a deep sense of inner strength or personal control, even in the midst of major trauma, that experience becomes the core of a mature sense of personal empowerment and control. An individual who has control is certain he or she can exert a powerful influence upon the course and destiny of his or her own life and the circumstances that surround it. Recent research shows that this factor of control, empowerment, or self-efficacy may be the ultimate determinant in human health and even aging.

Participants in the present study who had personal, medical, career, or financial setbacks turned them around by exerting control and creating a positive advantage, even though the process was long, often painful, and not clearly understood at the time. Essentially, one of the skills they learned was an acute ability to remember past successes while in the midst of their difficulties, a perspective that helped them avoid becoming lost in or encumbered by anxiety. Building upon positive memories, they proceeded to exert control, no matter what the crisis.

These individuals know how to use control effectively in the sense that they know which strings to pull and how to accomplish tasks. However, they employ this control within the context of strong inner values, ethics, constraint, and compassion, which shift the control decisively away from subjugation, negative manipulation, and Machiavellian authority. Most importantly, this ability to exercise control has a major positive influence upon mind-body interactions with regard to chronic diseases, ranging in these interviews from a potentially debilitating bone disease to advanced coronary heart disease.

Elaborating upon and supporting the interviews is a growing body of mind-body research confirming the influence of mind in swinging the balance between health and illness, life and death. Furthermore, findings from over ten years of research with both animals and people clearly indicate that the presence or absence of control is a major causal factor in health, illness, and even the aging process. In a classic study by Dr. Ellen J. Langer and Dr. Judith Rodin when they were at Harvard University, a group of elderly convalescent-home residents were given more choices about their living conditions and more control over day-to-day events in the community. After eighteen months these residents showed a significantly greater improvement in health than the residents who were not given such choices. Compared to a 25 percent mortality rate in the nursing home in the eighteen months before intervention, only 15 percent of the residents in the intervention group died. In the same period the mortality rate among the other residents in the home was 30 percent. Similar interventions among elderly persons have yielded positive results, as have interventions in other organizational contexts such as hospitals. Studies like these demonstrate a rather paradoxical quality of control. It is delicate in the sense of seeming to require little effort either to deny or to elicit, yet once it is elicited even in deceptively simple tasks, it appears to exert a very powerful influence upon such formidable occurrences as chronic illness, depression, and even death rates.

Exerting personal control is a vital element in sustaining optimal health. People who relinquish control revert to the classic state of helplessness and hopelessness, which every clinician recognizes as a risk for disease. In contrast, research by Dr. Martin Seligman at the University of Pennsylvania has shown that people who exert positive control in their lives exhibit the characteristics of optimists. They are optimists in the sense that they see success in both career and personal life as due in large measure to their own efforts and skills. Furthermore, they tend to see crises or challenges as temporary, limited to the immediate situation, and the result of the random events of changing circumstances, other people's actions, or just bad luck. Pessimists attribute crises or challenges to causes that are long-lasting, perhaps permanent, and are their own fault because of an inherent, unchangeable character flaw. Pessimists do not see themselves as being able to exercise control. They see their lives as being shaped by good and bad circumstances and luck beyond their control.

Seligman has documented major health consequences resulting from these diametrically opposed orientations. Collaborating with researchers at Stanford University in 1988, he completed a study of 122 men in the San Francisco Bay area who had been interviewed on videotape eight years earlier after having a first heart attack. The researchers analyzed the interviews for pessimistic versus optimistic styles and followed up on the men to see who was still alive. Of the sixteen most pessimistic men, fifteen had died. In a more recent study Seligman and his colleagues conducted research on thirty-four women in a National Cancer Institute chemotherapy program after a second diagnosis of breast cancer. They were interviewed, and the tapes were analyzed to see if the women's pessimism or optimism bore any relation to their medical outcomes. Since their breast cancers had metastasized before they entered treatment, the women only lived an average of one year. However, the optimists lived two to three months longer than the pessimists. Exercising control is a fundamental prerequisite to developing optimism, and both have demonstrably powerful influences on mental and physical performance, overall health, and even longevity.

Among the studies that have begun to define the positive influence of control on mental and physical health is the work of Dr. Suzanne Kobasa at the City University of New York. Her early research focused on a group of executives in the Illinois Bell system over an eight-year period while the company was dealing with the AT&T divestiture. During this difficult time in the company's history Kobasa found that some of the executives experienced unusual levels of stress and became ill, while others subject to the same external pressures remained healthy. These healthy executives manifested a quality that Kobasa termed "hardiness" and exhibited three characteristics that distinguished them from those who could not withstand the stress. These factors have been termed the "three C's": perceiving changes as *challenges* to be mastered; making a *commitment* to the self, work, family, and personal values; and developing a sense of personal *control*. Later research indicated that the two dimensions of control and commitment (which are discussed in the next chapter) may be most predictive of good versus impaired health. Most importantly, Kobasa and a growing number of researchers have found evidence that these abilities, which may in fact exert a greater influence upon health than purely physical or genetic factors, can be learned.

Literally every participant in my research indicated that the mature form of control that helped them face challenges as adults was built upon a series of encounters with challenges throughout their lives. When John Sculley, chairman and CEO of Apple Computer, was approached by Steven Jobs to join Apple, Sculley was president of Pepsico. He was happy in his position there and had actually never heard of this small California computer company that had the audacity to try to persuade him to give up his prestigious position. However, he was intrigued when Jobs asked him if he would "rather sell soda water all his life or change the world." Sculley agonized over the challenge, which became a focal point in his self-exploration. During that search he examined his personal values and goals and weighed the risks of leaving his established career for an unknown company. He was intrigued by Apple's dynamic track record and captivated by its vision and the dedication of its employees. He remembered his own childhood passion for electronics, which he had abandoned when he entered the business world, and it was this memory that helped him recognize that his own true values were reflected in the fledgling company. Being an astute businessman, Sculley did not rely solely upon sentiment or intuition in reaching his decision; he also negotiated $1 million in severance pay just in case the position at Apple did not work out. That guarantee turned out to be unnecessary.

That decision to leave Pepsico for Apple in 1983 was pivotal in Sculley's life. When I spoke with him in his high-tech office in Silicon Valley, I learned that he possesses a tremendous discipline derived from early childhood experiences and values. At age fifty-four he maintains a vigorous fitness regimen that keeps him looking years younger, and his office walls are lined with such demanding books as Ilya Prigogine and Isabelle Stengers's *Order out of Chaos* and Julian Jaynes's *The Origin of Consciousness in the Breakdown of the Bicameral Mind.* He believes that what he's learned from past successes has prepared him, when facing a crisis, to resolve problems calmly and rationally.

Shortly after joining Apple, Sculley found himself dealing with the worst crisis in the company's history, the departure of founder Steven Jobs in 1985. Reflecting on this crisis, he remembered, "I was to discover at Apple that I had to go back to my roots—all the way back to my childhood and to my family values. There were television crews going up and down the hallways, people crying, and newspapers and magazines writing that Apple was going out of business. Ironically, though, it was a very calm time in my life, because I went back and applied lessons that I had already learned. While at Pepsico I had started companies in Brazil, so I knew what it was like to work in roller-coaster environments and what it was like to put in tight controls. I also knew what it was like to work in a creative environment. But of all my resources, the most useful was my set of values. I built the conviction that I could control and direct Apple through the crisis on my set of values."

For most of those I interviewed, crises in business built and strengthened their sense of personal control. Looking back on his thirty-five years at Chase Manhattan Bank, David Rockefeller recounted what he learned from the necessity of crisis management as president and chairman of the board: "Of all that transpired in that thirty-five years, some occurrences do stand out as the most challenging. In my early days in the International Department I was concerned about the need to change the managerial structure and system of the bank. I was first challenged by that. Not surprisingly, the biggest crises came when I was president and chairman. There were a couple of episodes in the mid-seventies when the bank had serious problems—back office management, heavy loans in the real estate field, and substantial bond losses. As the chief executive officer I bore the responsibility for these problems. It was an intensely critical period. I suppose that period was the most traumatic and difficult for me, particularly because the media exaggerated the problems, as they often do. That didn't make life any easier for me, but the situation as a whole made me aware of how I deal with certain problems. And I realized I had to work harder to pull the company through. I don't have much doubt that one learns more from adversity than when times are easy." For those who have the competence and tenacity to achieve such high positions, an ability to exert control and resolve inevitable crises is vital to success and instrumental in maintaining both mental and physical health.

Among the individuals I interviewed, Saul Zaentz, founder and chairman of the company, formerly Fantasy Records, now the Saul Zaentz Company, which produced such classics as *One Flew over the Cuckoo's Nest* and *Amadeus*, epitomizes the willingness to take risks and rely upon one's own internal resources. Since he and his former wife, Celia, formed his company, he has refused to take the company public in order to preserve his control and the freedom to create without outside interference. He explained, "People in the film industry think we're crazy to refuse the blandishments to go public, since we could get enough money to be set for life. We have always resisted that because we know we can run our own company. I don't want a stockholder asking me why I did something a certain way. If you're a public company, you are constantly being questioned; for example, some friends of mine who went public say they are always explaining to analysts why the company didn't do as well as they expected. Personally funding all our films is a calculated risk, but I am willing to take it to retain control. For me the rewards are so much greater. I make the films that I want to make and I don't have to answer to anyone. After *Cuckoo's Nest* we heard that from one of the big studios; some big guy asked, 'Why does the hero have to die? He should live, and the nurse should die!' But that was not the picture we wanted to make. With *The Unbearable Lightness of Being* the president of the studio said, 'Saul, I know it's naive, but why do they have to die?' I said, 'It is another picture if they live. But it's not this picture. Not the one we want to do.'

"We have gotten offers from people who want to invest money in the company—a lot of money—and sure, that would take all the pressure off us, but then we would have to go public in three to five years.

Those people are in the money business. We have to make money to exist, but that's all. We don't have to make money to prove that we can make money. Right now we can walk into each other's offices and say, 'Do you think we should do this?' We can argue about a good picture instead of what we have to do here to be sure we meet stockholders' earnings. We end up with what we really wanted to do, not something dictated by a return of ten point eight percent on our investment. We want to make good pictures. For us what really matters is a certain amount of pride—that what we've created is not just a picture that made money, but a good picture!"

For each participant I interviewed, the tendency to exert personal control in challenging situations seems to have its roots in their experiences as children and adolescents. At some point in their early lives they were required to carry out a personal responsibility for someone in their family, neighborhood, or community. These tasks, termed "acts of required helpfulness" by Dr. Emmy E. Werner, resulted in positive changes in the young helpers, which stayed with them through adulthood.

A Republican representative from Rhode Island, United States Congresswoman Claudine Schneider became responsible at a very young age. At eight years old she was assigned tasks in her father's men's clothing store. "As soon as I was tall enough, I stood behind the counter," she recalled. "One of my early responsibilities was to watch for shoplifters. Also, I was in charge of gift wrapping on Christmas, Father's Day, and other busy holidays. As I got older, I was responsible for taking the money from the store to the bank. Then I was expected to open the store in the morning, turn off the alarms, get the money, and put it in the cash register. At the end of the day I closed the shop down. It was a lot of responsibility for a high school kid, but my parents always told me I could do whatever I wanted to do. That was a very important lesson; they never set limits on me. That was one of the best gifts they ever gave me, because even today, I often feel unstoppable."

Adulthood presented Claudine Schneider with a diagnosis of Hodgkin's disease and, thirteen years later, divorce. When an individual is faced with a debilitating or even life-threatening disease, the ability to shift the interaction between mind and body in a positive direction becomes vital. Serious illness becomes an occasion to confront loss, grief, personal limitation, impotence, and isolation, as well as established roles and expectations, goals and strategies, values and meaning. Every participant in my study experienced at least one health crisis that both challenged and strengthened their determination and control. A great deal of scientific research has shown, especially in the area of heart disease, that intangibles such as a sense of purpose play an important role in preventing and recovering from major episodes of disease. Disease is a force for change, and serious disease often effects profound change in those who suffer it.

It was early in 1973 when Schneider was diagnosed with Hodgkins disease, a form of cancer. At first she was overcome by the fear that she would die, but then she began to remember how she had faced earlier life traumas and challenges. Schneider remembered, "My first reaction was, Wait a minute, I'm too young to die. But then I thought, What have I done with my life? I haven't made a contribution . . . I can't go anywhere yet. I cried for three days. I felt sorry for myself. I was scared and angry and going through all the traditional emotions, and then I decided, I'm in charge and I'm not gonna die! I just knew it. It was an inner knowing and sense of control. Once I made up my mind, I knew that my will to survive was so strong that there really wasn't any chance I wouldn't combat the disease. I wanted to live so badly still; there was too much that I wanted to see, and do. My whole life had been a fairy tale up till then. I had good parents; they never abused me or gave me a rough time. I had a good family; I enjoyed school; everything was pretty good. Then suddenly my life was on the line and the doctor was telling me my odds were fifty-fifty. I immediately started radiation but no chemotherapy.

"I realized that the radiation wouldn't be enough and that I had to make myself better. I started doing deep breathing exercises. As I inhaled, I would imagine all of the cancer cells breaking up, and then I would breathe them out. Every morning and every evening before I went to bed, I would enter into a state of relaxation and work with my visualization. I would envision myself eliminating waste from my body. In this way I was working with both the medical system and my system to get rid of the cancer cells."

Through this combination of therapies, Schneider has remained in remission from her Hodgkin's disease, but that is only one of the serious challenges she has successfully overcome. Looking back at the experience that launched her into public life, she mused, "First I found out I had cancer and a fifty-fifty chance to live. Then I found out that a nuclear power plant was under construction in my backyard and that the federal government supported it, the state government supported it and the utility company supported it. To that I said, 'Okay, look out, here I come!' and stopped the nuclear plant in its tracks. It's been the same throughout my life. It's almost as though I thrive on challenges." Out of her activism as a concerned state resident she achieved the recognition and widespread public support that led her career in national politics. She now focuses her efforts in office on environmental issues, particularly ocean conservation and energy efficiency.

As if conquering cancer, stopping the construction of a nuclear power plant, and achieving high political office were not enough, her response to divorce illustrates the means by which she and others in this research have learned to handle personal crises positively. According to Schneider, "Clearly, the second most powerful thing to happen to me in these last years was my divorce in 1985. The divorce process caused me to really look at myself and at relationships. During that time my sensitivities were heightened and I developed an awareness of more metaphysical things. Although I did what I could to maintain my control, there were forces beyond my perception and beyond my understanding that were there to support me. During the day I appeared to be in control, but at night, in my exhaustion, I would suddenly understand what I really needed. It was a paradoxical time of being both in control and not in control. From that state I gained greater insight as to how to regroup my strength and how to go on. I needed to analyze my strong points and assess how my life was unfolding. . . . There, in a state of helplessness, came all of the ideas and solutions I needed." For virtually all of the individuals in my research, Schneider's paradoxical experience of being simultaneously in and out of control is familiar, albeit uncomfortable.

As riveting as these insights are, they might lack substance or acceptance if they were not consistent with a growing body of research and clinical data demonstrating the pervasive influence of personal control. Control is a major causal determinant of health in both mind and body. There are many terms both in professional and public literature that are used to describe this aspect of personal control, including *the will to live, self-efficacy, internal locus of control, learned optimism*, and *empowerment*, to cite but a few. Certainly there is substantial research underlying each of these terms, but there is a tremendous amount of overlap, and *control* clearly covers the common ground.

CONTROL: BETWEEN MIND AND BODY

Control is the vital link between mind and body. It is the pivotal point between psychological attitudes and our physical responses. Asthmatics sneeze at plastic flowers. People with multiple personalities exhibit one personality that is diabetic and another that is not. Researchers have documented the "anniversary phenomenon," whereby individuals with advanced or terminal illness will themselve to live to see a graduation ceremony, a birthday milestone, or a religious holiday. Women with breast cancer who were involved in a psychotherapy support group lived twice as long as a matched group of women who received physical care but no support. Episodes of extreme emotional arousal, either positive or negative, can precipitate a sudden, fatal heart attack. Over thirty-six hundred cases of spontaneous remission in diseases ranging from terminal cancers to organ regeneration have been verified in the world's medical literature. Carefully conducted research has demonstrated that trained individuals can voluntarily control such "involuntary" bodily functions as the electrical activity of the brain, heart rate, sensation of pain, bleeding, and even the response of the immune system to infection.

A vital mind-body model describes a dynamic interaction between internal and external stressors and a person's internal and external responses to them. An internal stressor might be a particular fear, such as a fear of spiders, while an external stressor might involve actually confronting a real spider in the house. An effective internal response to the spider might be to eliminate the fear through psychotherapy, while an effective external response would be to call an exterminator. Whether the challenge is inside or outside, it triggers a major positive or negative interaction between the mind and body. Which comes first is often impossible to determine; nevertheless, this interaction is a major, in some cases the exclusive, determinant of a person's health or illness.

Through research, therapeutic strategies have been developed or rediscovered to elicit and sustain a person's ability to buffer or eliminate the detrimental effects of stressors on the mind-body system. These include various stress management techniques; high-technology interventions using biofeedback instruments; very low-technology practices using therapeutic massage, hypnosis, and autohypnotic methods; brief psychotherapy emphasizing specific changes in behavior; physical activity and exercise; applications of visualization and guided imagery; and systems of meditation that are thousands of years old. Most important is that all of the above can be used in conjunction with virtually every form of medical and psychological treatment, ranging from drug therapy to aid recovery from surgery to surgical intervention to reverse major coronary heart disease. These approaches challenge simplistic concepts of causality yet withstand rigorous scientific examination.

For over fifty years Western science has accumulated findings that verify what every one of us experiences every day—that mind and body are in inextricable interaction. Now the question is not *if* but *to what extent* the mind holds sway over the body and the biochemical, electromagnetic, and immunological connections forming the links in the causal chain. Such psychological factors as control, as well as emotional states ranging from love and compassion to fear and hostility, trigger powerful reactions in the body, which in turn both directly and indirectly affect blood chemistry, heart rate, activity in the stomach and gastrointestinal tract, activity of the immune system, and every other cell and organ of the body.

In any system of such vast complexity, certain questions remain unanswered. What constitutes the average, normal, or baseline measure of these influences? At what point do factors of research and statistical importance become significant at the practical, clinical level? And ultimately, how can these findings be made available to individuals seeking care beyond the limitations of pharmacology and surgery?

It is a widely accepted fact, as summarized by Dr. William H. Foege at the Centers for Disease Control in Atlanta, Georgia, that as much as *two thirds* of all disability and death up to age sixty-five would be preventable in total or in part if we were to apply what we now know about the effects of a hazardous lifestyle on premature illness and death. According to the Office of Technology Assessment of the United States Senate, very few surgical procedures have ever been scientifically evaluated. Clearly, mind-body approaches need to be evaluated as well, but it is necessary to avoid a double standard, especially when the side effects, complications, and mortality incidence resulting from mind-body interventions are virtually absent in comparison to the consequences of drugs and surgery. Most importantly, mind-body research and its clinical applications are not antagonistic toward or antithetical to appropriate medical care. The issue is not mind-body approaches versus pharmacological and surgical interventions; rather we must determine what the most health-giving and cost-effective combination is for the individual.

Unsubstantiated, extreme, and dangerous claims are often made. As in any consumer judgment, be wary of claims that are too good to be true, because they usually are. Today legitimate mind-body approaches are widely available from licensed clinicians, in university and private clinics, as well as in hospitals. They are also an integral part of health promotion programs offered by corporate giants including AT&T, Johnson & Johnson, and IBM, to name a few in a rapidly growing list. There are thousands of self-help groups and programs that emphasize restoring personal control, such as the Wellness Community, founded by Dr. Harold Benjamin in Los Angeles, where actress Gilda Radner sought help during her terminal cancer. One of the best-developed and -documented research and clinical programs is the Stress Reduction Clinic directed by Dr. Jon Kabat-Zinn at the University of Massachusetts School of Medicine. His innovative and effective approach is described in his excellent book *Full Catastrophe Living*, which provides practical guidance for the reader. Such approaches are used as effectively in corporate boardrooms as in private medical practices, empowering individuals by providing them with insights and skills to exert control and make more informed choices. In traditional care the patient is a passive recipient of instructions and is usually given something from outside the self to treat the illness. Mind-body approaches, in contrast, encourage the individual to work with the clinician and with the medicine, as in overcoming nausea during chemotherapy, to search for the meaning of the illness, and to exert active control in undertaking psychological and behavioral changes needed to restore health or, in other instances, to face death with equanimity and peace.

It is important to remember, however, that all too often the relaxation or meditative techniques used in such approaches are confused with an abdication of social responsibility and a withdrawal from community involvement into an inner world of fantasy and narcissistic indulgence. While this may be the case for some patients and practitioners alike, it is clearly not the thrust of either the research or the clinical applications. It is most categorically not true for the participants in my study. Perhaps one of the most popular demonstrations of the power of an inner, meditative practice in changing a person's outward life is in the moving, biographical film *What's Love Got to Do with It?* about Tina Turner. Through the support of a friend, a Buddhist chant, and sheer will, the middle-aged Turner moved from an abusive marriage to the most successful phase of her career. Mind-body approaches are part of a person's general orientation and lifestyle, yet it is impossible to follow the chain of events that influence the mind-body system without recognizing such powerful factors as personal control, the presence or absence of social support, the unequivocal negative effect of poverty and unemployment, the consequences of physical and sexual abuse in childhood, the effects of carcinogenic agents in the environment, and the threat to health from ozone deterioration and the poisoning of the world's oceans.

Such issues need to be acknowledged as part of any mind-body interaction occurring within the fleshy boundaries of an individual person. Private thoughts, feelings, beliefs, and other influences upon the body extend far beyond that body's particular time and space, spreading outward into the collective and communal world of which we are an integral part.

YOUR HEART SHOULD NOT ATTACK YOU

Two years ago I accompanied one of my medical school cardiologists to see a man from Greece who had flown to the United States for a bypass surgery after suffering a near-fatal heart attack in Athens. With the help of a translator the cardiologist was explaining to the forty-two-year-old man and his wife what had happened and what the next stage of treatment would be. During the interval of time required for the translator to convey this information, the man's wife had a sudden flash of insight. She abruptly turned to her husband and in a tone mixed with reprimand and love admonished him (in her native Greek), "Your heart should not attack you!" That is literally what happens to thousands of people every day. This man had a notable absence of any known risk factors, but had in fact recently suffered a series of business setbacks and financial crises, which were further aggravated by the discovery that his lifelong business partner and friend was guilty of embezzlement and fraud and had consequently fled to Yugoslavia. Again and again the Greek entrepreneur related that he suddenly felt out of control, deserted by his friend and isolated from his wife, whom he did not want to burden with his fears for their future economic security. Amidst his emotional turmoil, he had ignored the warning symptoms of shortness of breath and chest pains until he collapsed at his office.

While the underlying and often undetected precursors of a heart attack may be anatomical, the events actually precipitating it frequently involve loss of control, social isolation, and emotional trauma. Control especially is a major factor in the mind-body interaction that either increases or decreases a person's susceptibility to heart disease as well as a vast array of other chronic and acute diseases.

Cardiovascular disease remains the number-one cause of morbidity and mortality for both men and women in the United States. Out of the fifty-three participants in my study, twenty-seven experienced some degree of heart disease risk or incidence ranging from elevated cholesterol levels or blood pressure to recovery from a stroke or bypass surgery. As I noted earlier, Norman Cousins and John E. Fetzer died from heart attacks. Their personal confrontations with heart disease will be detailed later in this chapter.

Less than half of all the heart disease in the United States is explained by the combined effect of all known risk factors. Furthermore, international studies have found that rates of heart disease vary from country to country and that this difference cannot be explained either by traditional risk factors or by genetics. Men in the classic Framingham Heart Study conducted in Framingham, Massachusetts, were twice as likely to develop heart disease as European men with identical risk factors. Men living in America are five times more likely to die of heart disease than men living in Japan. Studies ranging from research with 3,809 Japanese-Americans living in San Francisco to the studies of the community of Roseto, Pennsylvania, indicate that the presence or absence of social support, or a connectedness to other people, is an independent and powerful influence upon heart disease and mortality.

For both health professionals and the public, the initial discovery of mind-body influences upon heart disease came from the work of San Francisco cardiologists Dr. Meyer Friedman and Dr. Ray Rosenman in 1974. Since then the major elements identified by Friedman and Rosenman—particularly hostility and cynicism—have been studied intensively. Research by Dr. Charles D. Spielberger and his colleagues has refined these findings even further to differentiate hostility from the more general emotion of anger. Hostility results in behavior that is directed toward destroying objects or injuring people. The relationship between hostile behavior and heart disease is a complex one and has been the subject of hundreds of research papers in the past two years alone. At present the evidence indicates that the overt expression of hostility and cynicism appears to be a causal factor and potent predictor of coronary heart disease.

These findings dovetail with what we know about the biochemical pathways within the body that appear to mediate between specific emotional responses and their negative impact upon the heart and entire circulatory system. The first is commonly known as the fight-flight response. Fight-flight is a sequence of electrical and biochemical events in the body that literally prepare an individual to respond to stress—that is, either to fight or to run away. The medical term for this reaction is the sympathetic, adrenal medullary response. Under conditions of stress, this system results in a virtual barrage of biochemical and physiological changes, such as increased blood pressure, cardiac output, heart rate, blood flow to the skeletal muscles, and secretion of catecholamines and testosterone, which affect the heart. A second major neuroendocrine pathway, dominated by secretions from the pituitary gland, is identified as the pituitary adrenal cortical system. This system becomes activated particularly when an animal or person experiences a loss of control or feels helpless. Under these conditions, there is an increase in adrenocorticotropic hormone (ACTH) and corticosterone, a decrease in gonadotrophin, and increased vagal, gluconeogenesis, and pepsin activity. These biochemical changes are generally associated with depressed and withdrawn behaviors. Both of these systems have a negative impact upon the heart and circulatory system, especially when the source of stress is pronounced and prolonged.

There are thought to be at least six ways that specific forms of stress and specific aspects of hostility trigger these two systems: 1) direct injury to the arterial wall caused by turbulence in the blood and repeated or sustained increases in heart rate; 2) disruption of the brain's control over heart rate, which can cause a fibrillation leading to sudden death; 3) toxic effects on the arteries from the stress hormones catecholamines and corticosteroids; 4) Possible indirect influences of these and other stress hormones to increase platelet aggregation or clotting, which in turn could block arteries and/or increase levels of fats in the blood; 5) release of hormones that induce a vasospasm or sudden constriction of coronary arteries, especially those that have been narrowed by plaques; and 6) a newly discovered direct influence of these hormones on thrombosis, or the sudden rupture of sites of injury in the arteries. Together these biochemical mechanisms are beginning to show us how subtle such psychological factors as the presence or absence of control and such emotional states as hostility can trigger a chain of electrical, biochemical, and immunological events that can lead to the development and progression of heart disease. Such influences also begin to explain the sudden death from a heart attack in an individual with few if any previously known risk factors.

Our ability to translate mind-body interactions into the complex biochemical and physiological events that affect the heart and circulatory system is becoming much more precise. Although the actual knowledge of these disease-inducing causal chains is very broad, a few specific instances will represent the evolving field. Research by Dr. Tom Clarkson and his colleagues at Bowman Grey School of Medicine has focused on monkeys reared in a socially stable versus an unstable environment. While the two groups were on identical diets, rates of coronary blockages were twice as high for monkeys raised in an unstable environment, especially for the dominant male monkeys. Chronic stress increased the permeability of the monkeys' arteries to cholesterol and their levels of high-density lipoproteins (HDL) decreased. Of particular interest is that the monkeys in both the stable and unstable conditions who reacted to stressors with an unusually or highly "reactive" heart rate were found to develop heart disease twice as often as those who had a lower or more average heart rate. These findings are very significant, since there is a great deal of research indicating that hostile or cynical individuals react to stressors with higher sympathetic nervous system responses, including unusually dramatic increases in heart rate, blood pressure, epinephrine, norepinephrine, and T-wave amplitude suppression on the electrocardiogram. If these findings are characteristic of an individual's ongoing, daily response to stressors, then such excessive responses and chronic increased secretion of stress hormones would lead to heart and arterial damage in everyday life.

Research tending to confirm this hypothesis has been conducted by the cardiologist Dr. Robert Elliot. He has found that some people overreact to stress with an extreme increase in cardiac output accompanied by extreme constriction of their blood vessels. These individuals have been dubbed "hot reactors" and, like the monkeys in Clarkson's research, are at the highest risk from stress-induced death due to heart disease. Another significant line of research is that of Dr. Redford Williams and his colleagues at Duke University. The Duke team placed people under mental stress by having them do serial subtractions of thirteen from a large number to compete for a prize. Under these conditions men with high hostility scores showed greater secretion of epinephrine, norepinephrine, forearm muscle blood flow, and cortisol than men classified as having low hostility. When the researchers added a distracting harassment to the arithmetic task, the high-hostility men showed larger increases in muscle blood flow and blood pressure than did low-hostility men. Such an increased and prolonged sympathetic arousal, ranging from extreme anger to overexertion in exercise, could also induce a ventricular fibrillation, myocardial infarction, and sudden death in susceptible individuals.

One recent study has confirmed that a high score in emotional arousals is an independent predictor of sudden cardiac death. A large group of postcoronary men were given a vigilance task of watching a television monitor and pushing a button when a particular pattern of letters appeared. High-hostility men exhibited a higher level of testosterone, which, combined with other factors, can lead to coronary heart disease. Finally, several studies have found that hostility is associated with an increase in mortality from all disease, not just heart disease.

Very recent research has forged a critical link between the diverse elements of control, stress, and heart disease. Although this connection may appear self-evident and there is an abundance of personal testimonials to its reality, scientific confirmation of the linkage has remained elusive. In 1990 Dr. Peter L. Schnall and his colleagues at the Cornell Medical College published the results of a breakthrough study in the *Journal of the American Medical Association*. For this study the research team coined the term "job strain" to identify stress caused by work, specifically a type of stress that occurs when a job has high psychological demands and low decision-making latitude. This kind of job requires working hard and fast but allows little control, autonomy, or discretion over the tasks. Obvious examples are secretarial work, information processing, telecommunications, and related pink- and gray-collar jobs. Researchers conducted a case control study of seven work sites in New York City and found that job strain resulted in higher blood pressure and an increase in the mass of the left ventricular area of the heart, a common site for a heart attack. This study is highly significant in linking a specific type of stress and loss of control with an increased physical risk for heart disease. It has been found that working women who work outside the home actually have higher rates of heart disease than either working men or women who stay at home. It is also clear that women tend to hold a disproportionate number of jobs that fit the job strain description perfectly. This fact would indicate that women who work as waitresses, computer operators, bill processors, bank tellers, and retail clerks are at high risk. Given these findings, it appears that programs to provide both men and women with increased control and influence over the conduct of their work would reduce their risk of heart disease. Such measures include more control over workload and the timing of breaks, more input into work group procedures, and similar changes to provide individuals with meaningful, realistic opportunities to be in control of the demands of their employment.

These studies suggest that negative emotional states could exert both a direct and an indirect effect on the heart and other organs, leading to degenerative diseases and increased mortality. However, it is possible to change many of these negative states into health-inducing states. In the Recurrent Coronary Prevention Project conducted by Dr. Meyer Friedman of Mt. Zion Hospital in San Francisco and his colleague Dr. Carl Thoresen of Stanford University, over one thousand men who had already had a heart attack entered a program to reduce their time urgency and hostility. After the program the men had a 45 percent lower recurrence of both fatal and nonfatal heart attacks compared to men who had undergone standard cardiac rehabilitation. Of major significance in this research is that low self-esteem was targeted as the root cause of hostility and cynicism. These emotions and negative behaviors are an individual's reaction to internal feelings of helplessness, worthlessness, hopelessness, and anger toward a world in which they feel themselves to be isolated and alone.

THE WISDOM OF THE HEART

Clearly, a sense of isolation, hostility, and loneliness is the opposite of a sense of control, connectedness, and involvement with life. It is precisely this sense of control that is evident among the people interviewed in the Sound Mind–Sound Body study. Following a heart attack in 1980, Norman Cousins wrote *The Healing Heart*, the story of his recovery. During one of several interview sessions he summed up his experience: "When I had a heart attack at the end of 1980, the cardiologist told me that my chances of living out the year without bypass surgery were not as good as they should be at my age. He was very apprehensive, but I wasn't. I wasn't arrogant, but I had been around this track before, and lacking the fear that illness produces, I didn't become panicky, which often intensifies the underlying condition. Fear and panic create negative expectations. One tends to move in the direction of one's expectations. My experience in the tuberculosis sanitarium as a child was a great asset in overcoming my fear and remaining self-reliant despite the gloomy predictions of my doctors. I wasn't frightened by the cardiologist's prediction and actually tried to reassure the doctors. . . . What I suggested was reasonable. I said I would not reject the surgery altogether, but I would define my regimen of rehabilitation. It was up to me to take control and set the direction for my recovery. I told them they could monitor it week by week, and if there was no improvement, we still had the option of surgery. But if, in fact, there was improvement, we could measure it and continue on that course. They accepted the proposal. There was basic improvement. It was a joyous experience—not just because I like the idea of winning, but because it gave me access to new experiences and new options. I probably wouldn't even be at the UCLA medical school today if it hadn't been for my illness in 1964, which I chronicled in *Anatomy of an Illness as Perceived by the Patient*. So I owe a great deal to my illnesses. They have served me well." By exerting control over the potential panic in his own mind, by working with his cardiologists and not against them, and by making the necessary lifestyle changes, Cousins transformed a life-threatening occurrence into one that was life-affirming.

For John E. Fetzer a major heart attack became an occasion to reinstate rather than abdicate control. Such a response was not unusual for a man who in the 1930s arrived in Kalamazoo, Michigan, with his wife, Rhea, "a second-hand car, some radio equipment, and about one hundred fifty-six dollars" and who became one of America's wealthiest men in the Forbes 400. His long career in telecommunications began when he purchased a university radio station and started WKZO. In the process of setting up the station, he secured a landmark Federal Communications Commission decision that permitted the station to overcome signal limitations and broadcast in the evening. That decision paved the way for modern radio programming and ushered in the golden age of radio.

During the course of developing radio and then television, Fetzer became sole owner of the Detroit Tigers baseball team and undertook many other business endeavors, but possibly his most challenging achievement was his personal confrontation with mortality. Following a near-fatal heart attack in 1980 at the age of seventy-nine, he exhibited the control and tenacity necessary to survive and literally to thrive on the adversity. Fetzer recollected, "I had a heart attack. A young physician blithely told me that I would have a second attack within a year and it would prove to be fatal. To that I said, 'Young man, I beg your pardon. That's not my style. My belief system simply won't accommodate that.' Then I gave him an elementary lesson in energy medicine, which probably did me more good than it did him. In fact, he probably didn't hear me. But the truth is that I recognized the necessity for change and immediately took control of myself. I inaugurated a program of positive energy, beginning with a big *E*, knowing that the proper use of energy is in the creation of a dynamic force field which describes and prescribes a state of health. With that decision I took control and assumed full responsibility for my recovery. I added a big *A* for attitude."

During the next eleven years Fetzer also transformed his orientation from archetypal capitalist to visionary philanthropist. Building upon the Fetzer Foundation, which he had founded earlier, he established the Fetzer Institute in 1990, housing in it a magnificent building of his own design in Kalamazoo. When John Fetzer died on February 20, 1991, a month short of his ninetieth birthday, he had achieved his final goal of establishing an endowed research institute to carry on inquiries into the nature of mind, body, and spirit. In a eulogy the current president of the Fetzer Institute, Robert F. Lehman, observed that "John Fetzer, like Norman Cousins, took a commonsense view of health. If depression, despair, panic, and rage can produce adverse physiological changes, why shouldn't we look at the possibility that hope, faith, purpose, the will to live, and most of all, freedom and love, can bring beneficial changes to one's health?"

Reflected in these personal strategies for overcoming the challenge of heart disease is a focus on prevention and intervention. Moving beyond the traditional risk factors (blood pressure, weight, smoking, cholesterol), such innovative approaches place a strong emphasis on the mind-body interaction. These strategies center on "learned optimism" (to borrow a term coined by Dr. Martin Seligman of the University of Pennsylvania), enhanced self-esteem, and a sense of connection to people and the world as a whole.

Their effectiveness has been shown in major studies by Dr. Dean Ornish and Dr. Shirley Brown of the Preventive Medicine Research Institute. These studies have shown actual regression, or reversal, of stenosis (coronary artery blockage), in a group of forty-eight patients who were randomly assigned to the treatment or control group after they underwent angiography to determine the extent of their severe coronary heart disease. Based on reducing multiple risk factors, the program consisted of a low-fat vegetarian diet, stress management training (biweekly yoga and meditation training in groups and one hour daily practice individually), moderate exercise (walking), and smoking cessation. Overall, 82 percent of the patients in the experimental group evidenced an improvement in their condition . Most significantly, the degree of regression of the stenosis was found to be related to the degree of adherence to the interventions. This group also showed significant increases on a "sense of coherence" scale, a measure of a person's sense of life's meaning, and reductions in anger and hostility. Control group participants did not evidence any changes. These are the first studies to show that nonpharmacological lifestyle interventions can result in a reversal of advanced heart disease.

It is very difficult in a multiple risk factor study of this type to separate the pure mind-body components of the intervention from those that affect traditional risk factors, such as lowering cholesterol through a change in diet. However, great emphasis was placed here on the stress management component, which served to integrate the dietary changes and exercise regimen within a larger context provided by meditative awareness and the development of social support. Inherent to any stress management strategy is restoring and enhancing an individual's sense of control over his or her life. Participants in the intervention group used stress management techniques including hatha yoga and various relaxation, visualization, and meditation practices. Such interventions are ambitious in scope and demanding of the participants. That the studies were successful suggests that reducing heart disease by means of a strictly psychosocial/behavioral approach may be possible if sufficient motivation and commitment are maintained. The minimal level of intervention required to produce regression of heart disease remains to be established by further study, and long-term outcomes are under current investigation. But most important, these studies suggest that adopting a comprehensive lifestyle regimen can prevent heart disease in healthy individuals at risk of developing it.

Other mind-body approaches to heart disease were tested at the Stanford University School of Medicine by the cardiologist Dr. John W. Farquhar, founder and director of the Stanford Center for Research in Disease Prevention. In a report published by the *Journal of the American Medical Association*, Farquhar and his research team demonstrated that a low-cost, community-wide health education program could reduce levels of cholesterol, blood pressure, resting pulse rate, smoking, and deaths from heart disease. Such findings raise the utility of behavioral, mind-body interventions to a new and very meaningful level, beyond individual practices and toward the entire psychosocial environment.

In 1994 Dr. William L. Haskell, Dr. Edwin L. Alderman, and Dr. John W. Farquhar and their colleagues reported the very important findings from the Stanford Coronary Intervention Program (SCRIP). This research project was the first large-scale, randomized trial to determine the effects of a four-year multifactor risk reduction program using both aggressive lifestyle changes and cholesterol-lowering medications on the progression and regression of heart disease in men and women. This risk reduction program was designed to be practical for all participants and generalizable to most adults. Patients who had mild to moderate heart disease were recruited. After computer-assisted quantitative coronary arteriography, patients were randomly assigned to the usual care of their own physicians or to an aggressive multifactor risk reduction program conducted by the SCRIP staff. The SCRIP program included a diet low in fat, cholesterol, and sodium; regular exercise; stress management; smoking cessation; weight loss when indicated; and use of combination drug regimens for lowering LDL cholesterol and raising HDL cholesterol. Of the 300 patients, follow-up arteriograms were conducted on 274 (92 percent), the highest retention of subjects of any of the arteriographic studies to date. Initial data analysis indicates that this project was very successful, with highly significant reductions occurring in many major risk factors in the experimental group but not in the group that received usual care. The risk reduction program led to a 50 percent reduction in the rate of progression of heart disease, more frequent regression, and fewer heart attacks or strokes.

Impressive findings such as these do a great deal to advance our understanding of the potential effectiveness of lifestyle and mind-body interventions in preventing the development or facilitating the regression of coronary heart disease. Despite such impressive findings, existing data on lifestyle interventions are still not adequate to convince much of the general public and established medical community of the efficacy of such interventions. Furthermore, the data do not provide the information necessary to design aggressive risk reduction programs that are likely to be adhered to by a large segment of the general population. A significant possibility exists that the lifestyle approach to managing heart disease may still lose out to the invasive approach currently favored by many physicians, especially surgeons, cardiologists, and many internists, or to the pharmacologic approach vigorously promoted by the pharmaceutical companies and a large segment of the medical community. Major clinical trials using the lifestyle approach need to be conducted. Effective means of aggressive lifestyle modification for the general public need to be developed. And a national advocacy group for the lifestyle approach needs to be organized with the primary objective of influencing public policy on how to cost-effectively reduce the current human and fiscal burden of coronary heart disease. Through such measures both individual and collective control can be exerted to reduce heart disease as the number one cause of disability and death in the world.

SITTING IN THE DIRECTOR'S CHAIR

Developing control as a personal strategy is not accomplished through simplistic, how-to nostrums. Generating an inner direction is a matter of exerting a focused, mental discipline to find these options and choices that occur in the mind second by second, and in behavior minute by minute. The founder of modern psychology, Dr. William James, once roused himself from a major, debilitating depression when he recognized that he had a choice between one thought and the next. Throughout the Sound Mind–Sound Body interviews, participants articulated this ability to influence profoundly the course and direction of their lives by consistently exercising such infinitesimal choices as the first step toward making further choices, which in turn would lead to different and more effective behavior. By examining the insights of several of the study participants, it is possible to understand how they, and anyone, can achieve this power of choice and begin to exert control.

In November of 1985, Brandon Stoddard became president of ABC Entertainment in Los Angeles. While in his previous position as president of ABC Motion Pictures he released such highly acclaimed films as *Silkwood* and *Prizzi's Honor*, when he assumed his new position, he became responsible for all ABC Entertainment programming—including early morning, late night, children's programs, and made-for-television movies, novels, and miniseries. You are probably familiar with his work in *ABC Novels for Television*, which included such award-winning series as the ground-breaking *Roots*, followed by *The Winds of War* and *The Thorn Birds*. Those three productions were the most popular miniseries in television history. Perhaps his most controversial production was *The Day After*, which depicted the horrific aftermath of a nuclear war. Several sponsors withdrew their advertising and threatened to undermine the financial viability of the program, while the public response to the advance publicity ranged from condemnation to the highest praise.

In a rare departure from major network guidelines Stoddard appeared on ABC Television to introduce the broadcast of *The Day After* and stated his personal belief that such an issue needed to be aired and considered by the general public. Speaking out about his personal convictions won him praise from all quarters, and *The Day After* became one of the two most watched motion pictures made for television in the medium's history.

Stoddard's bold exercise of personal control and perseverance was born out of his teenage experience in New Haven, Connecticut, when he witnessed his father defending the Communists' right to free speech. Later in life it was through his confrontation with divorce that Stoddard gained insight into developing a personal strategy for exerting control. During his divorce he had experienced a "major loss of control" and found that "under those circumstances you try to feel something inside yourself, no matter how big or small, that you think is really you. Whatever the hell it is, it doesn't make much difference. Then you've got to act upon it, you know, make a choice. Again, it doesn't make any difference how big it is. It could be . . . going to the cleaners. Some feeling inside me said, 'Go to the cleaners.' I went to the cleaners; I got there; it was a good experience. You have a sense of control as soon as you've taken the first step—even if it is to the cleaners.

"It's a system that I used postdivorce in trying to pull my emotional life back together. Up to that point I thought I could think my way through anything. I have a high I.Q. and I am a fairly good problem solver, but I couldn't think my way through my divorce. I used to think that my mind ran ninety-eight percent of my life, but after the divorce I switched that to two percent."

Again, it is ironic that personal control stems from a loss of control, where reliance upon an inner feeling or deep conviction becomes the key to resolving a crisis. Similarly gifted with the ability to reach inside and find the means to exert control when faced with a challenge is actress Lindsay Wagner, whom most people know as the bionic woman, a television character she made famous from 1975 to 1978 and for which she won an Emmy. Wagner has been a vegetarian since the early 1970s, and she practices her meditation and visualization to help her cope with her demanding schedule. Despite these habits, she underwent a period of crisis during the *Bionic Woman* series, and the insight she derived from that period helped lay the foundation of her ability to exercise control.

At her home in Malibu Wagner reflected back to her first major role. "Their expectations of me were unreasonable because I was not physically capable of what they expected me to do. It was an action show that was physically demanding to begin with—lots of running and outdoor sequences, lifting, and things like that, plus the long hours, which were totally ridiculous. Also I was the sole focus of the show, so I appeared in every scene. I was not athletic prior to this at all, so I was not prepared for the physical demands. At the same time they were working the crew as hard as me. People were getting sick because the stress was just too much. I didn't feel I had the right to do something about it, until I reached a point of feeling pressure from all sides. I was really worried about the crew members, so I would often do things to help them or take care of them. I can see now that I was trying to live up to being the bionic woman, but I was literally dying.

"I finally realized that my body was screaming, 'Stop!' And I realized that if I wasn't working those crazy hours, they couldn't work the crew the way they had been, so all I had to do was say no to improve the situation for everybody. It was as simple as that.

"My priority became my mental and physical health. I decided if it meant that they were going to let me go, then it didn't matter. Inside I had a conviction that the right thing would come along, once I chose to put my mental and physical health first instead of everything else. Suddenly everything got better. Once I finally took that stand, they didn't fire me, and we got a decent working schedule. People who were quitting because they couldn't take the pace came back and became excellent crew members. . . . I learned from that experience, and now I assert my personal control whenever necessary."

Taking control involves risk. Daring to change requires courage in the face of possible failure. In hindsight it is easy to see that both Stoddard and Wagner made the "right" decision, but they couldn't be sure of the consequences at the time. Making such decisions seldom seems courageous at first, but think about civil rights pioneer Rosa Parks, who made a personal decision to take control by refusing to sit in the back of a bus. She set off consequences that shook the nation and continue to fuel the ongoing civil rights struggle.

This fascinating notion of innately knowing what is right has been independently confirmed by the research of Dr. Anne Colby and Dr. William Damon of Brown University: "Throughout history, extraordinary individuals have personified moral values for the rest of the human race. From the time of the prophets to the modern age of Gandhi, Mother Teresa, and Martin Luther King, Jr., certain individuals have come to stand as 'moral exemplars' for vast numbers of followers. One interesting feature of this phenomenon is that such individuals often represent ideas that are controversial and even unpopular in the broader context of the times. Despite this, the eventual impact of such people on the course of society is beyond question.

"From my interviews I found that the moral exemplars of my study all expressed profound certainty about the decisions they made based on personal choice and control. Even during times of great personal risk or threat to their lives, they experienced little fear or doubt in making these decisions. When making choices and taking action, these individuals did not consider what the possible negative consequences to themselves might be. They could not seriously consider doing anything other than following their convictions. Because they were simply taking action or exerting control consistent with their beliefs, they did not see their acts as courageous. Once they made a decision, their subsequent actions were characterized by certainty and direction. The decisions were not based on inflexibility or on any religious or political dogma that might preclude reflection or consideration of opposing points of view. Their well-considered resolutions to exercise control came out of a deep, intuitive sense of conviction and purpose, after all of the rational alternatives had been explored and exhausted."

What social consequences would result from a multitude of individuals experiencing and acting upon such inner convictions and assuming greater control and responsibility over the direction of their lives? Those who are self-directed do not seek external, material solutions for what they know to be internal, psychological conflicts. Advertising preys upon fears of loneliness, isolation, depression, and pain and promises remedies in a better toothpaste, automobile, or laxative. Journalist Lynn Payer focuses on the consequences in the current medical system of surrendering personal control to outer solutions in her controversial book *Disease-Mongers: How Doctors, Drug Companies, and Insurers Are Making You Feel Sick*. Her book asserts that the current medical system "medicalizes" all of modern life, ranging from common fatigue to childbirth to death, through self-serving, economically driven exploitation. Overmedicalization of our society is a critical issue, but a book review in the *New England Journal of Medicine* raises the issue of a lack of personal control, self-efficacy, and inner confidence on the part of patients, observing that "it takes two to tango. Plastic surgeons could not convince women to have breast implants if they felt secure about their self-image. If patients were not so entranced with the illusion of a technological fix for anxiety, the pharmaceutical companies would not profit so handsomely." When individuals can clearly differentiate between an inner conflict (or lack of personal control) and a misdirected need temporarily to resolve discomfort (via drugs, surgery, an automobile, or other material soporific), then the positive impact on society as a whole is profound. At present the medical system reflects the values of the people it serves. When a greater demand for personal control is manifest, then a major transformation toward a true health care system will be at hand.

PERSONAL STRATEGIES FOR DEVELOPING CONTROL

Out of these interviews and a growing body of research anyone can derive a personal strategy for developing or enhancing control. In the previous chapter we saw that it is possible to gain positive attitudes and skills from having experienced childhood trauma. Control is a dynamic, ongoing, lifelong process that involves an interplay among rational thought, intuition, convictions, and external circumstances, as well as among individuals and the people in their lives. It is not a fixed, static end-point.

Quite a lot is known about how people can take control and make sustained changes over many years. Individuals are most likely to change when they believe that they are at risk of developing a problem or want to improve their condition, and when the change is within their ability and resources to accomplish. Although there are competing models of how such changes take place, the classic work to date is that of Dr. Albert Bandura at Stanford University. His concept of "self-efficacy" is very similar, if not identical, to the concept of control in this chapter. Self-efficacy and control are such pervasive influences in chronic mental and physical diseases that the Office of Prevention of the California Department of Mental Health gave a grant to me and my colleague, Dr. Steven E. Locke of the Harvard Medical School, to develop an annotated bibliography on this topic. Published in 1992 under the title *Personal Efficacy: A Research Database*, it contains over one thousand annotated references in areas including children's health, alcohol and chemical dependency, mental illness, human aging, stress, social support, and a range of chronic physical diseases.

Bandura's work has determined that self-efficacy is influenced by four main factors: information and persuasion, observation of others, successful performance of the behavior, and physiological feedback. In the practical translation of each of these factors below, I have taken the liberty of substituting the word "control" for "self-efficacy" to maintain consistency. "Information" in the "information and persuasion" factor refers to the bewildering amount of information individuals receive, both through the mass media and other sources, which guides their behavior. On the national level the impact of this information is evident in such important changes in risk factors as decreased smoking and lower levels of cholesterol related to dietary changes. Despite the importance of the mass media, health professionals remain the most credible source of information and are often seminal in encouraging people to begin the health change process. "Persuasion" refers to the advice health care providers give, or do not give, to their patients. In addition to imparting information, providers play a critical role in creating positive, and presumably realistic, expectations in their patients about the rate, magnitude, and effects of change. Such expectations have been shown to influence strongly patients' behavior. "Observation of others," Bandura's second factor, takes into account that many important lifestyle changes are undoubtedly influenced by watching others. Some have argued that the value of group programs for alcoholism, psychotherapy, or heart diseases may derive from the opportunity for patients to observe how others are doing. "Successful performance of the behavior" is another practical skill. Past experience and current experience guide the actions of everyone.

Unfortunately, individuals are more likely to focus on past failures than on successes. For instance, smokers may conclude from past failures at quitting that they may have trouble quitting following coronary artery bypass surgery or a heart attack. In fact, most smokers are able to quit following such an event. Many lifestyle change programs request that individuals review their previous attempts at changing behavior to decide what they can do better or differently the next time. Finally, "physiological feedback" simply means that the successful performance of an act results in taking the next steps. Progress on an exercise treadmill is a good example of something that can have a strong effect on a person's sense of control and subsequent behavior. A health care provider's counseling and feedback following a treadmill test help the patient return to routine activities. With our increased knowledge of how to elicit control and sustain change, it is becoming increasingly possible to break down human complexity into sequential steps that can demonstrably improve and accelerate the experience of control as an integral, ongoing aspect of everyday life.

Drawing upon the research to date, as well as on the personal strategies of the individuals from the Sound Mind–Sound Body study, it is possible to cite specific, practical steps for developing an enhanced degree of positive control. Although these steps may appear to be simple, carrying them out requires patience and practice. An intellectual grasp alone is woefully inadequate; the act of exerting control and its consequences are what is essential.

• Define the problem or challenge as clearly and honestly as possible. The challenge can be anything from wanting to develop an athletic skill to being faced with a major decision regarding career, finances, health, or personal relations. Define the issue in a simple, first-person sentence without qualifiers, as in the familiar acknowledgment of Alcoholics Anonymous, "I am an alcoholic."

• One technique recommended by Dr. Suzanne Kobasa is termed "reconstructing stressful situations." For this step think about a recent past episode of distress. Write down three ways it could have gone better and three ways it could have gone worse. It is important to realize that this past event did not go as badly as it could have. It is even more important to recognize and appreciate that you did influence the outcome to a significant degree and that you will be able to think of ways to cope better in the future.

• Examine the options for resolving the situation. Write down a list of the things you could do about the problem. Include even those ideas that seem silly or impossible, and especially those that might involve major changes or risk.

• Consider the consequences of each option. Write down the pros and cons of each option and what might happen if you tried each of them. Remember, insights and solutions often arise spontaneously and in unexpected forms once the obvious, rational, immediate options have been considered to the point of exhaustion or even desperation
.

• Think about specific incidents in the past when you successfully overcame a crisis or made an important choice that had a positive outcome. All too often the first response to a challenge is to become entangled in the diffuse anxiety that failure is likely. In reality the fact that you have arrived at this juncture in your life and are facing a formidable challenge is a confirmation of your past successes.

• If a possible solution to the immediate problem seems too formidable to undertake, break it down into smaller steps that you can accomplish gradually and cumulatively. This strategy will enable you to gain an increasing sense of confidence that it is possible to begin a successful course of action.

• Vicarious experiences of watching, remembering, or learning about others exerting control, ideally a peer or someone with similar characteristics to you, can help you exert control in similar situations. This is termed *modeling* behavior; you model or imitate psychological or behavioral strategies used by other people, such as the individuals interviewed in this chapter.

• Take the important first step in exercising control by choosing one option actually to try. This first option may succeed totally, in part, or not at all. As with any skill, control requires practice, so don't be self-defeating by expecting the first attempt to be perfect or to achieve the exact results you anticipated. No matter what the outcome, you have taken the first step in developing or enhancing personal control.

• Whether or not the first step was successful, review what you did. If necessary, you might repeat or fine-tune it until you are satisfied. Complex problems that may have gradually developed over many years often require exploring multiple options.

• Building upon a technique created by the psychologist Dr. Eugene Gendlin, you might gauge the success of this first trial through a method dubbed *focusing*. Focusing is a means of recognizing signals from your body that something is right or wrong. All too often we become so used to tension headaches, knots in the stomach, or racing, anxious thoughts that we ignore the subtle variations in these signs of how well we are coping. Pick a particular physical sensation, such as a tightness in the neck, and see if it increases or decreases after you try one of the options. Increases in tension might not be a bad sign since it will sharpen your focus on a tangible, physical indication of how well you are doing with exercising your new options.

• Resolution of the situation is not a purely individual, isolated undertaking. Be sure to talk about the situation and your attempts to make changes with those people who are involved. In one 1991 research study this strategy was preferred in resolving difficult situations. So keep the channels of communication open and be sure to listen to others.

• Another technique developed by Dr. Kobasa, *compensating through self-improvement*, was also evident in the personal strategies of the people in my study. Sometimes, despite your best efforts, you are subject to situations—illness, divorce, or the death of a relative—that are overwhelming. It is essential to distinguish between what you can and cannot control. If a crisis is beyond your control, you can deflect its impact by taking on a new challenge. Choose a new task to master, like learning to swim or learning a foreign language, to reassure yourself that you are still the master of your own fate. One individual in my study had never learned to drive. When he was confronted by an insurmountable loss, he learned to drive for the first time in his early sixties. That sense of control compensated for his sense of being adrift, and he credits that experience with saving him from a relapse into alcoholism during this crisis. When all else fails, play a new game.

• Finally, if your exercise in control has been successful, new challenges will inevitably arise. Control is an ongoing, lifelong orientation. When the next challenge arises, return to the first step and work through the stages again. With practice and over time, these steps will become virtually instantaneous, as with any practiced skill. Then you will know that control—the certainty that you can influence your life's direction—is firmly established.

Control is a skill that can be developed and enhanced. An optimistic orientation is not a panacea, but even when a situation is in fact hopeless or an illness is inevitably terminal, there are options to be explored. In later chapters these skills will be expanded upon and others introduced, since the ability to manage stress, to visualize future outcomes, to remain engaged with other people, and to experience challenges far beyond individual circumstances through altruistic dedication to others are all part of the farther reaches of health yet to be explored.

CHAPTER FOUR

Sound Mind, Sound Body

From 1980 to 1990 the number of stress disability claims paid to California state workers increased by over 800 percent! According to the California Workers Compensation Institute in San Francisco, these paid claims represented less than 10 percent of the total number of claims filed during the last decade. These figures are compelling evidence that stress has become one of the major afflictions of civilization and a telling indictment of our current lifestyle.

For centuries doctors and scientists have attempted to determine a direct causal relationship between emotions, behaviors, and mental attitudes on one hand and human health and illness on the other. In the second century A.D. the Greek physician Galen noted that "melancholic" women seemed to have a higher incidence of cancer. An eighteenth-century physician writing about the great European plagues of 1763 observed that "those whose minds are depressed by fear are most frequently attacked when epidemic or contagious disorders occur." When the eminent Harvard University biologist Dr. Walter B. Cannon discovered the body's innate fight-or-flight response in the 1930s, the importance of the mind-body system became a cornerstone of Western medical science. Eastern cultures have literally hundreds of meditation practices that extend back over two thousand years. Although these practices have been known and used by millions of people in virtually every culture, our quest to verify mind-body interactions through modern scientific methods has been rekindled. This indefatigable search is beginning to yield some fascinating and promising discoveries.

Intangible influences of the mind upon health and illness have been either excluded or underestimated in the traditional materialistic and dualistic scientific model. Consequences of this oversight are profound. Materialism asserts that there are two basic domains of reality where the nonmaterial does not really exist with the same importance as physical matter. Dualism is the tendency to divide the world into two parts, such as good versus evil. Value judgments inherent in dualistic thinking, which emphasizes polarities and separateness, have had a pernicious effect upon both modern science and our definitions of health that have separated mind and body. We have embraced separateness to such an extreme that we have separated ourselves from nature, from other people and cultures, and from parts of ourselves. In his insightful book *The Passions of the Western Mind*, Richard Tarnas writes about the historical circumstances that have given rise to this particular form of thinking. Perhaps it was helplessness before the Black Death and other diseases, or the terror of the natural world and the need to master and dominate it, that led to the scientific, empirical, essentially male, extreme materialist philosophy. Together, materialism and the dualistic view of the world and ourselves have generated a kind of species arrogance or monumental hubris. As a result of this arrogance we have lost our relationship to nature, split our own beings into compartments, and forgotten our deeper connections to each other, which constitute a sense of the sacred. Throughout the research and interviews for this book the process of confronting and resolving the splits engendered by materialism and dualism was the basis for the evolution of the participants' optimal health.

Whatever the roots of the dualistic, materialist mindset, we are now faced with a different set of circumstances, requiring a new integration of mind, body, environment, and spirit. Increasingly, the necessity of including the intangible, even the spiritual, dimension of health is becoming recognized. Writing in the *Southern Medical Journal* in 1986, Dr. John F. Hiatt of the University of California School of Medicine in San Francisco articulated this new model. Drawing upon both his research and his clinical practice, he concluded that "the spiritual dimension is that part of the person concerned with meaning, and is therefore a principal determinant of health-related attitudes and the world view of both physician and patient. . . . this dimension can and should be reintegrated into health care models and practice." Virtually every participant in my research acknowledged this necessity and used their stress management strategies as the first step, both personally and professionally, in reaching deeper insights and a sense of purpose in their lives.

Surely the most important development in understanding the interaction between mind and body has been the virtual explosion of research in psychoneuroimmunology. As noted in chapter 2, this relatively new field attempts to encompass the domains of *psycho* (the mind and emotions), *neuro* (the brain and central nervous system), and *immunology* (the body's cellular defenses against abnormal internal cells or external invaders such as bacteria or viruses). Psychoneuroimmunology research opens a window onto the complex psychological and behavioral factors that influence the onset and course of stress and immune-related diseases. Correlations between high levels of stress and myriad health problems have been found, including cardiovascular disease, high blood pressure, headaches, back pain, ulcers, anxiety, insomnia, sexual problems, chronic fatigue syndrome, depression, increased accident rates, alcohol and drug abuse, suicide, increased susceptibility to infectious disease, autoimmune disorders (such as lupus), and even the common cold. This new research is a growing testament to the mind-body connection in health and disease.

Unfortunately the exciting findings of the psychoneuroimmunology research remain underutilized. There is always a time lag between a scientific discovery and its human application; although the lag is often attributed to a lack of conclusive data or the need for further research, it is attributable as well to a number of other roadblocks. Among these are an outmoded scientific model, diminished government funding for research, vested economic interests in a disease management industry, and barriers that keep the patient from making independent choices. These same influences created the thirty-year delay from the linking of cigarette smoking to lung cancer to the current proliferation of bans on smoking. It is true that further research is needed. However, it is neither prudent nor possible for clinicians or the general public to wait for decades before using appropriate medical interventions.

A great deal of data revealing the relationship between the central nervous system and the immune system have resulted from the work of Dr. George Solomon of the University of California School of Medicine in Fresno and Dr. Robert Ader of the University of Rochester School of Medicine. Their pioneering research has shown that there are numerous connections between the two systems (e.g., the presence of nerve endings in the thymus, lymph nodes, spleen, and bone marrow), which suggest a complex, communicative, and interactive system between the brain and the immune system. Additionally it has been discovered that cells of the immune system respond to chemical signals from the central nervous system. To date, the two best overviews of the immune system for general understanding are by Dr. Myrin Borysenko, formerly of the Tufts University School of Medicine, in the *Annals of Behavioral Medicine* in 1987, and Dr. Steven E. Locke of the Harvard Medical School in the *Comprehensive Textbook of Psychiatry* of 1989. Given these direct links, psychological and social factors may well have an effect on the immune system.

Any state of health or disease is the result of a complex interaction among such influences as genetics, age, sex, personality, social support, diet, environment, bacteria, viruses, carcinogens, medical care, socioeconomic factors, and a host of others, many of which are yet to be discovered. Although the focus of this chapter is to explore the mind-body interactions evident in psychoneuroimmunology, I am in no way discounting the importance of these other factors.

For the purposes of this chapter *stressor* refers to the challenge faced by an individual, while *stress* refers to any possible response to the challenge. Early in 1987 a major conference of psychologists and immunologists met for the sole purpose of defining a common ground in terminology, research procedure, and measurement in the mind-body arena. Ironically, their first stumbling block was defining the word *stress*; they reached the unanimous conclusion that any absolute definition was impossible. Despite this seeming impasse, it was agreed that stress is not what happens (that's the stressor) but how a person reacts to what happens.

Stress in itself is neither good nor bad. It is a mechanism built into our organism, not for the purpose of making us sick but to enable us to respond more effectively to challenges. My intent is to focus on the practical and effective ways the individuals in my study handle stress and the background behind these strategies. Every person I interviewed had experienced highly stressful events. What is unique about these successful men and women is that they have either unconsciously or deliberately created techniques to manage the inevitable stressors of their lives, techniques which enable them to go on. For many participants the goal of developing such a skill was not to obtain health. Instead the goal was, for example, to head the entrepreneurial development of a new computer business, or to adapt to the demands of making a sound stock market analysis, or to be a more loving and attentive spouse, or to attain myriad other goals where health was simply a means to a better life, not an end unto itself. In a culture that manifests a preoccupation with health and eternal youth that rivals its fixation on money and power, this distinction is important to bear in mind.

One of the world's best-kept secrets is that most truly successful people are not overburdened by stress. Nor do they achieve success at the expense of their physical and emotional health. In fact, many individuals in high-demand situations actually thrive on stress. A 1982 Gallup poll found that only 8 percent of the top executives in the Fortune 500 companies reported stress to be a problem. By contrast nearly 60 percent reported that they were sometimes or often actually exhilarated by stress. In spite of the accumulating evidence to the contrary, the old myths continue to be promulgated, warning us that professional success is not compatible with health and happiness.

Stressors can actually assume a positive role in a person's life. Stressors can prepare us to deal with emergencies and provide an opportunity for accomplishment that leads to gratification and an enhanced sense of control and productivity. Again and again the individuals in my study demonstrated a healthy way of utilizing stress. What they all have in common is an attitude that allows them to perceive a stressor as an opportunity for learning and achievement. They also possess a disciplined self-awareness and the flexibility to handle appropriately excessive amounts of stress. Furthermore, they uniformly learned to exert an appropriate level of control. To date, numerous studies conclude that uncontrollable stress produces negative consequences while controllable stress is not destructive and may actually be health-enhancing. One 1992 study by Dr. Judith Rodin and her colleagues at Yale University subjected adult men to uncontrollable versus controllable noise. Under this all-too-common circumstance, the men subjected to uncontrollable noise showed a reduced level of natural killer (NK) cells for as much as seventy-two hours. Men who perceived they had control over the noise showed no such reductions. Exerting control and perhaps simply believing you have control appears to be an important influence in stress management and overall health. Certainly for my research participants control was consistently cited as essential to their personal stress management strategies.

All of the participants indicated that they have individual methods for managing the inevitable stress of their very demanding personal and professional lives. Among these stress management techniques were deep breathing, listening to music, long walks on the beach, traditional meditation and yoga practices, Christian prayer, biofeedback, visualization, and the silent repetition of a meaningful word or a mantra. They all emphasized that these personal strategies were simply tools or training exercises for developing a consistently positive attitude toward themselves and the world around them. It is this attitude that is the real stress management, not the techniques themselves. There is a Buddhist koan that says we should not confuse the finger with that to which it points. The same applies to stress management strategies, which should not be confused with the ultimately important inner state to which they lead.

When the actress Lindsay Wagner said, "Actually, I tend to take any crisis as an opportunity or challenge," she was expressing an attitude common among everyone in the study. "I do believe," she continued, "that the things that we must confront, that we interpret as unpleasant, really are put there for our growth. When I say 'put there,' it's not as though there's some deity sitting up on a cloud somewhere dealing out difficult situations; I mean that we attract the things that are going to take us to the next level. It's an evolution in some way that will keep bashing away at the areas we need to look at in ourselves. Life will do that to us until we finally get it. Break loose of that challenge and move on to the next ones that we have yet to release or learn about in order to grow. That attitude really helps in a time of crisis because it helps me move through it instead of getting stuck with it and feeling victimized by it. Being a victim means consequently repeating it because I'm going to draw it again. Very often I've found that I've shared this feeling with other people who have had similar experiences. We seem to have a set of negative habit patterns that are ours to utilize this time around. When you think you've really got it, when you finally break through one of them, then you feel like you have a handle on it at last. Now that's not going to happen again. But what I've found is that I seem to be peeling away layers or veils. So even though I have been able to get a hold of this particular habit pattern, on a very gross level, and those kinds of things don't happen anymore, then there are other things that I start looking at. Sometimes I start manifesting other negative types of experiences and have found that it's kind of the same pattern. It's a more subtle experience with the same type of thing. . . . Those are the real challenges and stresses, but they always propel me forward to the next lesson in life. So I am actually very grateful for the crises and challenges."

Through her ongoing practice of meditation, Lindsay Wagner has enhanced her ability to address these challenges. During periods of particularly stressful circumstances, she said, "I spend a lot of time in meditation. . . . I know there's an answer there, but I also know I may not be able to see it clearly in my conscious mind. Very often the first thing to come out of my meditations is the question, What is your priority? Finding out your priority is the real challenge! Then commit to it and follow it through by expressing your feelings and, most importantly, by taking the appropriate course of action. Everything else will follow in its place and time." Wagner practices what she preaches. She has applied this attitude to resolving several life crises, including early childhood trauma, bankruptcy, physical illness, and on a more positive note, the decision to have a child as a single parent with a demanding career.

Stress management strategies used by Wagner and the other prominent individuals became their means for achieving a productive orientation toward the day-by-day, minute-by-minute challenges of their lives. This ongoing orientation was a means of personal growth that helped them attain true health: a sound mind in a sound body. Using what we can learn from this study, together with what we now know about how the mind and body respond to stress, we can go on to develop a model for optimal stress management. Ironically, while the scientific literature detailing the interaction between mind and body, and specifically the role of stress, is becoming increasingly more sophisticated, the actual means to manage stress remain disarmingly simple. In fact, many are so simple that some of us have been lulled into a false sense of security, somehow believing that merely knowing *how* to handle excessive stress is the same thing as doing it. In addition people are bored with traditional—and sometimes literally ancient—stress management techniques.

In a society where fad diets and new workout methods come and go like hit movies, we are not geared toward sticking to a simple method that works. Perhaps this is how can we account for the alarming rise of stress disorders when information and advice about stress and stress management abounds in publications ranging from the *New England Journal of Medicine* to *Ladies Home Journal*. Why do so many people smoke, and why is smoking on the increase among working women as well as male and female adolescents when it is now over twenty years since the Surgeon General's unequivocal report linking cigarette smoking to lung cancer and a host of other life-threatening diseases? Part of the answer is as straightforward and simple as the stress management techniques themselves: we must actually *do* the techniques for them to work. It is a dangerous delusion to substitute knowledge for practice. This is the essence of the disparity between unprecedented stress disorders and a virtual inundation of relaxation techniques provided by health professionals as well as the popular media.

FINDING A PURPOSE IN LIFE

Relying on stress management techniques alone to accomplish therapeutic goals is shortsighted. We must also take a good look at what drives us in our daily lives. Virtually every individual in my research project is driven by a deep and abiding sense of purpose, which fuels and is fueled by that sense of control we discussed in chapter 3. This strong sense of purpose is like a guiding light that comes from within, from their innermost intuition. They feel they have a role to fulfill in the universe. This role is their life's true work, and there is no turning back. It is not their egos that motivate them but rather this personal mission to serve a greater cause. Out of this pervasive sense of purpose they develop an unwavering commitment to their values.

Unique stress management techniques used by these individuals are simply tools for reinforcing their overriding sense of purpose. By harnessing stress and keeping their life's purpose solidly intact, they have the strength to face challenges and take on new commitments. I emphasize that the specific techniques they have chosen are not as important as their ongoing process of meeting and resolving life's many challenges. One of the earliest clinicians to recognize the central importance of purpose was the psychiatrist Dr. Victor Frankl. He was one of the first proponents of the idea that purpose was integral to health, having observed that "man should not, indeed cannot, struggle for identity in a direct way; he rather finds identity in the extent to which he commits himself to something beyond himself, to a cause greater than himself." Through his internment in concentration camps, Frankl came to believe that the goal of human life, for both the individual and the collective group, is to find meaning and order in the world. This goal includes a social sense of purpose as well as an orderliness in a person's inner and outer environment. More recently this sense of purpose has been found to be a major influence upon psychological and physical health as well as actual life expectancy. This finding is most intriguing because it indicates that purpose may exert a sufficiently powerful influence over body chemistry to postpone death, at least for a brief time.

In 1990 Dr. David Phillips, a sociologist at the University of California in San Diego, conducted a series of studies to examine the long-standing belief that people can postpone their death until after a significant event has passed. This occurrence has been termed the *anniversary phenomenon*. An often-cited instance concerns Thomas Jefferson. As he lay dying on July 3, 1826, Jefferson reportedly awoke and asked his doctor, "Is it the Fourth?" To which the doctor answered, "No, but it soon will be." On the next day, the fiftieth anniversary of the founding of the United States, Jefferson gave up his grip on life and died.

In his first study Phillips looked at the death rate of Jewish men around the important religious holiday of Passover. He analyzed 1,919 deaths in the three months prior to and following Passover. What he found was very striking. In the week before Passover the death rate fell 23.2 percent below the norm and rebounded to 24.4 percent over the norm in the following week. For his second study Phillips turned to the Chinese to see if the phenomenon carried over to an entirely different culture. For the Chinese the Harvest Moon Festival is analogous in importance to the Jewish celebration of Passover. However, in the Harvest Moon Festival, the senior women in the family play the central role, unlike at Passover, where men predominate in the ceremony. During the Harvest Moon study, Phillips examined 1,288 deaths among elderly Chinese women. Paralleling his previous study, the death rate for the women fell 35.1 percent below the norm before the festival and rose back up to 34.6 percent above the norm after the festival. In neither of the studies were the findings explained by such reasons as delaying surgery during the holidays. What seems to underlie this phenomenon is the individuals' strong desire to participate in these significant and symbolic celebrations. These findings suggest we take a closer look at the biochemical changes in individuals before and after important events to determine what the biological basis of the anniversary phenomenon might be. Phillips's studies and others like his provide real-life evidence that a strong sense of purpose and a firm commitment to a particular goal exerts a powerful influence upon human physiology.

In interviewing the Sound Mind–Sound Body participants, I frequently found that their physical health indeed reflected a sense of purpose. In addition the resulting commitment they felt appeared to lay the foundation for altruistic and selfless actions. There was one individual in particular who spoke movingly about the development of his purpose in life. At the time of his interview James Autry was president of the Magazine Group of the Meredith Corporation in Des Moines, Iowa, a Fortune 500 company. With about eight hundred employees the Magazine Group is the largest division of Meredith.

Among the many magazines published by that division are *Better Homes and Gardens*, *Ladies Home Journal*, *Country Home*, and *Sail*. Autry, an accomplished publisher, is also a published poet and author as well—a rare combination. His first book of poetry, *Nights under a Tin Roof: Recollections of a Southern Boyhood*, was published in 1983 and is now in its third printing. Most recently he was interviewed by Bill Moyers for his *Spoken Word* television series. The title of Autry's latest book, *For Love and Profit*, could be a pithy summary of his life. Having grown up in Memphis, Tennessee, the son and grandson of Mississippi Baptist ministers, he conveys a deep connection with his Southern upbringing and family values. He is a business maverick who has not only succeeded in the boardroom but also gained praise from the general public. Both his career and his personal life have benefited from the firm convictions and sense of purpose he developed and honed in the crucible of several family crises.

When Autry found out his brother had leukemia, he began to give him books, tapes, and other materials that focused on having a purpose and not giving up hope. Remembering that time, he said, "I pleaded with my brother to read the books and listen to the tapes. I didn't know if it would work because I really didn't know much about ideas. Anyway, he read the books and was back to work by December, which was when he was supposed to be dead. He lived two and a half years beyond that—a joyful life until he finally gave in to that galloping leukemia. . . . But even when he found out that he had only eight more weeks to live, he started a journal that was a complete celebration of life! The same week that my brother was diagnosed, one of my best friends for twenty years was given the same diagnosis. They corresponded with one another but my friend was dead within a few months. . . . I thought, What's going on? Something is going on here. That put me much more in the investigative mode about purpose and mind-body and the interconnectedness of life. . . . Then all these connections began to fall into place, and I felt certain that there was some purpose in all this."

As this sense of purpose grew in Autry's psyche, he married his second wife, Sally Pederson, in 1982. During the 1960s Autry had attended church with his two sons from a previous marriage, but it was not until his second marriage and a return to his church that he began to experience a new dimension to his sense of purpose. Looking back, he recounted, "In the sixties we were going to church and my two sons were singing in the choir and all that, but I wasn't paying attention; it meant nothing to me emotionally. . . . But when I returned to church, I would find myself crying. I'd be in tears and I'd hear messages that were very important to me. . . . Then I started reading some books on Western and Buddhist teachings. Something clicked, something about an interconnectedness between all people and all of life's events. It was and is through this feeling of interconnectedness that I came to realize the purpose of my own life." That realization did not result in a sudden change in Autry's life, but it did influence how he managed his employees as well as how he raised his autistic son, who became a "profound teacher" to Autry and his wife.

Not only does having a deep sense of purpose help people to cope successfully with stress, it appears to grow even stronger with the mastery of each new challenge. Research has documented that purpose is beneficial to psychological health, in alleviating such conditions as depression and anxiety, and to physical health, in contributing to recovery from heart attacks and cancer. It has also been shown that individuals who express their purpose in life through altruism are unusually healthy and recover more quickly and fully from both major and minor illnesses. Unfortunately such findings are often interpreted as indicating that the mind-body field is about gaining mental control over physical functions or fixing the body by using the mind. That misinterpretation does a disservice to this complex domain, where intangibles such as purpose are found to play a profound role in achieving optimal health.

Some of the most articulate statements about the mind-body field have been made by Dr. Rachel Naomi Remen, a practicing physician whose research has focused on cancer patients and the clinicians who work with them at the Commonweal Center in Bolinas, California. Early in 1993 Dr. Remen's innovative and moving work was featured in the Moyers PBS television series *Healing and the Mind,* which focused on the mainstreaming of mind-body interventions. Reflecting on the simplistic idea of using the mind to fix the body, she has stated, "This makes sense to people, and they are interested because the mind is a simpler, safer, cheaper, more efficient, more affordable way of healing the body than, let's say, surgery. So the whole purpose of the field may be coming to be seen as the manipulation of the body by the mind to attain physical health. And I'm not at all sure that understanding how to manipulate the body . . . with the mind is a large-enough purpose for the field. . . . Health is not an end. Health is a means. Health enables us to serve purpose in life, but health in and of itself is not the purpose in life. One can serve purpose with impaired health. One might even regain health through serving purpose."

Although a sense of purpose certainly does not guarantee uninterrupted health, it does give a more profound meaning to the challenges of life. In the Sound Mind–Sound Body study, the actor Dennis Weaver talked about living according to a deeper purpose while in the midst of adversity. Weaver first became widely known as Chester in the classic series *Gunsmoke*. Not satisfied with this initial success and eager to extend his creativity, he progressed beyond his supporting character role to become the star of *McCloud*. In that series he played a contemporary but unconventional New Mexico deputy marshal fighting crime in the streets of New York City. That role earned him three Emmy nominations and a perpetually recognized public image. An extremely diverse actor who has defied typecasting, he has played a terrorized cross-country driver pursued by a truck in Steven Spielberg's classic *Duel*, as well as a real estate salesman turned cocaine abuser in *Cocaine: One Man's Seduction*. Weaver is also known for his commitments to world peace, ending hunger and homelessness in America, drug abuse prevention, and the pursuit of his personal and spiritual growth.

In 1983 Weaver, the actress Valerie Harper, and several concerned community leaders founded LIFE (Love Is Feeding Everyone). This nonprofit, community-activated food recovery and distribution program gathers surplus food from supermarkets, produce outlets, food drives, and bakeries and distributes it to social service agencies, churches, and neighborhood groups through centers in South Central and East Los Angeles and the San Fernando Valley. Recipient of the 1986 Presidential End Hunger Award, Weaver serves as LIFE's president and remains active in virtually every phase of the organization's growth. LIFE, which began by helping four hundred needy people daily, now provides food to more than seventy thousand every day. LIFE, which is planning national expansion, serves as a role model for similar start-up programs throughout the country.

Looking out over the Pacific Ocean from his home in Malibu, Weaver spoke with intense conviction about his motivation. Dedicating his time to the hungry and homeless rather than making another film is not even a choice. It is a mission. In a clear and unwavering voice he said, "I have few crises in my life, few problems. I just don't think of things as major crises like some people do. I feel that love is the strongest force in the universe and that we're all being drawn back to that understanding or knowingness of the love, to that presence of God within us. At the time I didn't recognize it, sometimes, but everything that happens to me has purpose, a reason for happening, and happens for my eventual good. Therefore, if the end is a state of oneness with the universal consciousness, then all of the steps, all of the moments back to it, have to be good. . . . Rama Krishna said we'll be saved, it's just a question of when." Such broad statements might be dismissed as mere philosophizing, if it were not for Weaver's way of applying these beliefs to both the minor inconveniences and the major challenges in his life.

Musing over a relatively minor mishap, Weaver noted, "The time lag is getting shorter between seeing something as a problem or a crisis and being able to see it as a step in my own evolution. Much, much shorter, because I know that something good is going to happen. Right now I have a bum shoulder because I fell skiing and I've got bursitis. Something good is going to happen from that. I'm not sure what it is, because my vision and my wisdom are very, very shortsighted. It's like a jigsaw puzzle with hundreds of pieces. When you scatter them all out, and none of them are together, none of them make any sense. But as you start fitting them together, they begin to make more sense, and then when you complete the picture, you understand each piece's purpose and why each is shaped the way it is. It's the same with life. We will understand why each moment is as it is when we step back and look at the bigger picture. . . . Another nice thing about that philosophy or attitude is that it keeps your spirits up. It creates a kind of cheerfulness that I feel very strongly is an important part of my health."

The effects of being driven by a greater purpose do indeed extend beyond individual health to such issues as global ecology, world hunger, and a more equitable, humanitarian economy. But now let's focus on how purpose and commitment to a greater cause influence a person's orientation toward the challenges in life and personal health. As we have seen, the way a person responds to stressors is now viewed as equally important as, if not more so than, the stressor itself. Considerable scientific evidence demonstrates that an individual's strategies for coping with stress may determine ultimate mind-body health. In fact, it has been shown that poor coping skills can actually lead to a weakened immune response. This relationship has been effectively described by Dr. Richard Lazarus and Dr. Susanne Folkman of the University of California at Berkeley in their definitions of stress and subsequent coping behavior. Stress, they say, is a "relationship between the person and the environment that is appraised by the person as taxing or exceeding his or her resources and endangering his or her well-being." They define coping as "constantly changing cognitive and behavioral efforts to manage specific external and/or internal demands that exceed the resources of the person." What is particularly important about the Lazarus and Folkman research is that it provides the conclusive link between the old thinking that simplistically related major life events to disease and the more complex mind-body research. Mind-body research has illuminated the importance of purpose and conscious will. Our attitudes, perceptions, and personality directly affect whether a stressor is able to manifest itself in the body, and because stressors may strongly influence immune function, it is our psychological state that may play the ultimate role in determining health.

A wide variety of psychological characteristics that affect biochemical response have been identified, including mood, personality characteristics, coping style, hardiness, sense of purpose, suppressed anger, hopelessness, psychological vulnerability, inhibited power motivation, defensiveness, inattention to distress, frequency and intensity of daily hassles, and the presence or absence of social support. Clearly the same external event is perceived differently by different people, and individual responses to stressors are equally variable.

Some personality factors have even been correlated with specific diseases. For example, rheumatoid arthritis has been linked to perfectionism, compliance, subservience, nervousness, restlessness, reserve, and anger. Cardiovascular disease has been associated with the Type A personality, marked by hostility, social isolation, loneliness, lack of trust, and a tendency to be a "hot reactor." In fact, the purely biological risk factors for heart disease are inadequate to explain the disease or its treatment. Recently both Dr. Ray Rosenman, coauthor of *Type A Behavior and Your Heart*, and Dr. Paul J. Rosch, president of the American Institute of Stress in New York, have written influential articles indicating that mind-body interactions may play an equal role in both preventing and treating heart disease. While acknowledging that cholesterol is a major risk, they point out that reduction in dietary cholesterol is not always associated with reduced blood cholesterol. By contrast, studies that reduce Type A behavior as well as studies of propranolol, a beta blocker, have achieved protective effects, probably by lowering stress-induced levels of catecholamine, which is known to produce cardiac damage and has been linked to sudden death. Such findings and challenges as these provide the basis to create prevention and intervention programs that integrate both the mind and body dimensions of health. Cancer has been correlated with nonassertiveness, the inability to express emotion, and a sense of hopelessness. With regard to the reputed "cancer-prone" personality, though, it must be noted that the studies to date suggest only preliminary evidence of the existence of such a complex.

At the University of Chicago, psychologist Dr. Richard Shekelle followed the health histories of 2,020 middle-aged Western Electric plant employees and found that those who had been depressed were twice as likely to die from cancer. Depression is the emotional condition most linked to cancer incidence, but this one-dimensional explanation has not been substantiated. Although depression does suppress certain immune system activity, there are no studies linking that degree of suppression to cancer incidence. One of the most respected analysts of this data, Dr. Bernard H. Fox of the Boston University School of Medicine, wrote a brief, critical review of the literature linking major depressive disorders to cancer in the *Journal of the American Medical Association* and considered the evidence inconclusive. In 1987 a study in the same journal reported that married people were less likely to be diagnosed with cancer, and much less likely to die of the disease, than unmarried or divorced individuals. In another set of studies both stress and various personality characteristics were demonstrated to predict cancer. These studies were set up so that the subjects' psychological differences were identified prior to the onset of the cancer symptoms, lending credence to the notion that personality factors are associated with cancer onset.

In the past several years only one study has failed to find a relationship between psychosocial factors and health outcomes. In 1985 Dr. Barrie Cassileth failed to find a relationship between psychosocial factors and cancer survival in a cohort of 204 patients with unresectable cancers. The investigators concluded that while psychosocial factors may relate to disease onset, "The biology of the disease appears to predominate and to override that potential influence of lifestyle and psychosocial variables once the disease process is established." While this appears to be a reasonable conclusion from their data, other investigators have reported a strong relationship between psychosocial factors and cancer survival. Indeed, the Cassileth study has been criticized for a number of reasons, including a poor selection of psychological and social measures, questionable validity of the measures that were used, and probably most importantly, a sample size too small to produce statistical power.

On a more positive note, a 1985 British study of women with breast cancer reported that those women with a "fighting spirit" who were actively involved in treatment and felt in control of their disease were more likely to survive and less likely to experience a recurrence than those who felt helpless and hopeless. Also encouraging was a seven-year follow-up of breast cancer patients by the University of Pittsburgh School of Medicine researcher Dr. Sandra Levy and her colleagues. This 1988 study found that those patients who had expressed more "joy" at baseline testing lived longer, had fewer metastatic sites and longer disease-free intervals, and lived longer with recurrent disease.

The question of the link between emotional states and the onset and outcome of cancer remains one of the most intriguing medical issues. Rather than focusing only on cancer itself, researchers are now just beginning to ask how a positive attitude can diminish the impact of such a dreaded disease. Literature on this subject strongly suggests the importance of how people cope with stress.

BEING IN THE NOW

For decades researchers have studied how negative emotions affect the mind-body system, but the Sound Mind–Sound Body project is one of the first studies to show that purpose and other positive emotions actually benefit health. Yet while the individuals in the study consistently pointed out this relationship in their own lives, all showed that they were not particularly preoccupied with the status of their health. Instead they all spoke spontaneously about their focus on the immediate challenges of their lives. When asked about long-term goals or objectives regarding their health and/or profession, they actually seemed bewildered. Attention to the present time seems to be the means by which these individuals manifest their personal control, sense of purpose, and ability to manage stress in matters of both health and career.

Surprisingly, this characteristic was articulated most clearly by the founder and chairman of a major architectural and construction company, where long-term, strategic plans would be expected to rule the day. On a warm spring afternoon in New York City I interviewed John L. Tishman, chairman and chief executive officer of Tishman Realty and Construction Company. Since 1948, when he joined the organization that now bears his name, Tishman has been the prime motivating force behind its commitment to and commanding role in the advancement of modern building technology. He is recognized as an expert in the construction of complex, large-scale projects, particularly those incorporating state-of-the-art systems or requiring the application of new construction techniques. Over the years Tishman has been personally in charge of such landmark projects as the World

Trade Center in New York, the John Hancock Center in Chicago, the Century City Theme Center in Los Angeles, and the Walt Disney Company's EPCOT Center in central Florida. More recently he guided his firm in the renovation and restoration of Carnegie Hall. Clearly this is a business in which an individual's sense of purpose would be expected to take the form of a structured plan, but that is not the case at all with John Tishman. He has never tried to program his life. Looking back over his career, he reflected, "Fate just moved me; I have never had a plan. A lot of young people who have strong family ties are more or less programmed to follow in a set, programmed track from early on. I hear about young people who have a 'plan'— when they're thirteen years old. They go through high school and college, and they're on a track that may have been designed by someone else or in fact by them. But I must say, I never had a program. Actually, I went to the University of Michigan because my best friend's father had gone there."

"Since I had some mathematical prowess, I was heading toward engineering, but it was primarily because my best friend's father was an electrical engineer. I had no father, no one who was telling me, 'Follow me.' I had no profession. So we went off to college together. How it happened I don't know. I just slid into it; there was never any plan. Even now I don't have any plan. However, I do know that if you let yourself go, things will carry you along. I can't tell you how many people have interviewed me through the years about business matters, asking, 'What is your strategic plan?' and I'd say, 'I don't have one.' Whatever I can do, I'm doing, and tomorrow will bring something else that has to be done. Actually I'm very intense and sometimes overworked, but I love it and I don't have any plan."

While this attitude of living in the present moment may appear contradictory in individuals with a strong sense of purpose, it was an unwavering theme among virtually everyone in my study. They have a Zenlike orientation to being in the now, as opposed to dwelling on the past or fantasizing about the future. Their sense of mission and their careers go hand in hand. When describing their work, they often use the word *fun*, and they usually have no concept of what the future will hold. Enjoying what is happening *now* in their lives is a means of keeping them in the moment, thus making them more productive. This present-time orientation releases their minds from all concerns except the one they are facing at that moment. Approaching an isolated matter without the clutter of background chatter creates a positive and pragmatic mood in which every circumstance can reveal a silver lining. In essence, this is a healthy way to solve any everyday problem, whether it be talking over a sensitive matter with a spouse, dealing with a dilemma at work, or handling a harried sales clerk or bank teller.

This orientation is particularly evident in individuals involved in successful financial management. Among them is attorney Wayne Silby, who while in his mid-twenties started an investment firm that grew into the Calvert Group of Funds, now valued in excess of $1 billion. When Silby founded the Calvert Fund, he was the youngest CEO of a mutual fund group in the country; it has now grown to become one of Washington's largest. In 1977, when few people had heard of money markets, he pioneered an innovative investment approach that resulted in Calvert's First Variable Rate Fund. This fund became the highest-yielding and among the safest money funds in the country. Under Silby's youthful leadership, the Calvert Group fostered many of the new management values that were to become widely shared among his generation, the so-called baby boomers. His idea for the Calvert Social Investment Fund was a natural merging of his financial acumen and his experience as a member of the sixties generation. A model for how one can successfully express personal values through investment choices, the fund was recognized by the *Boston Globe* as "the fastest growing and most respected comprehensively screened mutual fund around, the acknowledged flagship of the industry." Silby enjoys pointing out that he and his colleagues selected the logo for their fund by throwing Chinese coins according to the *I Ching*, an ancient Eastern book of wisdom. When the coins landed, the pattern that emerged was the symbol meaning "the Creative."

In addition to speaking at numerous New Age conferences, such as the Telluride Festival of Ideas, the Omega Institute, and the New York Open Center, Silby has also been a speaker at the White House Conference on Productivity. In a related governmental effort he was part of a select group of fifty CEOs, most from Fortune 1000 companies, that engaged in a four-month teleconference on industrial competitiveness. He has made many other contributions to the private sector and was cited by President Ronald Reagan for his "energetic and farsighted community leadership." In 1985, as assets at Calvert climbed to over $1 billion among one hundred thousand investors, Silby moved out of day-to-day management to devote time to other innovative projects and interests.

Several years ago he sponsored a conference for one hundred select investors and entrepreneurs at which the spiritual leader Ram Dass and the consumer advocate Ralph Nader spoke. Out of this meeting Silby and several friends, including Joshua Mailman, founder of the Threshold Foundation, who was also a participant in my study, created the Social Venture Network to foster "socially responsible business." Among the network members are such like-minded people as Ben and Jerry of Ben & Jerry's ice cream, Rockport Shoes founder Bruce Katz, and Paul Hawken of Smith & Hawken (another study participant). Among Silby's many innovative ideas is to encourage financial institutions to speak out on economic policy issues. Management theorist Peter Drucker emphasizes in his writings that businesses themselves must meet their social responsibility and are accountable for the quality of life in the society in which they operate. Bolstering such theoretical views are recent court rulings and legislative directives charging American businesses with greater responsibility for their impact on the physical and social environment. The government's unbridled military spending is another concern of the Calvert Social Investment Fund, which is in the process of organizing a campaign with its own investors to address this economic and national agenda issue. Silby has been voicing his concerns about the nonproductive use of the nation's resources in the arms race since he served as an early board member of Business Executives for National Security.

With all of the demands on his time and attention, Silby is very disciplined about staying focused on what he calls the "bounce" of the moment. When I asked him if he followed his sense of purpose to determine his next steps, he said, "Actually, I really cannot project future plans. Life has such a way of bouncing that I want to be part of that bounce. I want to end up wherever life takes me, as opposed to letting my concepts of where I should be run my life. . . . I could say I want to run the first trillion-dollar security trust fund. That would be fun! Or be an adviser to politicians on basic economics or tax policies that really make economic and productive sense for the country. It would be fun to live in Thailand for a while or be the ambassador to Burma. Who can say? . . . I'm not a person that likes to just play in the meadows as such. I like to also see the other side of the coin, to see the dark edges of ideas or thoughts. Those edges are very much a part of what makes life interesting. For a curious person, making life interesting is living in the now. It's really almost a cliché—living in the now. But when you come down to it, now is really more interesting than whatever projections or conceptions you can make. Like everyone, I used to have a lot of fantasies. I still have some now and then. But more and more, especially with my meditation and other life experiences, just being in the moment is the biggest challenge. Anyway, all you really have is now."

IS MONEY THE PURPOSE?

In discussing their values, all of the participants stressed service to others as their highest aspiration and true life mission. They also emphasized material frugality, simplicity, and self-restraint. While discussing their life purpose, they never mentioned material security, wealth, or the conventional image of success. Money was not a goal in and of itself. Because these individuals have indeed achieved material success, it is all too easy to dismiss their socially conscious philosophies as nothing more than the posturings of Rolls-Royce radicals. However, that is clearly not the case. In fact, most participants attribute their success to being willing to take chances and live their lives in a way that is consistent with their deeper sense of purpose. Wayne Silby started his Calvert Fund with "a law degree, six hundred dollars, and a lot of conviction."

For too many people money is the only way of keeping score. For others the currency of self-esteem is job title, academic rank, or athletic statistics. The arena may differ for each of us, but the pattern is often the same. Sometimes we do get what we think will make us happy, only to find out it doesn't. In a 1981 poll conducted by *Psychology Today*, the respondents who expressed the greatest satisfaction with their financial situation were not necessarily those with the highest incomes. Rather their contentment revolved more around such psychological factors as self-esteem, satisfaction with their jobs, friends, and personal growth. Predictably, a majority of the respondents indicated that to feel truly successful they would need the security of adequate money along with love and meaningful work. A full 74 percent of the respondents also agreed with the statement, "In America, money is how we keep score." The respondents fell into one of two survey groups: the "money-troubled" and the "money-contented." The money-troubled—not necessarily the people with the lowest incomes—were defined by four characteristics: 1) they were frustrated with material aspirations; they wanted things they could not afford; they were in deep debt even with good incomes; they felt that their friends had more money and that they themselves deserved more; 2) they lacked a secure sense of self and felt dissatisfaction with friendships and personal growth. Ironically, the youngest respondents had the lowest self-esteem and were the most troubled in this dimension; 3) they were unhappy both at work and home; they reported dissatisfaction with career, love, and sexual relationships, as well as frequent domestic arguments about money; and 4) they had more fears, anxieties, psychosomatic disorders, and generally poorer health.

Conclusions of the survey focused much more on these negative traits of the money-troubled than on the positive characteristics of the money-contented. This zeroing in on the negative is the thrust of most of traditional research in psychology, medicine, biology, and related disciplines. Positive findings are usually deemed inconsequential. Generally it was noted that the money-contented "rule their money rather than let it rule them." Among the few characteristics attributed to these respondents were 1) a feeling that inflation had not substantially altered their standard of living in recent years; 2) a belief that their friends had about as much money as they did or less; freedom from debt; and a lack of desire for material possessions they felt they could not afford; and 3) fewer anxieties, phobias, and psychosomatic complaints, as well as more satisfying sexual relations and better general health. Overall this profile of money-contented people—again, not necessarily those with the highest incomes—is consistent to a large degree with the attitude of the truly successful individuals cited in this book. The *Psychology Today* survey indirectly confirms the notion that it is possible for individuals—regardless of their earnings—to attain the high-energy fusion of good health and career achievement.

Each of the Sound Mind–Sound Body participants answered my questions about the role of money with strikingly similar responses. Whether they had inherited money, as did Gordon Getty, Michael S. Currier, and David Rockfeller, or developed their success from very limited resources, as in the cases of John E. Fetzer, Saul Zaentz, and Laurel Burch, they uniformly agreed that money was not a principal objective in their lives.

In my interview with him at his studio in Berkeley, California, the film producer Saul Zaentz recollected the day from his childhood in Newark, New Jersey, when he first pondered the meaning of money. Telling me about "gambling on the street corner" as a young boy, when "money really wasn't the issue," he reminisced, "My oldest brother came out one time with a wonderful line. When he had bought a house for my family, somebody said to him, 'Jesus, you blew all that money on a house?' With a smile he said, 'Well, it's only money!' And in later years I always remembered what he said. It's true. That's all it is. I've always believed that but never really knew how deeply until later in my life. Now I feel I am really capable of understanding what he was saying, that it's only money. It meant nothing; it was just part of the game. Winning the bet was more important than getting the money. Playing the game, being able to outfigure somebody, out-think somebody, or outplay somebody if you're playing sports, is more important than the money. What money *does* mean is freedom. But then you have to make choices with that freedom. It puts pressure on you in many ways. . . . Once you have some discretionary money, then you actually have some added responsibilities."

Zaentz's responsibilities during his early adult years and marriage were of a more basic nature. Reflecting on his marriage to his former wife, Celia, he said, "She worked like a dog, even when we had kids at home. Celia was really an equal partner in our business. She was there through the bad times when we had no money at all. We went shopping at Goodwill for the kids to get shirts and gloves. It really was no problem with us. We were living in a place for fifty dollars a month rent. Even then I remembered my brother saying, 'It's only money!' "

Today, as the owner of Fantasy Records, a highly successful recording company, as well as his film company, Saul Zaentz Productions, Zaentz says his philosophy remains unchanged. Looking back over a successful year for his companies, he reflected, "We are very lucky to be a private company. We don't have to beat last year's earnings, and we're not subject to the constant pressure from analysts and stockholders to make money in the way that public companies must endure. We take on our projects one at a time. When someone asks me about financing our films, I tell them, 'You're sitting in the bank,' because we bankroll our films through loans secured by the building we're sitting in right now! After all . . . it's only money!" This attitude has contributed to the success of his film career by liberating him to focus on his creativity. With that creative energy he has produced such remarkable films as *One Flew Over the Cuckoo's Nest*, *Amadeus, The Unbearable Lightness of Being*, and *At Play in the Fields of the Lord* and has become one of the most respected contemporary film producers.

Designer and reluctant entrepreneur Laurel Burch shares a similar perspective. Although she enjoys her design work, she is still not attached to her business success and often quips that she still cannot read a ledger. Considering what material success has meant to her life, she thoughtfully comments, "Money and success are simply tools to access other things that I want to do, other things that I need to accomplish throughout different realms. Because of my background, I am now truly driven to become valuable in a global sense. In order to do that I need to gain access to other people so I can learn about and connect with them. It's something that is very important to me. It has to do with lessons and learning. A few weeks ago I went to the White House and met the President. That wasn't significant for the reasons that some people might think. I think it's wonderful, but that's not the inside experience. For me the real value is that it enables me to function in and be a part of the greater world in order to do the work that I need to do on this planet and in this lifetime in many different cultures and realms. . . . For me it is of the utmost importance to get to the very bottom and the essence of the human being . . . of all human beings. Something about my life purpose is connected with that, and with being a vehicle to connect people. . . . So to get back to the question of money and success and all that, it has been a vehicle through which I could have greater access to different people and different organizations. I don't want to be on the outside. I want to get on the inside of every different situation, because I want to understand and communicate with people. For me, the more I understand, the more valuable I can be in terms of the way that I use that knowledge and that information. It's a constant test of personal trust and integrity."

For Saul Zaentz, Laurel Burch, and every other participant in my study, these deeply held convictions and sense of purpose far surpass the pursuit of money, which is not an end in itself but a means to a greater end. By placing money and success in this framework, the participants set the cornerstone for their altruistic and philanthropic work. It is clear that they do not persevere under stress and pressures to earn a living but rather to learn to live.

When it comes to money-troubled individuals, there is the eternal nature versus nurture question of whether or not they are just chronically neurotic or because they really do not have enough money to make ends meet. While that is possible, the truly successful individuals in my work have demonstrated that they have *learned* to be the way they are. Healthy, contented, and successful, they came from the same kind of backgrounds as others who have become excessively preoccupied with material success and often succumb to illness and premature mortality. They have learned through trial and error, using flexibility, creativity, and growing competence and self-confidence, to become increasingly unshakable in their sense of direction and purpose.

As a former vice president of the Bank of California, the author of *The Seven Laws of Money*, and president of the Glide Foundation in San Francisco, Michael Phillips easily qualifies as an expert on the relationship between financial success and personal fulfillment. Striving to bring these two qualities into balance in his own life, he took an assessment of how he was living and decided to make a major change. Although he was not a participant in my current study, his independent statements are strikingly parallel and confirming. At the pinnacle of his banking career Phillips quit his position as one of the country's youngest vice presidents of a major bank. He had realized that his pursuit of money as a way of buying freedom and security was a self-defeating process. Instead he chose to lead a simpler lifestyle following the Buddhist principle of "right livelihood." Phillips told me, "Quitting the banking business was just the final step of a long process that began when one of my clients—who knew what I needed better than I myself did—sent me away on a cruise ship. I was thirty one years old, and I'd never had a vacation in my life. I was nervous, tense, and stressed—a typical superachiever. I'd never in my life been able to just sit still and do nothing. . . . Finally I was faced with the choice between going insane and just sitting in a deck chair and looking out at the ocean for several days straight."

On that deck chair in the middle of the ocean Phillips had the experience, albeit in splendid surroundings, of the enforced solitude that patients undergo while recovering in a hospital or during a long sick leave at home. At times like these an individual has the opportunity to consider the deeper purpose of life, a chance to take advantage of a breakdown and discover a breakthrough. Phillips realized, "It came down to the things *everybody* wants—freedom, respect, health, family security, and security in old age. I had been thinking that money would help me get these things. In fact, it was keeping me from getting them. What I was getting were hemorrhoids and stress ulcers." During the cruise Phillips made a significant decision: "I decided the best thing I could do was to start right now to do the things I really loved and to spend as much time as I could with the people I really cared about. Of course a person wouldn't necessarily have to quit his job to do that. He or she could just begin to realize that they were not working primarily for money and make decisions accordingly."

As a former banker, Phillips was not about to fulfill the naive and misdirected cliché of being poor but happy. He realized, like many other individuals in this book, that you can do what you want and get paid for it. Of course along the way there are risks, long hours, gnawing self-doubts, and lack of security. But to many people it is well worth it if the result is personal freedom and financial success. The daring composer John Cage was an inspiration for Phillips. Cage's early experiments with sound (nuts and bolts between piano strings, and the like) led to his broad influence in the world of avant-garde music and art.

From his present point of view Phillips sees money in a new light.

"I think our obsession with money verges on making it a religion. In the minds of many, money equals happiness, security, respect, and freedom, the very same things religions offer. I think that if people really believed you could take your money with you, the religion of money would compete successfully with Christianity."

This idea that an excessively irrational preoccupation with money in the United States is impeding rather than enhancing happiness was mentioned by most of the participants in my research. None of them would deny the importance of adequate income or divest themselves of what they had worked hard to earn, but all were convinced that more is not necessarily better. Cynics might sneer that it is easy for these successful individuals to make such pronouncements because they already have substantial incomes. Quite the opposite is true. The majority live in voluntary simplicity, well within or even below their means. In the final analysis these individuals could have easily chosen to spend their energies making more and more money, accumulating more material possessions, and aggregating the power and influence that even moderate wealth engenders. Examples of such unbridled acquisition are certainly an integral part of the American dream, from Horatio Alger to the rise and fall of the silver-baron Hunt brothers. At some point a choice must be made, and for many individuals the road less traveled has led to a fulfilling destination.

SOUND MIND, SOUND BODY

Good physical and emotional health are crucial components of optimal health. But for the Sound Mind–Sound Body participants, good health is only a vehicle that allows them to function to their fullest potential in the many endeavors of their lives. What these people are interested in is running their businesses, devoting themselves to their families, or pursuing other activities that are particularly rewarding to them. When they have endured a health crisis, it has often led them to think about what was really important in their lives and to make some radical changes.

There is no denying that some people have paid a price for the pressures of their jobs. In the early eighties the tragic suicide of Alvin Feldman, fifty-three-year-old president of Continental Airlines, following a long and bitter corporate takeover battle, a hijacking attempt, and his wife's death from cancer, illustrates the terrible toll that escalating stress can take on people living and working under unrelenting demands. Researchers studying the many instances of fatal heart attacks among relatively young, successful men and women have dubbed them examples of "unconscious suicide." Prosperous people in ill health have been a ubiquitous topic in business literature as well as popular fiction, a classic being F. Scott Fitzgerald's *The Great Gatsby*. Perhaps the theme owes part of its appeal to the all-too-common human tendency to knock the success of prominent people. There is a certain satisfaction in believing that those in positions of power are not really happy and healthy after all.

However, actual statistics quickly dispel that myth. Highly successful individuals are actually healthier than most other people. One of the earliest major studies on the subject was conducted in 1969 by Lawrence E. Hinkle, Jr., of the Cornell University Medical College. After examining the records of 270,000 employees of Bell Telephone, he determined that executives had fewer heart attacks than blue-collar workers. A 1974 study by the Metropolitan Life Insurance Company found that among 1,078 corporate executives from Fortune 500 companies, the mortality rate was only 63 percent of that among their contemporaries in the general population. In an ambitious long-range study begun in 1955, Charles Thompson has been tracking the health histories of some 15,000 executives from twenty of the largest Chicago-based companies. He has found their incidence of heart disease and their mortality rate to be surprisingly lower than the norm, especially among the top executives who, even though they are generally older, appear to be in better health than the middle managers. The health and longevity of these top executives may be due in part to their using preventive measures such as exercise, weight control, and reduction of cholesterol levels. It may also come from the basic physical and emotional fitness they must have had in order to occupy positions of responsibility in the first place. However, it is equally clear that in their positions as top executives many of these individuals are able to fulfill their sense of purpose, which may indeed contribute to the phenomenon of their healthier, longer lives.

Top executives can certainly attain a great deal of fulfillment from their jobs. But all too often their sense of purpose becomes clouded and their health becomes threatened as they are swept up in the pressures and responsibilities inherent in the nature of their positions. That is when one must take stock of a situation and decide to make a lifestyle change. When a person begins to adhere to a sense of purpose every day—every moment—mind and body will interact in such a way that there will be a subtle but profound positive influence upon health.

In the Sound Mind–Sound Body interviews, there was one individual who vividly recounted how he learned to integrate this ongoing process into his life. Anthony S. Tiano, president and CEO of KQED, San Francisco's public broadcast television station, described a crystal-clear scenario of how stress can be managed effectively by following a sense of purpose and paying attention to daily circumstances. After earning the obligatory M.B.A., Tiano spent over twenty years in various aspects of mass communications, ranging from radio and television spot sales to on-air presentations, production, direction, publishing, and management. He has worked to build a diversified communications company that provides some of the most extensive public media service in the United States today. With reductions in government support to public television, Tiano has succeeded in creating a successful mix of commercial and noncommercial programming. He believes this blend represents a model for leadership in the future of mass communications in a society that puts a premium on the free press.

Throughout Tiano's work there has been an overriding vision: "We often forget what an extraordinary right we have in the free expression atmosphere of the United States. I am still living with the wonder that I first felt in my high school civics class: we have a basic structure in our country which honors individuals' rights over government, and the opportunity to fulfill individuals' expectations is wonderful. Foreign travel reinforces this for me. . . . Once I was in Turkey when a Russian trawler ran aground. When I asked one of the Istanbul reporters about a story on the incident, he said, 'Don't worry, the government will tell us what we should know about it!' That made me see how much we take for granted." Out of his deep respect for the individual freedoms guaranteed under a democratic government, Tiano sees his role as president of a major PBS television station to be his way of ensuring and participating in the freedom of the press.

It might seem that a man of such outstanding professional qualifications and high ideals could carry on unscathed by the pressures of his executive position. In general Tiano has, but he did have a close call. In 1981 he returned from a two-week business trip with an exhausting schedule covering the major Eastern seaboard cities. His recollection of that trip was that there were "too many late-night rich dinners with people I did not know and in some cases did not like. Too much drinking and too many cigarettes—both of which left me with a hangover. Generally, by the time I got on the flight at Kennedy to come home, I was feeling anxious, pressured, and just plain worn out." And the red-eye flight on Sunday evening was not the end of Tiano's demanding schedule. That next Monday morning he had an important meeting with his board of directors. At that time the board and chairman were against his policies, a boycott was pending by several community groups, and there was considerable conflict among board members themselves, who were fragmented into special interest groups vying for disproportionate control over the programming of San Francisco's community television station.

During the meeting Tiano realized not only that he was hung over and jet-lagged, and disoriented from the previous night, but that he was very tired and couldn't concentrate. Afterward he took a good look at himself: he was chronically fatigued, depressed, irritable, overweight, and smoking and drinking too much. He was simply not enjoying his life, nor was he performing very well in the profession he loved. Then he made the decision to begin a regimen of physical exercise as his starting point for an overall health improvement program. Once he began regular exercise, he found that he had more energy; the exercise served as fuel that gave him a performance edge. Following his daily workout of aerobics and free weights, he found himself "more charged-up at the office. . . . Facts seem to stick better in my mind, and yet I am able to see the big picture. Exercise seems to break the worry circle for me, and I get so much done once I get to the office. My time in the gym is not time wasted because I seem to work so much more efficiently and effortlessly once I get here." With his usual refreshing honesty, he added, "You know, I really hate it when I am doing the workout—the sweat, the pain, the grunting and groaning—but I guess I'm really addicted to the feeling of being on top of things afterwards. . . . Now I realize I cannot afford to be in poor health, because my job is even more demanding now than when I started exercising six years ago!"

From this starting point with exercise Tiano was then able to stop smoking, reduce his "excessive" drinking, which he had not even realized had "gotten out of control," and stop keeping late social hours. Among the other changes he made was a firm decision never to take another red-eye flight. He and his wife also decided to alter their diets, eating less red meat and paying closer attention to their weight. One benefit of exercising that delights Tiano and many other people with a regular exercise program is that they can actually eat a great deal while staying trim.

Having made these major lifestyle changes, not only is he in much better health, but he also experiences an enhanced satisfaction with his life. He enjoys nearly everything he does. His activities no longer feel hollow and meaningless, and he doesn't feel constantly stressed. He is sharper and enjoys his business meetings. By giving himself permission to cut back on his social commitments, a tough decision for an executive whose main activity is socializing, he is now able to choose only the functions he really wants to attend.

Acting out of a deep sense of purpose and implementing real change in his immediate life, Tiano rediscovered the enthusiasm he had once had for the freedom of the press and his vital role in the business of communication. Perhaps the greatest benefit he derived from reevaluating personal health practices and professional performance was a restored outlook on life. An admitted Type A, he now characterizes his psychological orientation as "Zenlike. . . . I can see clearly what is and is not important in my life and in my work, and I see events in a long-range context. One thing I do now is to reflect back and ask myself, What was consuming all my time and attention one month ago . . . or one year ago? What was it? At the time it seemed like the most important thing in the world, and usually I can't even remember what it was!" With his new orientation, Tiano has developed a new management style that is consistent with his lifelong values and is infused with a new creativity.

He reflects philosophically about learning to respect his own process of aging and maturing. Rather than denying that reality by trying to outperform the younger executives at KQED, Tiano realizes that "I'm not necessarily going to feel great every day or make the best decisions all the time, but I do find myself in more crisis situations saying, 'I've been here before, and I handled it then, and I can handle it again.' . . . As I get older, I've had to become more efficient at management. With my involvement in the complexities of television, from fund-raising to cameras to lighting, I am trying to do my one thousand daily tasks just one percent better. At the same time I realize that I am never going to be good enough. . . . What keeps me going is the high from those fleeting moments of creativity where everything goes elegantly and beautifully right."

From a relatively undramatic moment of insight about his personal well-being, Tiano has reinstated a sense of purpose in his life and acted with courage to manage his stress and to implement the lifestyle changes that permit him to enjoy true health and success. At KQED he has developed numerous management practices that now pervade the work of other executives at the station. This "passing" of effective management styles is now becoming a common practice in companies around the world, fashioning a new and more viable corporate culture.

BETWEEN MIND AND BODY

To what extent do positive emotions and a sense of purpose affect mental and physical health? Research to date confirms the idea that attitudes, emotions, and behaviors do influence health, but the majority of the studies have focused solely on the negative emotions and effects. As mind-body researchers have been giving more attention to the effects of positive emotions and attitudes, possibly the most significant finding has been that individuals can actually choose the way they think. As we have seen from the Sound Mind–Sound Body interviews, these prominent individuals put the utmost value on following their sense of purpose, which engenders in them a powerful reason to think positively and to find their own ways to manage stress and get on with life. The following discussion of scientific findings will provide further evidence that these individuals have chosen optimally healthy ways to live.

In 1979 a study by the psychiatrist Dr. George Vaillant at Dartmouth Medical School reported that people with good mental health had a lower probability of becoming chronically ill or dying than those with a history of psychiatric problems. This finding held true even when both groups were parallel in terms of alcohol use, tobacco use, obesity, and ancestral longevity. Later investigations have demonstrated that even subtle psychological trouble can have a profound impact on the onset and outcome of disease.

Earlier the classic study by Dr. Caroline Bedell Thomas and her colleagues at the Johns Hopkins University School of Medicine showed that healthy adults appeared to have had positive relations with their parents during childhood, as well as strong self-esteem, an optimistic outlook, a relative lack of depression, and a marked ability to cope with stress. In contrast, the subjects in her study who had the opposite characteristics, and thus were judged to be of poor psychological health, had three to four times the cancer risk.

One deceptively simple study conducted in 1991 generated an inordinate amount of interest, if not controversy. A research team headed by Dr. Sheldon Cohen at the University of Pittsburgh School of Medicine published a study in the *New England Journal of Medicine* that proved a link between psychological stress and increased susceptibility to the common cold. After completing a questionnaire to assess their stress levels, 394 healthy men and women aged eighteen to fifty-four were given nasal drops containing one of five respiratory viruses. Placebo drops were given to twenty-six participants. Everyone was quarantined and monitored for two days before and seven days after the drops. Rates of infection ranged from 74 to 90 percent, while the occurrence of actual colds was much lower, at 27 to 47 percent. It was found that the higher the levels of psychological stress, the higher the rate of infection and clinical colds. This is one of the best studies to date indicating that stress suppresses the immune system.

Throughout these studies negative psychological and emotional attitudes and characteristics were shown to be detrimental to the immune system. But when will positive characteristics be seen as equally instrumental in benefiting human immunity and as being the basis for optimal health? This is ultimately the most challenging, intriguing, and significant question. Right now our knowledge about disease is infinitely greater than our understanding of health itself. The greatest potential for major discoveries in mind-body research will be in the attempts to restore, stabilize, or enhance optimal states of health and well-being.

Can conscious, deliberate choices and practices directly enhance immune function, thus preventing the onset or altering the course of disease? There are several behavioral interventions used today that imply, but do not prove, such an influence: clinical biofeedback, meditation, autogenic training, Jacobson's progressive relaxation, hypnosis, general relaxation, the relaxation response, behavior modification, and visualization techniques. Just as stress and the immune responses it causes cannot be simplistically reduced to a monolithic theory, it is equally ludicrous to consider such behavioral interventions, in all their subtleties and complexities, to be interchangeable. In the future the efficacy of behavioral interventions will be enhanced by a precise pairing of an individual diagnosis with a specific intervention. Because mind-body interactions are so complex, these behavioral techniques will be coupled with attention to such other dimensions as diet, exercise, social support, smoking cessation, cancer risk reduction, and the physical environment.

Among the several inroads that have been made into this area, stress management strategies and visualization techniques have shown positive immunological consequences. In a study by Dr. Nicholas Hall, people under hypnosis visualized their white blood cells as sharks attacking the germs in their body. Younger people and those who were easily hypnotized had a better response to this technique in general. In a study of geriatric patients, Dr. Janice Kiecolt-Glaser and her colleagues found that when the patients were taught relaxation and guided imagery techniques, their white blood cell activity went up and their antibodies to the herpes simplex virus went down, indicating better control of the virus by the immune system. Recently several clinicians have speculated that such interventions may prevent or at least delay the progression of AIDS in patients who have tested positive for the HIV virus.

In 1989 a landmark study by the psychiatrist Dr. David Spiegel at the Stanford University School of Medicine showed that group psychotherapy for women following treatment for breast cancer improved the quality of their lives and doubled their life expectancies. Like the British study mentioned earlier in which a "fighting spirit" helped women with early breast cancer, other studies have found that women who felt highly distressed, apathetic, and helpless were less successful in surviving the disease. Writing a 1991 influential annotated bibliography on the psychosocial aspects of cancer in *Current Opinion in Psychiatry*, Spiegel cites and analyzes the forty-two primary studies in this area. Overall, he concluded, "Recent studies suggest that psychosocial intervention may extend survival time among cancer patients." However, Spiegel and other responsible clinicians are quick to point out that their findings do not provide any specific answers for cancer patients. They note with guarded optimism that such findings merit serious consideration but caution that any definitive conclusion at this time is premature.

One of the most intriguing studies in the mind-body area was conducted by researchers at the University of Arkansas College of Medicine and reported in the *Annals of Internal Medicine*. Working with a thirty-nine-year-old woman who was an experienced meditator, they found that she was able voluntarily to inhibit her immune reaction to the chickenpox virus, and then return her reaction back to normal. This study is one of the most innovative research models to indicate that a practiced individual can regulate a specific immune response through meditation.

In 1991 the clinical psychologist Dr. John Schneider and his colleagues at Michigan State University reported an interesting study involving a group of students who were given a two-hour training session in guided visualization. The imagery sessions were focused specifically on teaching subjects to influence their own neutrophils, a particular type of white blood cell that enhances immunity. After the training the students outperformed all other groups in raising the adherence or "stickiness" level of their neutrophils through visualization. Greater adherence by neutrophils is thought to be linked to a superior ability to aid immune functions. Some individuals actually decreased the cell count of neutrophils by up to 60 percent, as well as decreasing their adherence levels. The result indicates both the potential power and the danger of the misguided use of mind-body techniques. In a subsequent study individuals were able to maintain a constant neutrophil level and increase adherence; no group was actually able to raise the neutrophil count. These studies confirm my observation that we do not enhance immune functions but stabilize them and allow them to function optimally.

Further analysis revealed that the poorest results were obtained by individuals who saw their minds as controlling their bodies, while the best results were seen in individuals who perceived themselves as being in partnership with their bodies and the neutrophils. Overall, the individuals who did best made less of a conscious effort and took a healthier, more playful approach to the visualizations.

In a related, though smaller study some participants were able consciously to increase or decrease the activity of their T-helper and suppressor cells, which are key cells of the immune system. The researchers concluded, generally, that the individuals who performed best were those who actually believed in their ability to influence their immune system or had considerable knowledge about the actual functions of the cells. They also determined that individuals needed to be trained in the use of a visualization technique that was stress-free and positive. These are important, albeit preliminary, findings, since they demonstrate that conscious visualizations focused on specific cells within the immune system can have predictable and measurable outcomes. From a purely scientific perspective the fact that these findings are highly specific and verifiable represents a very significant step forward in understanding the mind-body system in all its wonder and complexity.

These research designs and findings are consistent with the biofeedback studies I conducted with Dr. Joe Kamiya and Dr. Erik Peper back in the early 1970s at the University of California School of Medicine in San Francisco. In that research we provided the first unequivocal evidence that adept meditators could voluntarily control pain, bleeding, and infection from self-inflicted puncture wounds. It is essential to work with individuals who are practiced in mind-body techniques rather than relying on large numbers of inexperienced subjects. By studying skilled individuals who can alter their neuropsychological and immunological functions at will, we can learn how to teach others therapeutically to increase or decrease their immune response, depending on what is required in a particular disease. Development of such techniques, used in combination with basic preventive measures, could open up exciting possibilities for noninvasive and nontoxic adjuncts to traditional medical care.

An interesting study involving the effects of exposure to humanistic films on the immune system was conducted by David McClelland when he was at Harvard University. McClelland had a group of students watch a film about Mother Teresa's work caring for the sick and poor in Calcutta, India. After seeing the film, the students showed increased levels of serum immunoglobulin A (IgA), which is found in saliva, regardless of whether they outwardly approved of her work or not. It has been argued that salivary production is related to upper respiratory tract infections, but the actual clinical significance of this immune system variability is uncertain. Such studies show that information and suggestions that enter a person's psychological awareness on an unconscious level can enhance immune function regardless of whether the person is outwardly aware of an effect or emotional reaction.

All of the above studies have yielded valuable information on the complex connections between the human mind and body. Overall, it seems that research needs to take a broader approach. Since an individual's inner experiences can be discovered through structured interviews, studies should incorporate the individual's attitudes, beliefs, and personal strategies into their research. Granted, the task of assessing a person's pattern of dealing with the world is far from easy, but only by giving primacy to these strategies inside the individual mind can we understand and take advantage of the potential health benefits that lie therein.

Because the biochemistry behind mind-body interactions is so fascinating, particularly with regard to the positive emotions, there is concern that inquiry into this complex system may deteriorate into another mechanistic, reductionist enterprise. In pursuing how consciousness and the body interact, in discovering how emotions affect immune system cells, and in documenting dramatic recoveries from chronic disease, we may find knowledge of even greater importance eluding us. My interviews with the remarkable individuals in the Sound Mind–Sound Body study revealed that a sense of purpose, and the personal discipline to keep it in focus, were the main elements in their strategies for optimal health. They do not ask themselves so much how to live, as why.

CHAPTER FIVE

Friends Can Be Good Medicine

As the son of Russian-Polish immigrants, film producer Saul Zaentz grew up hearing stories of his Russian Cossack ancestors straddling rearing horses and brandishing razor-edged swords. As a teenager growing up in Newark, New Jersey, Zaentz spent most of his teenage years hanging out on the corner of Myrtle and Monroe streets with a few boys who lived in the neighborhood. And for over a decade now the Myrtle and Monroe guys have still gathered every three or four years to revitalize their friendships.

Like so many of the Sound Mind–Sound Body participants, Saul Zaentz has very strong feelings about how his friends and family have affected his life. No matter how great the moments of fame, or how bitter the frustration of failure, he frequently recalled how his social support systems helped him through life.

As I chatted with Hemingway look-alike Zaentz about his early years at the corner of Myrtle and Monroe, he told me that he cherishes his childhood chums more than the Oscar he was awarded for producing *One Flew over the Cuckoo's Nest*. "When I mentioned the boys of Myrtle and Monroe during my acceptance speech for the Oscar, I had no idea how much it would mean to them. Some of the guys who come back for the reunion are doctors and lawyers . . . some fly in from Miami, Chicago, and Paris, but others just walk across the same streets where we played as kids. They could have been anything they wanted to be or lived anywhere in the world, but they chose a different path. They are *not* living the lives of 'quiet desperation'; they are in fact very fulfilled by their families and friends. Some may have already reached the highest level they could attain in their professional lives, but often there's more pride, more love, and more integrity in these simple homes than in the million-dollar houses in the hills. At our reunions we get back in touch with each other and appreciate the differences in our lives by sharing stories and memories. It's like we are brothers, an extended family of some kind. That's what it is—a real family."

Whether their close relationship is with a group of friends, one friend or spouse, or even a pet, the other individuals in my study expressed like Zaentz an unswerving commitment to relating fully to others. Not one person said they suffer from being "lonely at the top"; it seems they have all retained an acute sense of what is most important to them and are unwilling to sacrifice their personal relationships for fame or fortune. It is probable that social support that stems from these close relationships contributed to their optimal health, yet this correlation clashes head-on with our society's single greatest and most insidious health misconception: that it occurs in isolation. Some people truly believe that they will become healthy by following perfunctory guidelines for diet, exercise, rest, and stress management, but as important as these factors are, even the full combination doesn't add up to optimal health. Of course the go-it-alone approach to health fits the modern American ethic of individualism perfectly and has incited our narcissistic preoccupation with looking young, thin, and beautiful. Not only does this mind-set reflect our culture's growing abdication of social responsibility and lack of compassion for others, but it is also a dead-end street—even for the individual.

There is mounting research that shows just how misdirected this individualistic approach to health really is. Until recently it was assumed that all persons were equally susceptible to illness, depending on a combination of traditional risk factors, like smoking and obesity, and stressful life events. But we are now discovering that many people pass through periods of intense stress and exposure to health hazards and remain untouched by illness. Like the groundbreaking studies conducted by Kobasa (chapter 3), which identified commitment and control as antidotes to stress, other studies have looked at additional resistance resources, such as social support, which have proven effective in buffering or eliminating the harmful effects of stress.

A sense of belonging and connection to other people appears to be a basic human need—as basic as food and shelter. In fact, social support may be one of the critical elements distinguishing those who remain healthy from those who become ill. It helps to prevent illness by maintaining homeostasis—our physical and mental equilibrium— and thereby protecting the immune system. Given the links between psychological, neurological, and immune responses, it is becoming increasingly clear that the presence or absence of social support has a profound influence on health and illness. But how can negative environmental stressors and positive psychosocial support systems directly affect the mind-body network? Research into this vital question is illuminating specific linkages between the mind-body system and physical and social environments.

Benefits of social support have been researched and documented thoroughly. Positive associations, such as a supportive community and close friends or family, have been linked to better health and therefore lower absenteeism from work, lower incidence of cancer, reduced risk and incidence of heart disease, and fewer and shorter hospital stays. In a study that followed sixteen families for one year, those that were closer knit had fewer cases of streptococcal infection. When an entire West Point cadet class was studied for over four years, those with closer interpersonal ties showed less susceptibility to the Epstein-Barr virus.

Conversely, the lack of social stability, often termed *social marginality*, has been linked to a variety of behavioral, physical, and psychological illnesses, including arthritis, tuberculosis, hypertension, schizophrenia, depression, coronary disease, as well as to higher general mortality rates. There are also appear to be negative physical effects stemming from the sudden loss of close ties. In a study of the connection between bereavement and death caused by heart attack, the rate of mortality was substantially higher for recently widowed spouses, particularly men. Research has also shown that, in general, married people are healthier than single people, and that divorce and marital difficulties can cause immune dysfunction.

Several extensive studies have come to be considered classics in this field of research, and some of the most compelling findings concern heart disease, cancer, and overall mortality. In a pioneering study conducted in Alameda County, California, researchers considered the presence or absence of social support as independent risk factors. After evaluating 6,928 men and women living in the neighboring cities of Berkeley and Oakland, they found that seven simple factors—including social support—exerted a powerful influence upon both the health and longevity of the Alameda residents. Building on the Alameda County study, Dr. James S. House and his colleagues at the University of Michigan conducted a study in Tecumseh, Michigan. Beginning in 1967, Dr. House and his associates gave psychological interviews and physical examinations to 2,754 adults from the ages of thirty-five to sixty-nine. The researchers traced these participants for ten to twelve years in order to determine their risk of death during that period. Along with all of the usual risk factors— blood pressure, age, cholesterol, lung capacity, heart rate patterns, smoking and so forth—they also recorded the individuals' social relations. What they found was that independent of all of the traditional risks, the presence or absence of social support exerted a powerful influence on death rates. Men who had weak social ties had a death rate two to three times higher than those with strong ties; for socially marginal women, the death rate was one and a half to two times higher. Two similar studies were conducted in Scandinavia, both yielding findings parallel to the U.S. studies. In eastern Finland the far-reaching North Karelia study followed 13,301 men and women, and in Stockholm, Sweden, 150 middle-aged men were observed for ten years. Again social isolation was found to be one of the best predictors of mortality. Looking for the basic mechanism by which social isolation might induce heart attacks, Dr. T. E. Seeman and Dr. Leonard Syme examined 119 men and 40 women who were undergoing coronary angiography (an X-ray of the blood vessels). As they reported in 1987 in *Psychosomatic Medicine*, the more people felt "loved and supported," the less evidence there was of coronary atherosclerosis. Once again, this result was determined to be independent of all other risk factors.

Although the presence or absence of social support is finally gaining recognition as a major contributing factor to optimal health, it was recognized decades ago by the pioneering physician Dr. Stewart Wolff. Wolff was one of the first researchers to document the finding, now often cited, that coherent social support is a major factor in individual health on a par with the more commonly accepted biological risk factors of blood pressure, cholesterol, bacterial and viral exposure, and aging itself. His seminal research discovered that the Italian immigrant community of Rosetto, Pennsylvania, had an unusually low incidence of heart disease despite the fact that the residents of Rosetto all had the comparable risk factors common to four adjacent communities. Apparently, the lower incidence was due to greater social support. Much to Dr. Wolff's disappointment, he later found that the Italians in Rosetto experienced gradual, inexorable, and negative changes in the intergenerational bonds of social support.

Members of the nuclear families began to drift apart, young people left the town seeking better employment opportunities, and the actual physical aspect of the town was transformed from neighborhoods of houses in friendly proximity to the manicured anonymity of suburbia. Within a few short years Wolff determined that the rate of heart disease in this population was rising simultaneously with the increasing fragmentation of their community.

Most recently Dr. Wolff presented his findings to a small annual invitational symposium in Montreux, Switzerland, which is organized by Dr. Paul Rosch, president of the American Institute of Stress, and includes international participants like Dr. Ray Rosenman, codiscoverer of Type A behavior and coauthor of the classic *Type A Behavior and Your Heart*; Dr. Richard Rahe, codeveloper of the Holmes-Rahe stress assessment; Dr. Lennart Levi with his pioneering work site research from the Karolinska Institute in Stockholm, Sweden; as well as senior researchers and clinicians from Japan, the former Soviet Union, and Africa. It was during the Montreux meetings of February 1993 that Dr. Wolff presented his most disturbing research to date. He reported that the incidence of all forms of heart disease and deaths from heart disease in Rosetto, Pennsylvania, is now equal to the rates in the four surrounding communities as well as in the United States at large. This increase in disease and death is despite an actual *reduction* in the known risk factors among the people of Rosetto. In effect, the now-disintegrated social support network appears to have contributed an independent positive influence in the past that perhaps outweighed the more commonly acknowledged biological risk factors. That protective influence of family, close relationships, and all that such values reflect, has been strained to the breaking point, with dire consequences for both individuals and their community.

From these and many other studies, it is clear that even the most dogmatic fixation on the traditional risk factors of disease is futile without looking beyond our biological boundaries and considering the quality of our connections to other people. Yet while there is fairly strong evidence for an association between social support and health, as well as a link between the lack of support and mortality, there is, as yet, no absolute evidence of causality. We cannot yet say that social support actually causes better immune function or that its absence can be considered a direct cause of death.

It is essential to cite such caveats and limitations for any single variable, be it psychosocial or biological, as all too often we embrace a newly discovered factor too enthusiastically and too quickly, which leads to unrealistic expectations, followed by disillusionment, cynicism, or even a total dismissal of the variable in question. This all-or-nothing cycle has held true for such "breakthrough" discoveries as interferon, for numerous innovative pharmacologicals and surgical procedures, as well as for supposedly new risk factors and their attendant interventions.

Therefore, it is imperative to exercise caution with regard to both the benefits of social support and the detriments of its absence. The leading researcher Dr. Leonard I. Perlin advocates a balanced perspective when considering the significance of social support. "Any set of circumstances," he says, "that promises to contribute to the prevention or alleviation of suffering or distress certainly merits close scrutiny. Yet the almost eruptive upsurge of research into social supports makes it imperative that we pause and take stock of what they can and cannot do and of the circumstances that regulate their influences on behavior and well-being. Clearly, we need substantial longitudinal studies linking social support, stress and coping measures, immunological parameters, subsequent health indicators, and control groups to clarify what appears to be an increasingly important insight into the complex interaction between mind, body, and the social as well as physical ecology."

Despite the fact that much empirical research is necessary to delineate further the relationship between stress, risk factors, social relationships, and health, we know enough about the benefits of social support to use this knowledge in assisting those who are most at risk of succumbing to illness. We should turn our attention toward designing preventive intervention programs—in both the community and the work site—that incorporate social support into programs to reduce those stressors that cause ill health. If we integrate social support systems into all aspects of daily life—from family gatherings and neighborhood get-togethers to mutual aid groups and career networking clubs—we will be weaving preventive medicine right into the fabric of our daily lives.

SHOWER THE PEOPLE YOU LOVE WITH LOVE

Every individual in my study talked about their relationships with other people—family, friends, and business partners—as an absolutely vital part of their lives. Each participant saw these connections as contributing to their self-fulfillment, career success, health, and to that greater sense of purpose that moved them to help others.

No matter how tough the pressures and demands of his acting career, Dennis Weaver has remained true to his family-oriented values. He explained, "Families are so valuable because they provide our first opportunity to expand our consciousness beyond ourselves. Then, once we really understand the value of sharing, the value of doing something together, the value of wholeness in the family, that begins to translate to the community, the nation, and the world.

"Our first movement into the outside world is toward our own family. We are all self-centered, and we all want to be happy individually. But we learn through the family that we can't be happy individually unless we share our happiness with others."

These words are not mere philosophical rhetoric but a reflection of Weaver's daily life and especially his family. When I congratulated him on his successful marriage of forty-five years, he was quick to add, "I can't say that we didn't go over a few bumps in the beginning. We certainly had our moments." But just as quickly he commented on his family's togetherness. "A couple of years ago my wife and I and our three sons formed a musical act so we could spend more time together. Both Robby, my middle son, and Rusty, my youngest, are musically talented. So is my wife. I'm not really musically inclined, so for me it has been very exciting to learn that you can do anything if you put your mind to it, devote enough time to it, and do so in the right environment. My family's musical talent encouraged me to write a lot of songs, which we've used in our act. We've played at rodeos and fairs—and even the Shrine and Long Beach auditoriums. It's a lot of fun and a great creative experience, but most of all it's great because we do it as a family."

The majority of the participants in my research reported that they derived their social support from their immediate family or one or two close friends. Even Gordon Getty, known to the world at large as the billionaire son of J. Paul Getty, attributes much of his success as both a businessman and a musical composer to his wife, Ann. In 1985 he engineered the largest corporate transfer in history with the Getty Oil takeover of Pennzoil, which ultimately sent Texaco into bankruptcy. While financial analysts praised Getty's feat, and he emerged in the press as a true corporate magnate, he shrugs off those accolades. More comfortable as a composer, he has received widespread acclaim for two of his major works: an opera entitled *Plump Jack*, adapted from Shakespeare's *Henry IV* and *Henry V*, and a song cycle called *The White Election*, inspired by Emily Dickinson's poetry.

On the surface Ann and Gordon Getty are a study in complementary contrasts. She is an outgoing Democrat, involved in community and social affairs, who exudes a joie de vivre that is downright contagious. By his own description, Getty, a Republican, is more of a "stick-in-the-mud" who would rather work on his music than attend a social event. Despite these differences, their marriage of more than twenty-five years, during which they have raised four children, is marked by mutual respect and love.

Getty was quick to communicate how important his family is to him and how supportive Ann is of both his business endeavors and his music. "When Ann makes a comment, I listen. She's very supportive, but she's also realistic. What's most important in our relationship, though, is that we share a love for our family and our children." When I asked what kind of legacy he would like to leave for his children, he responded, "Apart from the genetic legacy, I'd like them to be as proud of their father as I am of mine. I'd also like to leave them with a feeling of family solidarity. Family is very important to me."

Despite all the scientific unknowns surrounding the topic of social support, Getty's last statement sums up perfectly the unequivocal feelings all the Sound Mind–Sound Body participants expressed about their families, spouses, and friends.

Apple Computer's John Sculley has successfully managed to glean personal support from both his family and his career. Although he admitted in our interview that his position at Apple could consume "every minute of every day forever," he stated emphatically, "Family is a very big part of my life." He then went on to explain the challenge he faced being a young father and a high-powered executive with Pepsico. "I got married young, had two children, and then got divorced. I made an arrangement with Pepsi that no matter where I was in the world, every third week I would go and visit my kids in Los Angeles. In those days I was all over South America, Central America, and Mexico, so I would fly just to spend eight or nine hours with my kids. Then I would turn around and go back. Even coming from Japan or Europe, every third week I was always there for my children, knowing that if I didn't have a relationship with them when they were young, we would never have a relationship when they were older. That was a hard way to raise a family.

"Now my free time is spent almost entirely with my family. My wife is very much into nature and animals, so we have a ranch. We're not into a lot of social stuff. We tend to lead a very low-key life, but it's very fulfilling." To complement the closeness he enjoys with his second wife and his family, Sculley has a few supportive friends, which he made through his profession. "There are some people I especially admire," he reflected. "I may not spend a lot of time with them, but it's quality time. Laurance Rockefeller is one of them. I think he is the world's first venture capitalist, since he realized long before anyone else that the way to have an impact on the world was to invest his wealth in things that would make a difference in the future. Through VENROCK, the Rockefeller venture capital arm, he started with Eastern Airlines. Now he has helped launch biotechnology companies, computer firms, all kinds of things. But you never hear about his involvement in these projects. He is the quiet brother, but I think he is the most interesting. He's also very spiritual and cares a great deal about the environment. I guess I admire those people who are relatively quiet about their accomplishments and who look at the world through an intellectual lens and try to understand the meaning of things."

Even Charles Darwin, though obviously *not* a Sound Mind–Sound Body participant, mused about the effects of social support in recounting a memory his father had: "My father told me of a careful observer, who certainly had heart disease and died from it, and who positively stated that his pulse was habitually irregular to an extreme degree. Yet to his great disappointment, it invariably became regular as soon as my father entered the room."

In their article in *Science* magazine entitled "Social Relationships and Health," Dr. James S. House and his colleagues at the University of Michigan provided an insightful overview of the ways in which social support can affect an individual's health. "Just as we discover the importance of social relationships for health and we see an increasing need for them, their prevalence and availability may be declining. Changes in other risk factors (for example, the decline in smoking) and improvements in medical technology are still producing overall improvements in health and longevity, but the improvements might be even greater if the quantity and quality of social relationships were also improving." House went on to point out that more people in the United States and most other modern nations now tend to live alone, remain unmarried longer, have longer life expectancies (and thus more years alone after the death of a spouse), and have fewer (or no) children to visit or care for them. It is indeed ironic that just as research is confirming the importance of social support, the very ties that bind people together are becoming increasingly frayed or nonexistent.

Findings like these call for a redefinition of our concept of health within a much broader context. Truly to understand optimal health, we must consider the many ways in which individuals are linked—with their spouses, families, and friends, as well as with their emotional and physical environments.

Throughout my interviews I found that the most important form of social support was the relationship between spouses or between any two people who share their greatest intimacies with each other. My conversation with Dr. Dorothea R. Johnson was particularly enlightening on the subject of mutual support between husband and wife. Dr. Johnson began her career in occupational medicine with AT&T in 1957. Today, as the company's vice president for health affairs, she is responsible for developing health policy and practices that affect more than 300,000 employees, their dependents, and retirees, at a budget of over $1 billion a year. Considered one of the founders of the field of health promotion and disease prevention in the workplace, she is recognized as an international authority, and her pioneering programs, designed to assist employees and their families in "achieving and maintaining optimum health and performance," have touched every individual working in corporate health. With her unwavering commitment to improving the quality of life for all people, she has earned respect in the boardroom of AT&T as well as recognition from her peers, who elected her the first woman president of the American Occupational Medical Association.

Among her colleagues Dr. Johnson is known to have a ready smile, an insightful word, and an unshakably positive attitude about life. Even with the great demands of career, community, and church, Johnson is very close to her family. Her husband, Harry, is a retired clergyman, and their three adult children include a physician, a nurse educator, and an opera singer.

Johnson said lovingly of her husband, "Harry and I have been married for thirty-five years, and he's the best support I've ever had. He has always been one hundred percent supportive of me. We were married at the end of my first year in medical school, and he was in seminary at the time and working full-time in a steel mill. Even though I made more money than he did, it wasn't a problem. We share and share alike. He has a lot of interests all his own, like working with his hands and camping, but we complement each other. We talk about everything. He's always been so supportive of me.

"My kids are also a source of emotional support. We are really close and try to get together every year for a vacation. We've met at

Disney World between Christmas and New Year's ever since it opened in 1971. When the kids went away to college, they really looked forward to that every year. We spend at least a week together at the campsite in Disney World. It's a real nice, positive thing that our kids all grew up together, went to high school together, and now all come back together. Sometimes we have thirty-one people at our campsite. During that precious time, teenagers meet their cousins, and grandparents and grandchildren really get to know each other."

Whether it's an extended vacation or simply a birthday, anniversary, or holiday, the time spent together is a time for healing the self, the family, and consequently society. But social support doesn't mean that you're always on the receiving end; giving is just as important. And although some types of giving are easy and enjoyable, others can be demanding and difficult. Many of my study participants have given patiently and unselfishly to others who were in great need: a retarded child, an ailing or terminally ill relative, a friend in personal or financial jeopardy, and in four instances a severely disabled spouse.

For more than thirty years, John Tishman has compassionately cared for his wife. "She has been an invalid ever since our children left home. She has meningioma with multiple tumors in her head." Tishman's wife had four tumors removed. "Now she is brain-damaged. Altogether she has had fourteen craniotomies, and there are always more problems.

"Looking back, I realize I was never that close to my family. I have some cousins out there, a couple who are older or retired, and some younger ones, but I realize my real family, my true support system, is the family my wife and I created. Through all of this misfortune my kids and I have become closer and closer. My daughter is an artist and lives in Providence, and I'm really close with my son. Together we have been able to give each other the love and support necessary to go on, even when things seem bleak. But most important is that together we have been able to provide my wife—their mother—with the compassion and understanding that helps make her life worth living."

WORKING HEARTS

Social support is not confined to family and friends. In fact, there is some preliminary evidence that social support in the workplace may be of equal or even greater importance than support at home, since most of our waking hours are spent at work. Additionally, a great deal of the sense of personal identity, self-worth, and control is tied to career or professional status. For thirty-one of the participants in my study, business or career relationships were major sources of social support.

While they were developing the film *One Flew over the Cuckoo's Nest* in the early seventies, Saul Zaentz and his colleague Michael Douglas carried out a search for the right director. They agreed that Milos Foreman fit the bill, and ever since, Zaentz and Foreman have enjoyed an enduring friendship. Remembering when he first met Foreman, Zaentz said fondly, "We had been through a few directors and a few screenplay writers, and then we met Milos. He came out to the West Coast, and Michael and I talked with him for about four hours over dinner. He was exactly in tune with us, even though he didn't know it at the time. But that's part of Milos's courage: He'll always tell you how he thinks something should be. Where other guys' egos get in the way, what drives Milos is making the best picture. He is secure enough not to let his ego get bruised if someone disagrees with him. He's really a rarity. Especially now, after working with a few other directors, I realize how special he is."

Working together on that film, Zaentz and Foreman discovered that they shared the common vision that a film should have a strong footing in reality. Zaentz recalled from their first meetings together, "A lot of people don't see the vision behind the film. Directors have a tendency to glamorize a film. But Milos could see the vision and helped us articulate it. He talked about reality—that the picture should be real—which is exactly what we wanted. One day he came up to me and said something which I've never forgotten. He said, 'All symbolism and allegory come from reality.' Once he said that, I knew that this was the purpose of the film."

Out of their shared vision and the intensity of working together on Zaentz's first film—the subject of which was at that time controversial—an abiding personal and professional friendship has evolved. "We've spent a lot of time together as friends. Days, weeks, months, even years. We'd drive through countries together, literally eighteen hours a day. After all this time together, our friendship grows more precious and important."

An ancient Buddhist paradox of the "wisdom of insecurity" embodies one of the more subtle ways that social support that can occur at the workplace. In effect, the honest exposure of oneself in acknowledging a shortcoming or insecurity can be transformed into an asset. Among the many study participants who benefited from the wisdom of insecurity in their careers, Walter Landor expressed it particularly well. His international strategic design company, Landor Associates, is headquartered on board the magnificently restored ferry boat Klamath in San Francisco Bay and has offices in New York, Mexico City, London, and Tokyo. The largest firm of its kind in the world, it is known for developing corporate logos and executing sophisticated marketing strategies. You probably couldn't get through a single day without seeing a half-dozen Landor logos, ranging from Bank of America and Levi-Strauss to Seven-Up and Stouffer's Lean Cuisine. Landor Associates is well known for its ability to guide the client through an intricate decision-making process, which leads both parties to a clearer understanding of the company's mission and goals for its products and services. With the enormous turbulence in the current marketplace, keeping a positive corporate image in the mind of the general public is a most formidable task, both for the firm's American clients and foreign-based accounts.

Born in Munich, Germany, to Jewish parents, Landor was eighteen and spending a summer as an exchange student studying art at Oxford University, when he began to hear the words *Nazi* and *Hitler*. Not much later, his family was forced to emigrate to England. Although the turmoil of relocation occurred when Landor was already a young adult, it parallels the early life challenges that all of the individuals in my study endured. Like those other remarkable people, Landor was able to adapt to this trauma, which gave him a sharpened power of observation as well as a drive to achieve success.

"Early on I recognized that I actually wasn't a very good designer and that I needed someone to work in collaboration with me," Landor said. "I'm more intuitive, with more of an artistic than a business temperament. When I worked with others, I performed magnificently on the creative side, and then they perfected the design. . . . I am very aware of my faults and my weaknesses, and similarly, understanding my collaborators is very stimulating to me. I sense an almost immediate understanding of people when I start talking to them. By being honest with myself and *about* myself with others and treating my colleagues and associates fairly, I'm establishing a professional support system. When people you work with sense that you care not only about how they perform but also about who they are, they are more productive and happier in their positions."

Whatever topic Landor discussed, he always spoke with honesty and genuine humility. In fact, every one of the Sound Mind–Sound Body participants reacted similarly when I asked them to take part in the study. Their responses echoed Landor's: "Why me? I'm honored, but I'm not part of that group." In addition I found, much to my surprise, that they all removed themselves a certain distance from their own success. They may have just produced a film, developed a new drug, started a magazine, or created a work of art, but they always attributed the achievement to a fortuitous team effort. Lacking the need to aggrandize their egos, they felt no need to take all the credit themselves.

ONLY THE LONELY

For some people, being part of a social network may mean a busy social calendar, while for others it may mean time spent with only one individual. Intimacy may occur at home, at work, or both, but its absence or disruption is devastating to our mental and physical well-being. Research shows that people who are connected to other people, pets, and their environment are happier, healthier, and better able to manage stress, have fewer severe illnesses, and actually live longer. Single, divorced, and widowed individuals, unless they have at least one supportive friend, are at much higher risk than happily married people.

Yet there is a subtle factor that this tidy equation doesn't seem to take into account: a lack of connection to others in a social support system may be symptomatic of a lack of connection within oneself. When we're isolated from others, it's readily apparent to us; it's much more difficult to recognize that we are isolated from parts of ourselves. As discussed in earlier chapters, it is increasingly evident that such psychological factors as hostility, cynicism, and excessive self-involvement have profound negative effects upon both mind and body. These are isolating emotions because they poison our relationships with other people. However, such emotions are so difficult to see and acknowledge in ourselves that they are all too often denied and repressed.

Feeling apart from oneself, apart from others, and apart from a sense of meaning in life is a fundamental cause of chronic stress. It is not surprising, therefore, that the documented consequences of the lack or disruption of social support are virtually identical with the diseases associated with long-term stress.

Socially isolated people appear to be more likely to have self-destructive lifestyle habits, more depression, a greater incidence of suicide, and shorter life expectancies. Among people who share identical risk factors—such as specific health habits and emotional character-istics—those who are socially isolated are more susceptible to a wide range of illnesses, including heart disease, cancer, intestinal problems, skin diseases, arthritis, headaches, and even pregnancy complications.

There are two major theories about how insufficient social sup-port interacts with the mind-body system to cause both acute and chronic diseases. One theory is that social relations "buffer" or pro-tect an individual from the full impact of a stressful event. The sec-ond theory is that there is actually a direct positive effect of social support upon a person's health. These two explanations are not mu-tually exclusive. In his major review of this research, Dr. James S. House and his colleagues at the University of Michigan found "in-creasing evidence for the *causal impact* [emphasis added] of social relationships on psychological and physiological functioning in . . . studies of humans and animals." In other words, our positive connections to other people are a direct cause of our well-being, health, and longevity.

REVERSING HEART DISEASE

Perhaps the presence or absence of our connections within ourselves and to other people is the missing link that accounts for much of what remains inexplicable in our current, purely biological model of health and disease. There are several very recent studies pointing in that di-rection. A particularly intriguing and highly publicized study was published in *Lancet* in 1991 by a friend and colleague, Dr. Dean Or-nish, and his associates. Their study demonstrated that people could actually reverse advanced coronary heart disease through a program of aggressive lifestyle change. The twenty-eight people involved in the study participated in a demanding one-year program with a diet very low in fat (10 percent), cholesterol, sodium, caffeine, and alco-hol, plus moderate exercise, stress management through yoga class-es, and group therapy. Specifics of the outcomes of this study and each of the above components of the program are detailed in Ornish's book, *Dr. Dean Ornish's Program for Reversing Heart Disease*. The overall result of the study was that the patients actually experienced a decrease in the cholesterol blockages in their coronary arteries.

Reversal of heart disease had previously been demonstrated in studies on both animals and humans; however, all of the studies had used cholesterol-lowering medications to achieve the outcome. What made the Ornish study so significant is that it was based on lifestyle change only. Yet there have been criticisms and concerns over the limitations of his study, primarily focusing on how realistic or generalizable the results really are. Among these criticisms are: 1) the study included very few women, 2) the participants had virtually all of their food prepared for them for months at a time, 3) there were several hours of yoga classes each week, and 4) lengthy group therapy sessions were held twice a week. More technical issues were raised regarding the actual measurement of the degree of regression in the coronary arteries as well as the actual clinical significance of what was found. Further research will undoubtedly address and resolve these issues.

In the meantime, amidst the clash between publicity and criticisms, perhaps the single most important finding of the study is being overlooked. Conventional medical wisdom would predict that a reversal or progression of blockages in the arteries would be related to cholesterol levels. That was not the case. In the abstract of his published study, Dr. Ornish and his colleagues stated that "favorable change . . . was related to the overall adherence to the lifestyle program." Practically speaking, this means that the more the patients changed their lifestyles, the greater the improvement in their arteries, independent of their cholesterol levels. In fact, when people adhered to the program, they showed regression even if their cholesterol levels did not fall below 150 or even below 200. Although this result may seem surprising, it is backed up by data from studies that demonstrate that cholesterol-lowering drugs reverse heart disease in only a minority of people. Among the lifestyle changes that contributed to the improvement in Ornish's patients were the intensive twice-weekly group therapy sessions. The social support patients received from these group gatherings provided occasions for them to identify the isolation in their lives and create new, health-giving connections.

Taken individually, the findings from various research projects do not make a coherent picture. However, there are several recent studies that further illustrate the effects of personal and social isolation. Specifically considering heart disease, Dr. Robert B. Case reported a significant study in 1992 in the *Journal of the American Medical Association*. Case followed 1,234 people who were actually in the control group of another multicenter study. The patients ranged in age from twenty-five to seventy-five, and all were survivors of a heart attack. After following them for one to four years after the heart attack, Case found that living alone led to a 1.54 percent higher risk of having another heart attack than not living alone. This link was most pro-

nounced in the six months immediately following the first heart attack. During this critical period the people living alone were nearly
twice as likely (15.8 percent) to have another heart attack as those
who lived with someone (8.8 percent).

A pioneer in this field, Dr. James P. Lynch of the University of
Maryland Medical School, documented in his classic *The Broken
Heart: The Medical Consequences of Loneliness* that the heart attack
death rate of widows aged twenty-five to thirty-four is five times that
of married women of the same age. At all ages divorced people are
twice as likely to develop lung cancer or stroke. For divorced white
males, cirrhosis of the liver is seven times and tuberculosis is ten
times more common.

Lynch began his research with dogs; he found that their heart rates
became lower when they were being petted. Later research demonstrated that there are also benefits of a lower heart rate and blood
pressure to the person doing the petting.

Anyone who has a beloved pet can attest to the strong and enduring bond that comes from a connection with another living thing. Relationships between humans and animals have been shown to alleviate
a variety of illnesses, ranging from depression to arthritis, and even
to increase life expectancy. Since human-animal bonds are emotional in nature, and given that emotions and the nervous system may be
linked, the health benefits are understandable. An abundance of research has shown improved psychological and physical health among
elderly in long-term care and psychiatric hospital adolescents who
interact with pets, as well as notable acts of altruism among people
who have a connection with animals. Other studies have demonstrated that pets can be helpful for individuals suffering from autism
and neurological disorders, for relieving anxiety in cancer patients,
and even for the morale of health care staff. These positive health effects are thought to come from the responsibility people take for their
pets, the emotional bonds they develop, and their increased sense of
social connectedness.

Value of the interaction with animals—and even plants—has only
recently been recognized. It would be wise for the medical community to use this knowledge in creating new social and behavioral interventions for enhancing health. In one of many recent research
projects that produced such findings, Dr. Judith Siegel at UCLA
tracked approximately one thousand Medicare enrollees, more than
one third of whom had pets, including dogs, cats, birds, and fish. During a period of one year she interviewed the people about their health

every two months. The interviews clearly indicated that having a pet had a very powerful positive impact on the health of these elderly people. Overall, the pet owners had fewer doctor visits, particularly ones that were self-initiated. Interestingly, pet owners who underwent stressful life events did not seek out additional medical or psychological care. Under all circumstances, dog owners were the least likely of all participants to need medical care. In interpreting these results, Dr. Siegel speculated that the companionship of a pet supplanted the people's need for support from medical personnel. This is an extremely important study because it shows that people can have an effective and warm social support system even without close human companionship.

Published studies as well as popular books have suggested that psychotherapy and positive social support can also help cancer patients. It is already well known that two types of social isolation in women—having few close friends and feeling alone even when friends are present—are major risk factors for death by breast cancer. At the Department of Health Services in Berkeley, California, Dr. Peggy Reynolds and Dr. George A. Kaplan conducted a seventeen-year study of nearly seven thousand men and women. The subjects, who began by completing questionnaires in 1965, were followed until 1982. The women who reported little or no social support were twice as likely to die of all cancers and five times as likely to die of smoking-related cancers. Those who felt isolated had five times the risk of dying from hormone-related cancers, such as breast cancer. Whether or not the women were depressed did not predict later cancer death rates, so the operative factor seemed to be the presence or absence of social support. From these findings, the researchers concluded that social isolation appeared to exert a direct and causal influence on hormones, leading to an increased risk of cancer. Women with the most and the highest-quality social support, and who as well reported a feeling of connectedness to others, had the lowest cancer incidence and death rate.

Some of the most compelling research in this area was conducted by Dr. James S. Goodwin and his colleagues at the Medical College of Wisconsin in Milwaukee. In their landmark 1987 study published in the *Journal of the American Medical Association*, the team examined the relationship between marital status and cancer survival among 27,779 patients. Overall, the unmarried men and women were more likely to be diagnosed at a more advanced stage of cancer, were more likely to go untreated, and had a poorer rate of survival. It appears, then, that the absence of social support delays both detection and treatment, leading to an earlier death from advanced disease. Although this study suggests an indirect consequence of the absence of social support, it did not address the possibility of a direct influence upon the person's response to treatment.

Clearly the most important and rigorous study in support of this concept is the research of Dr. David Spiegel of the Department of Psychiatry at the Stanford University School of Medicine. In 1989 he published a rather startling study in *Lancet* that focused on the effects of group therapy on eighty-six women who had metastatic breast cancer. These women were randomly assigned to receive either no intervention or a year-long weekly group therapy program which included self-hypnosis for pain control. The outcome of the study was remarkable and unanticipated. The women in group therapy lived, on the average, 36.6 months, nearly 18 months longer than the women who received their usual care but no group therapy (18.9 months). This is a dramatic instance of the influence of psychological therapy and social support upon even a terminal disease. Despite these impressive findings, Spiegel is very cautious in drawing any firm conclusions. At the present time he is conducting further studies at Stanford to begin to refine these initial results into more effective interventions.

Although Dr. Spiegel did not measure the response of the women's immune systems during his initial study, it is a reasonable assumption that enhanced immunity played a role in the extended life expectancy. If that is the case, then a separate study with a very different group of people in Sweden lends a real insight. Social support and stimulation were measured in the real-life situation of sixty elderly people living in a Stockholm senior citizens apartment building. The staff in the building worked with half of the people to create a "social activation program." Activities for these people ranged from moderate physical exercise to having a role in decision making about their apartment building complex. Blood samples and psychosocial testing were performed immediately before the program began, at three months, and at six months for both the social activation group and the control group, who conducted their lives as they had before. The results were quite amazing. In the activated group, blood levels of three hormones (testosterone, dehydroepiandrosterone, and estradiol) all increased— a reversal of the usual decline of these hormones in advanced age. In the nonactivated group, blood levels of hemoglobin decreased, indicating a less efficient blood system for carrying oxygen. Hemoglobin remained constant in the activated people. Finally, height actually decreased in the nonactivated group while remaining the same in the activated people. This study, conducted by the internationally recognized Karolinska Institute of Stockholm, is significant for many reasons. It indicates that a moderate, realistic program involving social support, empowerment and control to make decisions, and modest physical activity can have a dramatic, positive effect on a person's mind, immunity, and overall physical health. Furthermore, this benefit can occur in as little time as three to six months, and in people over the age of sixty-five, when such improvements are often assumed to be difficult if not impossible to attain.

SOCIAL SUPPORT AND HEALTHY AGING

Healthy aging is not an obvious consequence of social support, but it is an area where we have some of the best research to date. All of the individuals I interviewed in the Sound Mind–Sound Body study looked young for their age and were vigorous and energetic, and those who were in their advanced years maintained very high levels of functioning. They all attributed these qualities to their interactions with family and friends and to their being involved with challenging social issues. While the futile search for the modern equivalent of the Fountain of Youth continues, perhaps the real secret is relationships with others and the world at large.

One of the most influential articles addressing this issue was published in *Science* by the epidemiologists Dr. John W. Rowe of the Harvard Medical School and Dr. Robert L. Kahn of the University of Michigan. The ground-breaking article drew a distinction between usual or average aging and "successful" or healthy aging. It criticized the current approach to aging for focusing on disease and on average health and ignoring the fact that there are vast differences in health among people of the same age. By contrast to this dismal "gerontology of the usual," Rowe and Kahn challenged researchers to look at people who are exceptionally healthy at a given age, or those who exhibit "successful aging." They raised the perpetual issue that there are no commonly accepted measures of how old people are, except for the number of years they have lived. However, they went on to point out, there are some scientific measures that do seem to indicate an individual's true biological age, which may be more or less than the person's chronological age. One such measure is an impairment of the person's ability to metabolize glucose, leading to an increased incidence of diabetes. Another gauge is a decline in bone density, or osteoporosis, which increases with age and leads to serious fractures and ones that do not heal, especially in women. Also, reduced intellectual abilities, such as failing memory, are considered to be accurate indices of aging. Having presented these specific scientific measures for true aging, Rowe and Kahn then boldly questioned just how inevitable and irreversible these declines really are.

A second question posed by Rowe and Kahn was that if these age-related declines are not inevitable, is their onset and progression governed by internal biochemical factors within the individual or by external and behavioral factors? Surprisingly, the research data overwhelmingly shows that these supposedly inevitable, irreversible, "normal," "usual" declines are most influenced by behavioral and social factors. This is good news for all of us. It also shows that the optimally healthy individuals in my study are on the right track by taking an active, intuitive role in their own health care.

As an example of behavioral influences, the decline in insulin metabolism can be reversed through diet and exercise. Studies indicate that when older men are physically active, their ability to use glucose is "identical to that of young athletes" and significantly better than that of sedentary men of the same age. For the supposedly inevitable advancement of osteoporosis, preventable factors have been found to be adequate calcium in the diet, abstention from smoking, and moderate alcohol intake. The cliché "Use it or lose it" appears to be true with regard to the decline of intellectual abilities. Not only are there vast differences between people who continue to challenge themselves intellectually throughout life and those who don't, but even as few as five brief training sessions have helped older adults greatly to improve memory for the use of attention, inductive reasoning, and spatial orientation.

If such vital functions can be prevented from declining and even be reversed and restored, and if this reversal is not due to biochemistry, what is the operative influence? Overall, Rowe and Kahn concluded, "Many of these associated changes that have been viewed as normal and natural are subject to purposeful modification and can lead to successful rather than usual aging. Desirable interventions might include modification of exercise and diet, training programs to prevent or reverse cognitive loss, and provision of social support for health care and reduction of stress at times of bereavement and relocation. Research that links the psychosocial and physiologic aspects of aging could help promote health and prevent disease." They also emphasized the body of research that found control, autonomy, and social support to be the major influences upon the psychophysiological and immunological factors associated with usual versus healthy aging. In considering social support, they cited it as having both a direct and indirect influence upon a person's health, by both reducing disease and extending life expectancy.

In conclusion, Rowe and Khan acknowledged that a "revolutionary increase in life span has already occurred." They added, however, that "a corresponding increase in health span, the maintenance of full function as nearly as possible to the end of life, should be the next . . . step." In my study I discovered that the participants consistently lived their lives in accord with such health- and life-affirming principles and practices. Most did so out of intuition rather than by conscious decision. Fortunately, their examples provide us with living prototypes demonstrating that we can now consciously choose positive health attitudes and practices.

GIVING AND RECEIVING SUPPORT

From my interviews it appears that there are three basic ways to find social support. One is to wait until it is given or offered. This most often occurs when we are totally dependent upon others, as infants or young children, but it can also recur during adult crises. A second alternative is somewhat more difficult but more reliable: asking for help and support. Many people are afraid to ask for help out of fear of rejection, embarrassment, apparent vulnerability, or shyness. The participants in my study often expressed these same potential barriers to connecting with other people. However, they learned to recognize honestly these limitations, consciously chose to take a risk in reaching out to others, and found that each attempt made the subsequent one easier and more effective. The last and perhaps best way to find social support is to give support and friendship, because when we give support we also receive it. Through a beautiful paradox of human nature, the giver seems to get more from the act of giving than the receiver gets from accepting. Connecting to others by giving love, friendship, and nurturance is the first step toward true altruism, or selfless service to others, which is perhaps the highest expression of optimal health in body, mind, and spirit. It is most fitting that the great scientist Albert Einstein stated it best:

> Many times a day I realize how much my own outer and inner
> life is built upon the labors of my fellow men, both living and dead,
> and how earnestly I must exert myself in order to give in return as

much as I have received.

Acting upon that deceptively simple challenge to "give in return as much as I have received" is precisely what makes social support work. Essentially, our balanced relationship with others and everything around us—family, friends, animals, plants, and the environment—is what gives us the power to manage our affairs and change our lives.

Start within your immediate family. It is important to remember that at every crisis point within the life cycle, there are choices and options that will either enhance or diminish the getting, asking for, or giving of support. Family members all too often find that even though they are physically in the house at the same time as others, they spend much of that time alone or feeling isolated. They may occupy the same room when watching television, for instance, but there is very little interaction, which is needed to strengthen and enrich their bonds to the others in the family. However, there are many ways to enhance this bond:

• Develop and practice family customs and traditions that have special meaning for everyone. This can mean celebrating holidays together, reciting a prayer or observing a moment of silence before dinner, being sure to remember birthdays and anniversaries, giving a pet or even a plant to a child to encourage responsibility, attending parents' night at school, taking a simple walk together, focusing on a colorful plant or bird to begin to appreciate nature's beauty together, or being involved in the hundreds and thousands of daily events that can provide meaningful times to share small but significant intimacies.

• Mealtimes are particularly important, since it may be the only time the family comes together during the entire day. At least two or three times a week get rid of distractions and give conversation a chance by turning off the ubiquitous television or radio. By reducing external distractions, you will find it easier to discuss what happened during the day, plan to go to a movie or take a short trip on the weekend, ask how a child is doing in school, or simply share the thousands of private—or not so private—moments that occurred during the day.

• Even during periods when the demands of travel or work or even illness make spending time together difficult, leave notes for each other, make a telephone call or even leave a surprise message on the answering machine, reward a chore or responsibility that was under-taken at home with a token or small gift that costs little but conveys appreciation and a clear message that the family member is not being taken for granted. Realize that physical presence is important, but continue the emotional bond even when time and other demands separate you.

• Family councils are increasingly common. This is a structured time, usually weekly, when family members commit a specific block of time to each other. While this can seem artificial or contrived at first, it is an exceedingly effective means for addressing problems or con-flicts, or for discussing matters of mutual concern. Above all else, any existing or incipient problems need to be talked through. Common family issues include relocating to a new community, concerns over a decline in an adolescent's scholarship or his or her responses to peer pressures regarding sexuality and substance abuse, and conflicts and misunderstandings between the spouses, which can and should be discussed in the presence of the children to serve as an effective mod-el of an adult way to manage inevitable conflicts in life. Topics to be addressed can include any issue that may have an impact upon the family as a whole. One of my study participants dubbed his family council sessions "kicks and kisses," a time when both the positive and the negative feelings in the family are aired. Although this structured time is particularly useful for talking about problems, it can also be an occasion for congratulating someone, noting an achievement or a chore well done, or accepting a new responsibility. It is a time to be explicit about positive feelings, to ask for help, or simplly to exchange back rubs at the end of a long week.

• Bedtime and playtime are particularly important between parents and children. Reading a bedtime story, or reading to and with chil-dren whenever the opportunity arises, is a time-proven expression of love and caring. People in their eighties and nineties often remember their childhood bedtime stories with an undimmed fondness. Physi-cal activities, board games, puzzles, or even video games all present an invaluable way to bond and exchange the gift of laughter.

• Pick a social issue or topic of concern and create a common focus for the family. Recycling bottles, cans, and paper can be an educa-tional as well as a bonding experience that not only costs nothing but may actually provide an allowance or small business experience for a youth. Taking part in Earth Day events, planting a tree, or creating a small garden are all means to foster appreciation for the environment and teach a child that a tomato does not arrive at the supermarket by magic. Responsibility for the care of a garden or a pet is one of the most invaluable social lessons that a youngster can experience. But what about those circumstances when social support in the family is nonexistent or disrupted, or when family relations are the very source of unmanageable conflict? A person can deliberately choose or create a support system as an adjunct to or replacement for the family support system. Following are some of the many instances of such alternative systems:

• "Self-care" support groups can be created by people in common stressful predicaments or in anticipation of stressful life events or transitions. Obviously, the model of the classic Alcoholics Anonymous program comes to mind, as well as the proliferation of similarly structured programs addressing adult children of alcoholic parents, weight reduction, and incest survival. These groups supplement or substitute for the ongoing network of social contacts that people ordinarily maintain in their daily lives. Often these programs assume a greater importance for the individual than their nuclear family, especially when that family is the cause of the trauma or insoluble stress. An example is the California Self-Help Center at UCLAI, which maintains an 800 number for residents of California to call for free referrals to one or more of over forty-five hundred self-care support groups throughout the state. They can tell you who to contact for concerns you may have about virtually any aspect of the human condition, whether you are seeking a caregiver for an elderly relative, treating a medical condition, getting premature infant care, dealing with a drug addiction, learning about gay rights, or handling bereavement. The center has also created a Common Concern Program, a series of twelve self-directed audiotapes that teach the listener the basic means of creating a self-care support group. Materials are available from the California Self-Help Center at little or no cost.

• Community-based support groups are often started or led by health professionals who may or may not maintain a continuous involvement. Many crises are time-limited events that are followed by an intensive and often extensive period of adjustment. Such events may include prenatal and postnatal periods and infant care, caring for a disabled or ill parent or spouse, caring for a child with a mental or physical disability, and cardiac or physical rehabilitation. In each instance the mental and emotional aspects of social support create a positive outcome beyond the specific clinical intervention or education. With the growing prevalence of chronic diseases in our increasingly elderly population, there is an increased emphasis on home and community care rather than hospitalization and institutionally based care. We should view the trend as an opportunity for the conscious creation of social support systems to address this growing need.

• Enrolling in continuing education or skills training programs can provide social support as well as restore and enhance an individual's sense of control and self-esteem. Such groups can be led by either peers or professionals; they are distinct from self-care groups in that there is a structured focus on a specific issue or set of materials to be learned. Among the many skills development programs providing peer support are those for developing stress management skills, teaching first-aid and CPR, managing conditions ranging from diabetes to AIDS, and assisting recovery from strokes or heart attacks. Their structure often includes pairing people as buddies in addition to the classes or skills training. Many excellent materials and organizational instructions have been developed for such programs. One source of such materials at little or no cost is the Health Promotion Resource Center (HPRC) of the Stanford Center for Research in Disease Prevention at the Stanford University School of Medicine. This approach teaches specific skills and knowledge to groups of individuals who share a common experience of crisis transition in their lives and need to learn new adaptive skills.

• Work sites provide an excellent potential source of social support. Many of the previous programs are offered at an increasingly large number of work sites. Often these health promotion and disease prevention programs focus on the areas of physical fitness, smoking cessation, weight reduction, stress management, cardiovascular risk reduction, hypertension and cholesterol screening, ergonomics, and back-saver programs for proper lifting. They provide social support by giving coworkers an opportunity to relate in an environment of relaxation and cooperation. Increasingly and wisely these programs are being extended to family dependents and spouses, to build an extended support system beyond the work site. Even for those individuals who work at home or in single-person sites such as a computer terminal or a truck cab, or who have a physical disability, technology in the form of the computer, fax machine, and the AT&T videophone is opening up new dimensions to the social network.

Where such programs exist, join. Where they do not yet exist, you can find such free or low-cost community providers as the YMCA, the American Heart Association, and the American Cancer Society to set up or access such social support programs for your business or employer. Guidelines for the self-development of programs are available at modest cost from the Washington Business Group on Health (WBGH) in Washington, D.C.

Throughout our lives there are innumerable day-by-day, minute-by-minute opportunities to participate in receiving and giving social support—even at the end of life. Noted physician and author Dr. Elisabeth Kübler-Ross has wisely observed that "dying is something we human beings do continuously, not just at the end of our physical lives on this earth. The stages of dying apply equally to any significant change, e.g., retirement, moving to a new city, changing jobs, divorce, in a person's life, and change is a regular occurrence in human existence. If you can face and understand your ultimate death, perhaps you can learn to face and deal productively with each change that presents itself in your life. Through a willingness to risk the unknown, to venture forth into unfamiliar territory, you can undertake the search for your own self—the ultimate goal of growth. Through reaching out and committing yourself to dialogue with fellow human beings, you can begin to transcend your individual existence, becoming at one with yourself *and* others. And through a lifetime of such commitment, you can face your final end with peace and joy, knowing that you have lived your life well." We can face death and terminal illness in many ways. At one extreme is isolation, despair, depression and fear, while at the other is equanimity, acceptance, resolution, and a connection to others sustained right up to the moment of death and transition.

During the course of my study Dr. Kübler-Ross's observation became all the more clear to me in a conversation with Paul Hawken, founder of the garden supply company Smith & Hawken and author of *How to Grow a Business*, as he described the death of his closest friend, Gordon Sherman, whom I had intended to interview for this research project. With unguarded emotion Hawken related, "Gordon was so very important to me, especially in the writing of my book. I wrote most of it with him next to me in the next room—dying [of leukemia]. We loved each other. Gordon was fearless. You don't see many fearless or courageous men or women who possess the power to achieve almost anything and do it all with such charm and humor. He would never bend the truth, and his flaws were so obvious that they didn't bother you. He was never ashamed of who he was.

"He died at home, but his wife was not prepared for it. She tried to call a private ambulance service, but she couldn't find the number, and so she called 911. Fifteen minutes later they finally showed up. But because she called, they had the responsibility of trying to re-suscitate him. But he was dead and his liver was engorged with blood. Regardless, the paramedics threw him on the floor and pounded on his chest. They gave him electroshock and respirators. While they were pounding on him, I tried to stop them, but they wouldn't listen, until finally his liver erupted and they stopped. Then they called Marin General Hospital so they could pronounce him dead. As they were finally leaving, I asked, 'Would you help me put the body back on the bed?' I knew his sons were coming right from the airport. They said, 'No, the coroner has to do that.' . . . At that moment, his sons were coming up the driveway. . . . I met them and asked them not to come in yet but to go comfort their mother in the kitchen. I told them he died peacefully, and then I went back downstairs to clean Gordon up. . . . When they finally saw their dad, I wanted him to be cleaned up.

"With all of that going on, I felt I never really had a moment to my-self to grieve, so it hit me doubly hard. I had no private time to say good-bye. He was so full of life right up to the end, and then he was gone."

As I listened to Paul Hawken's emotional description of his best friend's death, it seemed an epiphany revealing the endurance, depth, and vulnerability inherent in true intimacy. His story proved to me that the connections of compassion and love can transcend even death.

CHAPTER SIX

Your Grandmother Was Right:

Positive Prescription for Optimal Health

Imagine the headline: Three fully loaded 747 jumbo jets crash, killing everyone on board. Then imagine that happening every day for the next year! That is the toll smoking exacts in the United States, by contributing to an appalling 434,000 premature deaths each year from such smoking-related diseases as heart disease and lung cancer. If the cause of such preventable deaths were airline crashes, surely there would be a public outcry leading to steps to prevent such carnage. However, as Shakespeare's Cassius admonished, "The fault lies not in the stars . . . but in ourselves," and that is where we need to begin.

In the introduction to *Healthy People 2000*, Dr. Louis W. Sullivan, U.S. Secretary of Health and Human Services, unequivocally stated, "Personal responsibility, which is to say responsible and enlightened behavior by each and every individual, truly is the key to good health. . . . We have become increasingly health-conscious, increasingly appreciative of the extent to which our physical and emotional well-being is dependent upon measures that only we, ourselves, can affect." While emphasizing this vital dimension of personal responsibility, he stated with similar conviction that we must attend to the community and the quality of the environment; perhaps most importantly, we must "find the means to extend benefits to the poor, elderly, homeless children, as well as to all racial and ethnic minorities." Outlined in the 692-page document are objectives for the nation to achieve by the year 2000. The list of the ten most prevalent and costly diseases in the United States today begins with heart disease and concludes with endocrine and metabolic diseases (such as obesity). In *Healthy People 2000*, virtually all of the proposals to prevent—or even eliminate—these ten most common diseases, as well as many less prevalent ones, are based on moderate, commonly accepted, widely known, and easily undertaken practices:

Stop the use of all tobacco products.

Reduce blood pressure.

Consume moderate amounts of alcohol or none at all.

Reduce total blood cholesterol levels.

Manage stress.

Practice safe sex.

Exercise in moderation three to five times per week.

Place smoke detectors in your home.

Drive within five miles per hour of the speed limit.

Wear seat belts in cars and helmets on bicycles or motorcycles.

Maintain an appropriate weight.

Eat more fresh fruit, vegetables, and fiber.

Consume less red meat and poultry, substituting fish, lentils, and rice.

Take medications properly.

Participate in cancer self-exams and age-appropriate screenings.

There is nothing extreme, magical, or unattainable in this list, but adopting these practices—even gradually—can help prevent or eliminate a large percentage of disease for the vast majority of individuals in the United States and the Western world.

WHAT IS REALLY NEW?

Every television documentary producer, newspaper writer, book and magazine publisher, and researcher at major international scientific conventions always asks, "What is *really* new?" Each poses the question with the urgency and earnest gaze of confidentiality *entre nous* that has become a cliché in spy thrillers. Their expectation is always that there will be yet another "breakthrough" that can be translated into a sound bite on the evening news or a provocative headline in the morning edition.

In interviewing my subjects I also asked myself what was really new. The answer was that I had found absolutely nothing extraordinary about their health practices. What I discovered was the very *ab-*

sence of any extraordinary or heroic levels of personal practice or the use of unusual medical interventions. It is a cause for great optimism that even though these people do have virtually unlimited access to whatever kind of care they choose, their personal strategies for optimal health and their use of conventional and alternative care are both extremely moderate. It seems then that the beliefs, practices, and ultimate achievement of optimal health need not belong solely to this elite group of exemplary individuals. Instead, every characteristic I discovered in these participants represents potential for any individual, group, or community. Each practice can be learned, improved upon, and integrated into daily life. Although each interviewee took a somewhat different approach to optimal health, nothing that I found was remarkable or unattainable, given modest commitment and practice.

Two key findings resulted from my analysis of the interviews: that every personal practice and every use of the medical care system was done *in moderation*, and that each of these individuals were able to attain a state of mental and physical quiet whenever they chose to do so.

These characteristics common to all the participants in my study are even more significant when placed in the context of the health-related practices of average Americans. New research demonstrates that the established "normal" measures for weight, blood pressure, and cholesterol levels used by doctors and insurance companies to determine a person's level of health are in fact distinctly abnormal: some are too high (such as blood pressure and cholesterol), while others are too low, including the standard measures for vitamin requirements and lung capacity.

Optimal health practices are not a guarantee of uninterrupted health but a means to reducing known risks and increasing the likelihood of continued health. During the course of my study one of the medical directors of a major Fortune 500 company represented his company to my Stanford Corporate Health Program. Since he and I have been friends for many years, I knew that he never smoked, adhered to an essentially vegetarian diet, managed stress very effectively, sought and used appropriate medical care, had a happy family and three children with his equally successful wife, was at the peak of his career, and at the age of forty-seven had been running marathons for over ten years! Surely he fit the textbook prescription for a long and healthy life.

Late in 1993 my friend ran a full marathon but was off his pace because of a persistent cough that had intermittently bothered him throughout the previous six months. Assuming it was either an allergy or a minor cold, he shrugged it off until after the marathon. His wife finally urged him to have a physical to determine what if anything could be done to alleviate it. Since he had not had a chest X-ray in many years, he underwent one as part of the routine exam. Within hours of his appointment his internist notified him of an opaque area on his left lung, and within a few days he underwent surgery to excise an orange-sized tumor. To compound his condition, the internist discovered that some lymph nodes were also malignant. Subsequently my friend underwent radiation and chemotherapy.

Certainly this was an unpredictable trauma for both the individual and his family, especially given his own history of personal health and the absence of cancer in both his paternal and maternal family trees. True to his lifelong orientation, he addressed his illness straightforwardly and sought out a family therapist to work with him and his entire family to help them prepare for and adjust to the trying months ahead. Thanks to courage, insight, and an undiminished zeal for life, this young doctor is now in remission. While there are no guarantees—even when you do live a healthy life—his story illustrates that there is indeed a healthy way to have a disease. Today he remains cancer-free, and he lives every day as fully as if it were his last.

ANALYZING THE HEALTH PROFILES

In one part of my study I requested that the participants complete a Group Health Risk Management Report in addition to their self-report. The Group Health Risk Management Report was developed by General Health Incorporated, a wholly owned subsidiary of Johnson & Johnson Health Management Incorporated. This appraisal was used to provide objective data and compare the health risks, behaviors, and disease incidence for the study participants to those of a matched group derived from national norms. Each participant who completed the health appraisal received a personalized health report. To keep the reports strictly confidential, the individuals' names were keyed to a numerical code maintained by General Health. When the individual appraisals were completed, they were aggregated into a group report, which forms the basis of the findings I discuss below. In essence we wanted to know how the study participants' health compared to the health of other people of the same sex and comparable age, as well as how their specific health practices measured up.

Of the fifty-one active participants in the study, forty-eight completed the health appraisals; assessments were made for thirty-four men and fourteen women over the course of the four-year study. Given my self-imposed limitation not to analyze the reports individually, all data were analyzed as group data to preserve confidentiality. Although the data were analyzed by numerous breakdowns, including age, marital status, race, education, income, and other factors, the following findings are reported as averages for all participants.

Within the group there were four major categories: risk indicators, risk estimates, overall risk, and group risk summary. Three of the areas within the risk indicators category are the main focus of this chapter; they are demographic measures (such as age and sex), biomedical indicators (such as blood pressure and cholesterol), and behavioral factors (including exercise, smoking, and Type A behavior). Type A behavior is characterized by hostility and by an incessant time pressure or unrelenting sense of urgency, which have been linked to an increased risk of coronary heart disease. Of the thirty-four men and fourteen women tested, ages ranged from one individual under 30 to three men over 70, the average group age being 52.8 years old. Most participants were married, while one was widowed, five were divorced, and four had never been married. Race and ethnic background were limited, as the majority were Caucasian, with only three individuals being Hispanic. Regarding religious preference, an equal number reported being Protestant or having no preference, while ten reported being of the Jewish faith, two identified themselves as Roman Catholics, and six indicated orientations toward Asian meditative traditions. Every individual earned more than forty thousand dollars per year, which is the upper limit in the health appraisal report. In terms of education, twenty individuals reported earning graduate degrees, while twenty-two had bachelor's degrees, and six held high school diplomas.

Regarding health risks and behaviors, two types of analysis were performed. One type compared the group to another group matched for age, race, sex, weight, height, marital status, number of marriages, level of eduction, living environment (urban or suburban versus rural), income, and religious preference. The second type of analysis was performed to determine how the participants compared to more "ideal" levels of risk, that is, those possible to attain under ideal conditions. This latter analysis is extremely important as it addresses the problem of comparing the group analysis to essentially abnormal averages derived from the general population. Also, this comparison to an ideal goal, suggesting, for instance, the positive influence of a further reduction in cholesterol or an increase in physical activity, gave each individual a clear indication of what he or she could do to become even healthier.

In terms of the common biomedical indicators, the study participants turned out to be distinctly average. The group weighed approximately the same as its counterpart, with a wide range of 135–199 pounds for the men and 128–158 pounds for the women. Systolic blood pressure was 5 percent less for the participants, indicating a somewhat lower risk of atherosclerosis, kidney damage, and overall heart disease. During the interviews the participants uniformly showed a high degree of knowledge about the risk of heart disease. What is more significant is that this awareness obviously translated into personal strategies and actions, judging by the results of their cholesterol assessment. Overall, the Sound Mind–Sound Body participants evidenced cholesterol levels 14 percent lower than the mean of the matched group.

According to the Johnson & Johnson health risk appraisal, a "desirable level of serum cholesterol is 180 mg/dl." (Cholesterol values are expressed in *mg/dl*, or milligrams of blood fat per deciliter.) This desirable value, which is actually lower than the generally accepted 200, is the approximate value found in the study participants. In terms of a range of the participants' cholesterol levels, only two reported a reading above 260, while eight reported levels below 180, with the majority falling between 200 and 220. An analysis was also undertaken on reported levels of high-density lipoproteins (HDL), or the "good" lipids, which actually transport excess cholesterol out of the bloodstream and which at higher levels are associated with a lower risk of heart disease. Based on national data, the average values for HDL are 49.5 for men and 60.1 for women. Overall, the majority of male participants fell in the 46–55 range, and the majority of women fell in the 55–65 range, consistent with established norms.

Actually, the behavioral indicators were much more revealing. Information was obtained on two categories of exercise. One included specific activities, such as jogging, that could be identified as part of an actual exercise program. The second considered the less specific energy expenditures that can be part of routine work or recreation. For specific exercise activities, such as walking, swimming, bicycling, running, or aerobic calisthenics, over 83 percent of the participants reported engaging in two or more activities per week. At the low end, eight people reported at least one activity each week. To be sure, not everyone was an exercise devotee.

Developer John Tishman was actually "allergic" to exercise. He maintains that he does "nothing that is visibly good" for his health, and when we discussed his physical activity, he quipped, "Everyone kept telling me that I should walk to work, so we took an apartment one block away! I do not exercise, and I am against jogging; I watch all my friends drop dead from it. Fortunately I happen to have low blood pressure and almost never get sick. I am sixty-three , and I have never gotten into exercise. I tried swimming once, but I got psoriasis from the chlorine."

With regard to smoking, twenty-six participants (54 percent) never smoked, which is unusual since most grew up in a time when smoking was considered acceptable. Additionally, twenty-two participants (46 percent) were former smokers, so of the forty-eight participants who completed the health appraisal, there was not one single active smoker. Certainly this is an optimistic note, if their practices do indeed foreshadow a trend in the general population.

Alcohol consumption was moderate. Thirty-three percent indicated they were nondrinkers and 50 percent reported they were light drinkers, averaging one to five drinks per week. Seventeen percent classified themselves as moderate drinkers, consuming six to ten drinks per week, and none were categorized as heavy drinkers. This finding is also somewhat surprising given the frequent social obligations demanded by their careers. My subjects were also diligent about practicing road safety. Over 75 percent reported using automobile seat belts more than 75 percent of the time, which was above the upper limit set by the General Health appraisal.

Before concluding this brief assessment of physical risks, it is important to note that the vast majority of the study participants made extensive use of alternative medicine during periods of illness. Since there were no questions in the health appraisal on this area, it is not possible to provide statistics, but based upon the responses to the self-report, the majority of participants regularly sought such treatments as acupuncture, massage and therapeutic touch, homeopathy, herbal remedies, chiropractic, macrobiotics, and most frequently, mind-body practices, including hypnosis, biofeedback, and meditation. These findings, which were clearly confirmed in my interviews, are also dramatically emphasized in research conducted by Dr. David M. Eisenberg and his colleagues at the Harvard Medical School.

In January 1993 Dr. Eisenberg reported the results of his study of 1,539 adults who were asked about their use of sixteen unconventional medical therapies, including those cited by my participants. Much to his surprise, 34 percent reported using such therapies in the previous year. What was even more remarkable was that based on these findings, Eisenberg estimated that in 1990 Americans made approximately 425 million visits to receive unconventional therapies, exceeding the 338 million visits to primary care physicians during the same year! Expenditures for alternative therapies amounted to approximately $13.7 billion, with as much as $10.3 billion paid out of pocket with no insurance coverage. Use of such practices constitutes a major source of care and expenditure of money hitherto unrecognized.

In response to the growing demand for unconventional therapies, the National Institutes of Health established the Office of Alternative Medicine in 1993 to begin researching these widely used interventions. From the perspective of my research it is important to note that the widespread use of unconventional medicine by the study participants again emphasizes that they seem to be living prototypes of the future form of a true health care system. When individual health is restored to the center of health care, the artificial division between mainstream and unorthodox medical care becomes obsolete. All approaches require rigorous evaluation, high standards of clinical efficacy, and well-trained professionals, but one approach is not assuredly preferable to another based on politics, bias, and money but rather as a matter of choice.

Finally, in the psychological sector the factor of most interest was the measurement of Type A behavior. Given career pressure and the high level of performance demanded of the study participants, the relative presence or absence of Type A behavior is of great relevance. Only four participants (8 percent) scored at the level of "definite" Type A tendencies. Overall, the majority of the participants (71 percent) evidenced "some" Type A behavior. Rather than relying upon anger, hostility, and aggression to resolve the inevitable business and interpersonal conflicts, this majority of the group relied upon their creativity and ability to strike a flexible compromise.

Epitomizing this orientation was the late philanthropist John E. Fetzer. When he was embroiled in controversial situations, especially as the owner of the Detroit Tigers, he did not permit himself to resort to his admittedly Type A tendencies. "During baseball season, I would go to the league meetings, which were usually fraught with controversy. I seldom participated in the mudslinging but instead would step back, identify the issues, and begin developing a compromise. Generally I could draft a resolution that satisfied both sides and solved the problem.

"I believe problems are more easily solved that way than through confrontation. Confrontation doesn't hurt the other fellow a bit, it . . . only hurts you." Both in the short and long run this philosophy has proven successful—personally and professionally. Fetzer's approach to conflict resolution deepened during his recovery from a coronary. "Philosophically, my reaction has been shaped by many years of transcendental meditation. I started doing it ten or fifteen minutes at a time, but now my periods of meditation are sometimes much longer. Meditation is far more effective in relaxing me than going on a cruise or on a vacation. Relaxation is a state of mind, not just where you are physically."

For the majority of the study participants (71 percent), this orientation toward and adaptation to their aggressive tendencies was far more evident than the stereotypical misconception of the time-pressured, aggressive behavior supposedly conducive to success. Working *smarter* was clearly the solution among these individuals.

There were numerous other, more detailed analyses performed in the areas of risk estimates, overall risk, and group risk summary. These are much too detailed to include in this book, although the area of analysis that looked at "attainable risk" warrants mention. Attainable risk is the average risk the participants could achieve if they reduced the level of all their risk indicators to the lowest possible value or healthiest level. This information can be expressed in terms of average life expectancy. The average life expectancy of the participants is 82.2 years, or 2.5 years longer than the national average of 79.7 years old for a comparable group. Although this mortality risk is lower than average, it is still not the ideal level of optimal health that this group could theoretically achieve. There were several areas of risk where the group was very close to achieving optimal health; among them were low or ideal levels of risk for getting lung cancer and low risk for any other form of cancer. However, the participants could considerably improve their risks in most other areas, including having or dying from a heart attack, stroke, cirrhosis, and pneumonia, and especially dying from a motor vehicle accident, the risk of which could be reduced simply by following the *Healthy People 2000* guidelines for using seat belts 100 percent of the time and not combining drinking and driving.

As a whole, the group data in this study confirm that these individuals too are trying as hard as everyone else to maintain optimal health (with a considerable distance to go), and that they do not represent an unattainable ideal in health, career, or dedication to altruistic causes. They struggle with all of the same if not more challenges, obstacles, and crises as anyone, with the critical difference being that they have committed themselves to exercising choices that lead to behaviors that optimize their physical, mental, environmental, and spiritual health.

COMMONSENSE APPROACHES TO OPTIMAL HEALTH

During a meeting I had with Norman Cousins to brief him on the results of the study, he was particularly struck by the moderate personal strategies that were evident throughout both the data analysis and interviews. With his inimitable insight and good humor, he said, "You see, your grandmother was right!" To a great degree these practices *do* come from common sense, but the challenge is not simply to know what to do but to actually *do* it. According to *Healthy People 2000*, "Implementation of what is already known about promoting health and preventing disease is the central challenge. . . . Good health comes from reducing unnecessary suffering, illness, and disability. It comes as well from an improved quality of life. Health is thus best measured by a citizen's sense of well-being." It is this purely subjective sense of well-being that ultimately determines behaviors conducive to optimal health. Jogging out of the fear of having a heart attack, dieting to look attractive for a class reunion, or even volunteering to support a social cause because it is fashionable are woefully inadequate and temporary approaches destined to fail. To get at the more enduring yet intangible dimension of a deep commitment to sustained positive behavioral change, we must delve directly into the Sound Mind–Sound Body interviews.

Paralleling many of the same developmental crises experienced by other study participants and arriving at many similar inner convictions and health practices is the entrepreneur and author Paul Hawken. At the time of our interview Hawken was chairman and chief executive officer of the phenomenally successful Smith & Hawken garden supply catalog and stores, which he cofounded in 1979. Among his many other achievements he has published four books, including the bible of entrepreneurial businesses, *Growing a Business*, which spawned a seventeen-part public television series of the same name featuring such innovative companies as Ben & Jerry's Homemade, Esprit, and Quad Graphics.

Perhaps what is most significant about the book and the PBS series is that they emphasized the unconventional, even spiritual qualities that inspired the business founders. *Growing a Business* is often cited by new entrepreneurs as their inspiration not only to begin a business but to adhere to socially and environmentally responsible values.

Seeing Paul Hawken's tremendous success as an author and businessman, it might be tempting to assume he enjoyed a privileged upbringing or that his success was fortuitous rather than hard-won. In fact, Hawken's early childhood and adolescence were both traumatic and potentially destructive, but he believes these experiences were what provided the impetus for developing his present-day personal strategies for optimal health. Hawken's challenges began virtually from the moment of his birth in San Mateo, California, in 1946. He explained, "At the age of six months I developed severe asthma and was put into an oxygen tent. I have a twin sister, and since the doctors just assumed I would die, they actually told my mother, 'You're a lucky woman. You may lose one child, but you still have a healthy daughter.' Back then people just didn't question doctors, so my mother left the hospital and didn't come back for six weeks.

"Then one day the doctor called her and said, 'Well, he's still alive.' For those six weeks I had lived under fluorescent lights without being touched. It's really a wonder that I survived. Now that I have children of my own, I can fully appreciate the horror of leaving a six-month-old child under a bank of lights in a plastic oxygen tent for six weeks. Just leaving a child for the night, hoping he won't wake up and cry, is painful to me."

Hawken's near-fatal illness and confinement were only the beginning. At the age of nine, he recounted, "My mother was hospitalized and my father disappeared. . . . One day my grandparents were at our house, and the next thing we knew, we were being taken away and being stuffed in the back seat with the parakeet cages. We went to live on my grandparents' farm without even knowing what had happened until many year's later. Apparently my mother had a heart condition. Since we did not have much money, her condition just got worse. Before long she was sent off to a hospital. Visiting her was truly traumatic for me."

When Hawken finally left home at age twelve, he sought refuge with his alcoholic father, whom he described as a "violent and critical man." Finally, at the very young age of fourteen, he left home to live on the streets. He remembered particularly that "basements were always good." Fortunately he found his way to Nevada City in northern California. Even today Nevada City is a well-preserved, picture-postcard community, with a main street of Victorian homes that looks very much like it did during the town's heyday in the Gold Rush of the mid 1800s. This environmentally idyllic small town in the Sierra foothills was a refuge to young Hawken in the early sixties, just as it is now for many people from the San Francisco Bay Area seeking a better quality of life away from the big cities. There Hawken lived with a family; his "stepfather" was an accountant who took him on frequent trips to San Francisco. "We were a real family. We lived with his wife and daughters in the country. We even had horses." Despite his traumatic, potentially destructive childhood, Hawken has maintained a sense of identity and purpose. He nevertheless admits with unflinching candor that he is "a person with extremely low self-esteem. When I get up in the morning, every good thing that has happened in my life up to that point doesn't count. I have to start all over."

Like many of the Sound Mind–Sound Body participants, Paul Hawken possessed the remarkable ability to transcend childhood illness and trauma and incorporate positive health practices into the personal and professional aspects of his life. Faced with the responsibilities of running a rapidly growing and successful business, frequent travel, and a sixty to seventy hour workweek, Hawken knows he must pay attention to diet and exercise. "I don't drink alcohol, I don't drink coffee, I don't drink black tea, don't smoke, don't do drugs, or any of those things that suppress your immune system. I also exercise on a regular basis. I may sound like a cereal commercial, but I actually eat a lot of fiber and generally am very conscientious about what I eat. For me healthy eating is a conscious decision. If someone says have a piece of chocolate cake, I just say no thanks. There is no internal stress or struggle for me about being healthy. A lot of people try to be or are healthy but there is a real tension inside of them. There is a constant, nagging tension of what you should or should not be doing. Maybe the reason I don't feel this tension is because I started my health practices and diet so young. Many people start when things go wrong or when they get sick later in life. I just got a head start."

Because of his asthma Hawken was taking massive amounts of medication by the age of twelve, which made him feel "really jacked up. I was taking medications at three times the maximum dose, and I had three dozen doctors prescribing. Since I was always feeling so hyper and I knew I wasn't going to grow out of it, I realized it was up to me to do something about it. For years I tried different diets and kept going back for more testing. . . . I wanted to see the effect each food, each diet had on my lungs, but obviously it was my brain and lungs. More and more I became convinced I had a food allergy. Was I stubborn! . . . That was nineteen sixty-four or sixty-five, when people who went to health food stores were strange, but I finally found the right diet and the asthma ended. Not only did I do the obvious things like stop drinking milk, but I noticed that foods of specific benefit to the lungs were foods that grew in water. Lotus root and other roots like ginger that thrive in water or damp, foggy places are the things that enhance the lungs. Through many fasts and trial and error I discovered the optimal diet for me."

Out of the necessity of coping with his own asthma, Hawken's innate curiosity was piqued and sent him off on a trajectory that led to his first inklings about business. "My business interests were born from the realization that the food I ate made such a big difference in my health. Actually I was astounded by the magnitude of the effect. But for a year I still was sure it was psychosomatic, because I was just so stubborn! I tried to go back to hamburgers, milk shakes, and Coke, but it was just not possible." In 1967, seeking to refine his own dietary discoveries, he went to Boston to study with Michio Kushi, who remains the guru of the macrobiotic diet movement. At that time the small food co-op owned by Kushi and his wife sold very few products. Diving in with an astounding enthusiasm, Hawken transformed the tiny co-op, which was subsequently incorporated into the Erewhon Trading Company.

Mark Twain's prescription for longevity, "Have a minor illness and take good care of it," was echoed by another participant who asked to remain anonymous, a prominent motion picture director and producer whose health practices evolved from the same need as Hawken's—to cure his asthma. Growing up with chronic asthma, he continued to suffer episodes as an adult, especially during the intensity of making a film. "Inevitably, I would get a cold or the flu while working on a film. That always happens because you're exposed to so many people. I would develop a cough, which for most people goes away in about two weeks. But I would get a cough and it would last for three to six months. I started calling it 'director's cough,' because I'd be either coughing on the set or trying to suppress a cough."

Since he was unable to control this exposure to lots of different people, and medications were of no use, he learned to adapt to a series of colds and chronic lung infections, which only compounded his asthma. During one particularly acute episode, his wife noticed that his cough seemed even worse when he wasn't even speaking. After that, he noted, "I finally took the time to understand my allergies and change my diet. Slowly I began to realize that allergies are sort of like an addiction; they are a kind of poison to your system that your body actually thrives on. When I would write, I would frequently drink coffee in the mornings, and eventually I realized it was aggravating my asthma. Even after one or two cups of coffee I would begin to wheeze. That realization also made me aware that I was allergic to milk. I made a conscious decision to stop drinking coffee and milk, and lo and behold, the director's cough stopped!

"Then about a year and a half later we were on location in a desert and I had the chance to have a milk shake. Immediately I started to cough. Now I will have a frozen yogurt or tofu, or even a little bit of milk, but that is the limit for me. . . . Now I'm really sensitive to both the negative and the positive subtle influences on my health. . . . Now I stick to a very low-fat diet, even though I still eat some red meat. I work out with a trainer every day for an hour and a half, doing a combination of weights, stretching, and aerobics. And occasionally I go out and play tennis. Paying attention to my diet and exercise has really helped me, both when I'm working and in my personal life. I think that's what got me through the tough times of my divorce, which was actually the event which pushed me to get serious about taking care of my health."

Surely Dr. Dorothea Johnson of AT&T is one of the participants most personally and professionally knowledgeable in the field of health and one who derived her personal health strategies from positive, early life experiences. I was particularly interested to hear her respond to the question, "What is health?" After a long and pensive pause Dr. Johnson responded, "Health is becoming the best that you can be, physically, mentally, emotionally, and spiritually. It may not be the absence of disease; as you get older, there are certain disease processes which are virtually inevitable. However, you can be healthy in any state. There is a healthy way to handle a disease. Health is a mental thing, but it's also got to be spiritual and physical. It's also got to be emotional. . . . For me this kind of thinking goes back to my childhood. My father was a good role model. He exercised every morning and ate properly, and so did I. I never took any medications, not even aspirin. We were never allowed potato chips and stuff like that. So I really learned how to be healthy from my dad. When he was eighty-five, he was still diving and swimming and enjoying his life to the fullest.

"To this day I still eat properly. For breakfast every morning I have raisin bran, unless I am traveling and just can't get it. Then I try to eat just bran flakes or corn flakes. At noon when I eat in the executive dining room at AT&T, I generally eat a chunk of tuna or salmon, with lettuce, tomatoes, and sometimes cottage cheese. Also I drink two glasses of skim milk a day. Ever since I was a little kid, I drank skim milk, and I drank it all through my teen years because I had acne.

"As for vitamin supplements, I take a five-hundred-milligram C and B complex from Darby or Abbott, plus ten thousand international units of A. My belief is that A helps to prevent colds and viral infections, and it's good for the eyes. Now we are just discovering that beta carotene is an anticarcinogen, but I have been following this regimen for over twenty years."

Dr. Johnson exercises too. "I don't jog anymore because my knees really go, so I just run on the treadmill at about three and a half miles an hour three times a week. When it's nice, I walk outside, sometimes with my husband. We live on an acre and a quarter of land, so I pace it out, with one, three, five, seven, nine steps up to two thousand six hundred forty, which I figure is a mile because I take a two-foot stride. It keeps my mind busy. Instead of a mantra, I do the one, three, five meditation!"

Like Dr. Johnson, every individual in the study made idiosyncratic but informed choices from the various health prescriptives. These choices represented their unique adaptation of general guidelines to fit their particular lifestyles. Exercising choice appears to be as essential to optimal health as exercising the body.

Approximately ten years ago there was a front-page article in the *Medical Tribune* by a medical reporter who attended a meeting of the most prominent national authorities on cancer held at the National Cancer Institute. The writer asked each of the cancer authorities what they personally did to prevent cancer—not what they would necessarily determine from the scientific data, not what measures they believed effective based on the scientific data, not what they would tell their patients, not what they would advocate as a matter of national policy, but what they personally practiced. Ironically, their actual practices were as interesting individually as they were contradictory as a group. The experts' responses were as wide-ranging and unscientific as any that would be derived from interviewing a random cross-section of people in the health food aisle of any supermarket. A number of the prominent cancer experts, such as the late Dr. Lewis Thomas, author of *Lives of a Cell*, and a former head of Memorial Sloan-Kettering Cancer Center in New York, still smoked heavily. Predictably, Dr. Linus Pauling extolled the virtues of megadoses of vitamin C, which the others shunned. Regardless of specifics, each cancer expert, like the interview participants in my study, made individualized, subjective choices in devising his or her own idiosyncratic strategy for optimal health.

To illustrate further, let's briefly consider the health choices made by a representative sample of the study participants. For David Rockefeller a commitment to a systematic exercise program began when the medical director at the Chase Manhattan Bank convinced him that "the Bank's health would be improved and its efficiency would be enhanced" if they installed a cardio-fitness facility, which David authorized. He recalled, "Then I felt that if I was going to encourage others to do it, I had better set a good example. Close to fifteen years ago, I started going to the gym on a regular basis, exercising at least three times a week while I was at the bank. There is no question that this improved my general health, and I also think it has helped me keep my weight reasonably under control. Even as a child I had a weight problem. When I started the exercise program, I was about fourteen or fifteen pounds heavier than I am today. That weight fell off fairly quickly after I started exercising, and it has stayed off. Although I do not see a direct connection between my exercise and concentration on productivity, I really do not doubt that it has been beneficial."

Nobel Prize–winning physicist Dr. Murray Gell-Mann reflects, "As time goes on, I have had to become more aware of my health—but only recently. Now I try to keep my weight down, I eat a lot of oat bran, and I do exercise daily, but it's a minimum. Usually I ride an exercise bike for about fifteen minutes, but I am not the kind to run ten miles in the morning. Certainly I have never experienced the 'runner's high.' Well, maybe once or twice with young ladies when I was inspired to run five or six miles, but I can't help wondering if it was the ladies' company or just the lack of oxygen which made me feel high."

Another participant who recently began focusing on his health practices is the producer and screenwriter Norman Lear. "I exercise every morning and have grown fond of it because I love the feeling, not because I know it's supposed to be good for me," he admitted. "I do stretches and abdominal exercises and ride a stationary bike. Sometimes I even use weights. Generally I work out about forty minutes—and at my age, that's pretty good. I also try to make healthy food choices, but I think I love food more than anybody who ever lived.

"For me the real discipline is, paradoxically, surrender. Discipline is very much related to the ability to relax, to let yourself lie in the lap of that immense, universal intelligence, to banish all negative thoughts and just let go. That is my meditation. That's real health."

No matter what their starting point, all the individuals in my study attributed their choice of and perseverance in personal health practices to their desire to attain a state of mental and physical peace and equanimity. They reported feeling the positive impact of their healthy choices, without which they would feel out of balance and adrift.

STANDING AT THE STILL POINT

All of the study participants stated emphatically that health was not as much a mastery of physical fitness, proper diet, or even the "right" lifestyle, as it was a matter of mental and spiritual well-being. Their health had nothing to do with face-lifts, silicone breast implants, yo-yo diets, fashionable attire, or superficial fads. Optimal health is a means of fulfilling a deep purpose and life mission, not an end unto itself. Physical health is only one manifestation of a more profound inner state of mental, emotional, and spiritual equanimity, a state that is referred to within the Zen Buddhist tradition as "standing at the still point," but which is a universal experience.

Stress management strategies are not techniques for obliterating stress, but tools to help calm the body and mind enough to experience a sense of balance and direction. As chapter 4 emphasized, stress is not a function of a person's environment. The way we perceive the world determines how we react to the inner and outer challenges of that environment. Whether we perceive ourselves to be threatened or challenged, isolated and separate or connected and integrated, fearful or or enthusiastic is a function of a perceptual standpoint independent of the actual event. Choosing among those options is the ultimate challenge.

Yet how many of us make active, positive choices from among the vying and often contradictory health practice options, and why? To make these choices—and to make them wisely— individuals need to feel a part of, rather than apart from, everyone and everything around them. Such an experience is not a philosophical abstraction but is actually very common, except that the most frequent occurrences are often too fleeting to be recognized or fully appreciated.

Any stress management technique used to quiet the body and mind can also be used to sustain these fleeting intervals and permit an individual to experience deeper, more subtle, more enduring periods of equanimity. During such periods there is the inevitable realization that while on one level of reality we are separate, but on another we are not separate, not isolated, not alone. Essentially, an individual can have a double vision and be able to enjoy the diversity and richness of life while simultaneously remaining aware of and rooted in a profound sense of an underlying unity. It is vital to reside in this experience to examine options free of fear, compulsion, ambition, or predisposition, and to make positive choices while moving away from self-destructive patterns.

Every one of the study participants described this sense of inner balance to be a guiding force in choosing their personal strategies for optimal health. When asked about the practices he used to handle the demands of his career, Dennis Weaver responded, "Certainly, I maintain health practices and a diet that contribute to my physical well-being. But what's most important is that all 'well-beings' are hooked together. My physical, mental, and spiritual well-being are all connected. My spiritual health comes first, then mental and physical. For my physical health, the primary regimen is diet and exercise, but also the quality of the air, the water, and my total environment.

"My meditative and stress management practices are a big part of my health and my life. One of the major problems with us humans is that we always look outside of ourselves for fulfillment and the answers to our problems. We try to find happiness in material possessions or in our activities. Through my experience, I've learned that you will never find completeness outside of yourself because nothing complete exists outside of us. The greatest completeness I have experienced is within. I really think the inner search is something that has been ignored in this age of health, with its emphasis on scientific materialism. The general feeling is that if we can just get enough money, enough power, enough of a position, enough fame, then we'll be happy. But take a look at the wealthiest part of society. That section has one of the highest rates of suicides per capita, which suggests that you can search and search and search outside of yourself, but no matter what goals you attain, or how much you achieve, there will always be that feeling that something is still missing. What's missing is that connection that we keep striving for, that 'something else,' if you will, which is within our very own consciousness."

When I asked Weaver to elaborate on what he experiences when he is "standing at the still point," he responded, "It is what I call the presence of God, which is always within us. It is a very tangible, concrete feeling. There is nothing that will give you lasting fulfillment outside of yourself, because there's absolutely nothing that's ever-lasting. You cannot find permanent happiness in something imper-manent. However, the permanence we do have is within our own consciousness. That is why, for instance, Christ said, 'My Kingdom is within.' He also said, 'My Kingdom is not of this world!' In the Psalms it says, 'Be still and know that I am God.' It is professed so clearly, and not just in the Western religious tradition."

Although each participant had his own method of attaining a state of balanced body and mind, their inner experiences were essentially the same. Weaver explained, "My particular meditative practice is hatha yoga, which is one of Yogananda's techniques which has to do with concentration and devotion. The simplest way to explain it is that it is an experience of the peace and bliss of God's presence within. It is actually palpable during the breathing exercises, particularly at the supreme spiritual center of the body, which is in the forehead. Tech-nically, it has to do with the opening of the pituitary gland. There is the sensation of a glow, accompanied by a pull, which I call the pull of God's love. You focus on merging your attention and being into one with that feeling. You literally become what you are conscious of . . . so through the power of your attention you can direct your thoughts to the center of your forehead and you become aware of nothing but that. Physically you are focusing on and experiencing your higher consciousness. You feel a sense of well-being, a sense of peace, and there is a pure joy associated with it that has nothing to do whatsoever with what you experience through your senses.

"We can know the outside world through sensory experience. We can touch things, we can taste things, we can look at things, but the experience of that outward reality is such a gross vibration that it takes gross instruments to experience it. That is why we have physi-cal senses. But to experience the bliss of God's presence, the spirit within, requires the sixth sense, or what you might call the power of intuition, which is direct perception. It is a direct knowingness, *with-out* the aid of an intermediary, which is what the senses are. You know it because you're one with it.

"It is so uplifting and peaceful that it has a positive effect on every-thing in the world around you. The feeling just overflows into your external activity. There is such a feeling of love that you really want to express it outwardly. The LIFE program is an outward expression of this experience and feeling. Compassion is an expression of this love, and forgiveness is, of course, also an expression of it as well as a result of it. When you truly experience that inner connection to yourself and others, you inevitably feel compassion and forgiveness toward all people. Outward service to others, like through the LIFE project, or compassion toward the environment and animals who share our planet and destiny, concern for people, for the homeless, just naturally flow out of that experience." This orientation described so eloquently by Dennis Weaver is an inherent, albeit often overlooked, dimension of optimal health.

How intimately people are linked to their own inner state of balance—and in some cases to the people around them—may prove to be a better predictor of heart disease than cholesterol levels, diet, exercise, blood pressure, or even hostile behavior and its variants. While heart disease mostly strikes older individuals, some coronaries have stricken people in their twenties and thirties. Concern is now focusing upon premature heart disease among younger adults and even adolescents, and a number of key researchers and clinicians following the pioneering research of Dr. David McClelland, now at Boston University, are looking at people's excessive and inappropriate need to control themselves and others in a form of "power motivation." Some of the most recent and compelling evidence for the negative effects of an excessive drive for power comes from research with monkeys. Stanford biologist Dr. Robert Sapolsky has been observing baboons on the Serengeti Plain in Africa. His ongoing study of this troop of males and females has revealed that intimate, cooperative behavior by lower-status males may pay off in many ways. When these males "hung out with females," acting in a friendly and caring way, they appeared to experience less physiological stress than the more dominant males. Other researchers at the University of North Carolina have found that among macaque monkeys dominant, powerful males show less coronary artery disease under low-stress conditions. However, when subjected to major social stress by being put into a new group of unknown macaques, these dominant, power-oriented males struggling to establish status suffered considerably higher levels of coronary artery disease than their more submissive counterparts. It seems to be the same for humans.

This need to seize power and control virtually always conflicts with the need for intimacy. Every person needs to resolve the issue of getting ahead versus getting along. Unfortunately, the dominant mode in today's culture is clearly weighted on the getting-ahead side of the fulcrum, especially during tough economic times. As a result there is a decline in the getting-along dimension of intimacy. Successful living requires a balance between these two conflicting needs. Surely the participants in my study not only showed that such a balance is possible but also stand as living proof that getting ahead, being assertive, and working hard for power and success do not necessarily entail aggression, hostility, and loss of intimacy with yourself or others.

Among the leading researchers exploring these issues are Dr. Carl Thoresen of Stanford University and Dr. Meyer Friedman, codiscoverer of the Type A personality. Most recently their attention has moved away from the question of who gets heart disease to the question of what can be done to prevent the onset or improve survival for those who have already had a heart attack or stroke. At the root of their research is the theory that a misplaced, inappropriate need to exert power and control results in a chronic and incessant barrage of biochemical and immunological excesses in the body, as described in the previous chapter. These excessive reactions induce massive changes in the heart and circulatory system in a form of slow suicide. Provocative results have come from Thoresen and Friedman's ten-year study of heart attack survivors, the National Institutes of Health's seven-year study of over twelve thousand men at risk for heart disease, and numerous other investigations. From the National Institutes of Health study it's clear that although most of the male subjects were smokers with high blood pressure and cholesterol, those who were rated as more "hostile" during their interviews suffered 50 percent more deaths from heart attacks than the others. This finding was especially true for men younger than forty-seven years old. Similarly, a twenty-year study conducted at SRI International concluded in 1990 with the finding that men with high hostility, also rated from interviews, suffered 40 percent more deaths of all kinds (including 42 percent more cardiac deaths and 50 percent more cancer deaths) than those with low hostility.

Another related study conducted in Sweden examined the relationship of Type A behavior and social connections in over two hundred coronary patients. Those rated as "socially isolated" from a self-reported questionnaire died at much higher rates than those rated as "socially connected"—68.9 percent versus 17.3 percent. Such findings about isolated and hostile individuals led Dr. Thoresen to make the urgent observation that for them, "the human 'being' aspect of their lives is gone. There is only human 'doing.' No time to be present, to be here now. They are always processing the past or planning the future. They have little access to their feelings, to the present situation, especially how others may be feeling. This is not an obscure disorder, or an exotic problem. Many Americans live this way." These specific characteristics underlying disease diametrically opposed to the characteristics revealed in the health profiles and interviews of the individuals in my study: an orientation toward the inner self, toward others, and toward positive lifestyle practices. No disease-related characteristic is necessary for career success. Rather, virtually all will predispose a person to premature disease and death.

Today a great deal more is known about the negative attitudinal and behavioral predispositions to heart disease that compound the biological risk factors. An understanding of the positive end of the continuum—the optimal health end—is only beginning to emerge. From Dr. Thoresen's ten years of work with heart attack survivors, it is clear that "growth counseling actually saves lives above and beyond surgery and medication." Thoresen says the vital issues now are, "How can we recapture a much greater sense of shared beliefs, a sense of community and a tempered concern with personal gain? How can we foster a much greater genuine mutual respect for those with divergent interests and experiences?"

Answering this challenge is not a new problem. In 1835 Alexis de Tocqueville wrote in his classic *Democracy in America* that he was concerned how America would survive because individuals were so extremely individualistic, self-centered, and narcissistic. That challenge is more evident now than in the middle of the nineteenth century, but solutions are more at hand.

WHAT TO DO ON MONDAY

How is it possible even to begin to resolve such a formidable issue? Or as one of my patients asked, "So what do I do on Monday?" A great deal is possible. For better or worse, the initial steps are quite simple. Based on all of the available research to date, from my own clinical experience with individuals and groups of patients, and from the majority of practices described in the interviews, I believe the vital first step is to establish a method of quieting one's body and mind to attain an inner point of stillness, from which one can then begin to examine and change negative, destructive thoughts and behaviors. Unfortunately the means to finding this stillness are often presented as either of two extremes: as overly esoteric meditation practices or as an overly simplistic power of positive thinking or relaxation response. Neither extreme is viable, and both tend to turn more people off than on. Between these two extremes is a highly effective approach based on three steps: quieting the body, quieting the mind, and using this state of inner balance to picture or visualize choices. Intellectually understanding this process is easy; the essence of its effectiveness, and difficulty, is the doing.

At the same time that I was conducting the Sound Mind–Sound Body study, two colleagues and I were working under a grant from the Office of Prevention of the California Department of Mental Health. Our challenge was to conduct a thorough review of the clinical stress management research and, based on that critical review, to develop a simple but scientifically based self-care program by which people might achieve a quieting of the mind and body. My two seemingly different research projects reached a surprising point of convergence. The personal strategies described by the interview participants and the methods which were developed for the Department of Mental Health program turned out to be virtually identical. Most often the interview participants developed their strategies through trial and error or had radically adapted their formal training to their own idiosyncratic use. Despite the plethora of individual expressions, the common elements from their personal practices and from our review of the scientific literature were strikingly similar.

A self-care, stress management program developed from the literature review had to be scientifically based, safe, effective, and deliverable at a fifth-grade level of reading comprehension. Results of this two-year project were entitled *That's Life: Learning to Manage Life's Stress* and disseminated in a bound packet that included a self-directed workbook, an audiotape containing a simple relaxation and visualization method, and a stress sensor card to indicate an increase or decrease in blood flow and temperature in an individual's finger as an indication of relaxation. Initially we distributed the kit throughout the state of California by conducting a series of five separate orientation seminars for all of the more than fifteen hundred mental health providers in the five major regions of the state. Thousands of the kits were disseminated to and used by nurses, psychologists, social workers, psychiatrists, and physicians in settings ranging from a prison population of sex offenders to general medical practices.

Since the distribution of that program in 1988 and 1989, hundreds of letters from both practitioners and patients have given us feedback helpful in refining and enhancing the basic guidelines. Conducting both this stress management program and the Sound Mind–Sound Body study led me to formulate practical guidelines for a first step toward quieting the body and mind. By following these simple rules, an individual can come to stand at the still point, a necessary pre-requisite for choosing among personal health options as well as deciding how to reestablish a positive connection to others and the environment as a whole.

These guidelines are featured here without an explanation of the underlying science and neurophysiology. Complete details are contained in the 1992 edition of my book, *Mind as Healer, Mind as Slayer*, in *Full Catastrophe Living* by Dr. Jon Kabat-Zinn of the University of Massachusetts Medical Center, as well as in *The Relaxation Response* by Dr. Herbert Benson of the Harvard Medical School. Being familiar with the underlying biology is not necessary for effective practice, but a few insights are helpful. During the physical quieting step, the focus is on the two sensations of heaviness and warmth. *Heaviness* is the subjective sensation of muscles relaxing, while *warmth* is the subjective sensation of increased blood flow to the periphery of the body, into the hands and feet, as an indication of overall relaxation. By focusing attention on these two sensations, you are essentially asking or communicating with both the voluntary muscle system of the body as well as the supposedly involuntary, or smooth, muscles of the circulatory system. In both cases the purpose is to quiet the body and become fully free of the usual physical tensions and distractions that are an inevitable part of everyday life.

There are ten practical steps to quiet the body and mind:

• Choose a comfortable, armless, straight-back chair such as a kitchen chair. Sit comfortably on the chair toward the front edge so that your back is not resting against the back of the chair. This is a posture of balance, which will keep you from becoming drowsy or falling asleep as you practice this technique for longer periods of time. Just let your arms and hands hang straight down by your sides.

• Gently close your eyes and focus your full attention on the act of sitting in a relaxed and balanced posture. While in this position slide the left foot forward until you feel your weight shift to your heel. Then slide the foot back in toward your body until you begin to feel your weight pressing on the ball of your foot. Moving your foot in this manner, find the position in which your foot is flat on the floor with your weight evenly distributed on both the heel and the ball of your foot. In this position your leg should be extended in front of you at approximately a 120-degree angle. Then do the same thing with your right foot. There should be no tension in the legs, and the knees should be approximately one foot apart. Hold your knees in your hands and wiggle them so that your legs move without resistance.

• Now that your legs are in a stable position and you are balanced between the soles of your feet and the base of your spine, you can balance the upper part of your body as well. Moving the upper part of your body as though it were one unit, just lean forward until you feel your lower back muscles pulling. Then allow yourself to lean back in the chair until you feel your abdominal muscles pulling. Next, as you did with your feet, rock back and forth until you find the position where neither set of muscles is strained and the spinal column feels as if it is poised perfectly on the pelvis. Your torso is now in a state of balance.

• Next turn your attention to your head. Drop your head forward onto your chest until the muscles at the back of your neck pull. Then lean your head back until the muscles in front of your neck pull. Rock your head back and forth until it feels like a ball balanced on the end of your spinal column, which is in turn balanced on your pelvis.

• Muscles generally need to be tensed in order to rebound and relax maximally. Because back and neck muscles carry a great deal of tension, it is best to tense and relax these muscle groups. To do this, just imagine that there is a string from the top of your head to the ceiling and that this string is pulling you into an upright posture with both arms still hanging down to your sides. Then imagine that the string is cut and your head just flops forward like a rag doll. It is very important that you do not collapse over your throat, which would make breathing difficult.

• While you are sitting in this relaxed position, raise your left hand and let it drop on your thigh as if it were a dead weight. Do the same with your right hand, and let them both relax where they fall.

• Then just let your attention flow like water down into your left arm and hand. Silently say to yourself, "My left arm is heavy and warm." There is no magic in those words; they are simply meant to remind you to feel these two sensations. Repeat this phrase three times. As during any relaxation meditation practice, your mind may tend to stray as you attempt to focus on the exercise, but there is no need to be disturbed by this. Merely direct your attention back to the task at hand in a gentle manner, without getting upset at your vagrant imagination or trying too hard to hold your focus.

• Then let your attention flow up to your head and face, and silently repeat, "My face feels cool." This thought will direct blood flow away from the head and face out to the extremities, a signal to the body and mind to become increasingly relaxed. Again repeat this phrase three times. You might imagine a cool breeze blowing over your face from the ocean or from the mountains.

• Finally, let your attention flow down into your right arm and hand, and silently repeat, "My right arm is heavy and warm," three times. At this point you are physically relaxed and mentally alert. In order to make this state of quiet increasingly easy to achieve, it is helpful to take a mental picture of your position and the feelings of heaviness and warmth, so that the overall posture becomes clear and familiar. It is like creating a map of how to get to a familiar destination; the more you visit this place, the easier it becomes to find.

• Ending is as important as beginning. The duration of this exercise can range anywhere from two to fifteen minutes and will usually lengthen as you practice. Take a deep breath, and as you do, raise your hands up toward your chest. As you exhale, stretch your legs, stand up, or do whatever you want in order to feel how good it is to move after sitting still for so long.

All of us differ in our ability to relax, and the help of a trained therapist is always useful in monitoring progress and determining at what point to move on to the next step. Nevertheless, the sensations of heaviness will be very real to you when you are doing the exercises correctly; they will tell you that you are mastering the practice. The exercise sounds deceptively simple, but it can result in a pronounced positive effect upon your entire body and mind.

DIRECTING THE MOVIES OF YOUR MIND

Practicing this relaxation technique from three to as many as fifteen minutes a day is an effective means of creating a time to be free of the usual distractions and unexamined, automatic reactions to both inner and outer challenges. Increasingly you will find that it is easier and quicker to enter this state of physical relaxation, that you can remain still and undistracted for longer periods of time, and that your state of calm continues long after you conclude the exercise. All of these are indications that you are ready to move on to the next, more subtle step: quieting the mind. Many people in the interviews indicated that just focusing on such simple body sensations as heaviness, warmth, breathing, or heartbeat is enough to bring the mind to a gentle, undistracted, clear focus. Other individuals focus on a word, such as *peace*, or repeat a favorite phrase, poem, prayer, or mantra. No matter what your actual practice, if you still your mind and body, you become more sensitive and attuned to your own responses and choices.

Your time in a mentally alert, physically relaxed state can then be used in a productive manner. All too often we respond automatically to problems and challenges without even considering alternatives. The time available during periods of quieting the mind and body can be used to rehearse alternative thoughts or actions prior to actually having to carry them out. For the majority of individuals in my study this rehearsal involved envisioning actions different from their usual, habitual responses. One film producer referred to his skill in this area as "directing the movies of your mind." That is a most apt description; however, it need not be experienced exclusively in visual terms. A businesswoman participant in the study would enter a period of physical quieting and then "script" or imagine the specific words she and another party would use in an upcoming conversation. She would rehearse this discussion in very specific detail right down to the last sentence that she imagined the other person would say. She said that the actual negotiation would often progress with the other person saying exactly the words she had imagined. When she heard those words, she knew with certainty that the negotiation would prove successful.

Seeing visual images in the imagination may sound esoteric, but it is literally a second-by-second occurrence we experience every day of our lives. For many years I have used a one-second exercise to demystify visualization. Close your eyes and open them when you know the number of windows in your living room. How did you do it? For virtually every person the answer is the same. They "saw" their living room and "counted" the windows. That is visualization, and if you can do that, then you can practice the mental rehearsal of alternative, positive thoughts and courses of action to achieve optimal health.

There was only one time when this demonstration did not work. In the winter of 1990 I visited Moscow, Leningrad, and Tbilisi as part of an ongoing Soviet-American exchange program. Following one of my lectures in Moscow, the topic of subjective visual imagery arose, and I asked the audience of over three hundred very serious Soviet scientists in their black suits, white shirts, and black ties to try to visualize and count the windows in their living room. Much to my surprise they burst into highly uncharacteristic laughter. My translator leaned over and informed me, "They are not laughing at you, but we all live in state housing, so we all have only one window!" To which a bilingual Russian surgeon in the front row added, "Yes, and they are all the same size!" Although these Soviet scientists had some trouble with the concept of visualization, the participants in my study had none. The interviews revealed that for all of these individuals, rehearsing alternative responses and behaviors through visual imagery was a simple and effective strategy in their lives.

Here is an excellent four-step visualization that serves as a starting point for, or enhancement of, a person's ability to initiate positive choices. Start this visualization once you have become comfortable with sustaining a state of physical relaxation.

• As you enter into your state of relaxation, start to imagine a place, preferably outdoors, where you feel perfectly safe and where you will be undisturbed for as long as you like. This can be a place you knew as a child or a place you like to visit on vacation. It can be real or imaginary. Allow this place to become as vivid and real as possible. Starting with your visual sense, look out toward the horizon, then scan to the left and to the right. Ask yourself details: What time of day is it—morning, noon, evening, or night? Is the sky clear blue or cloudy? Are you in a deep and cool forest, an open field of golden grasses, on the edge of the ocean standing in the sand? Then have your other senses come into play. Using your sense of touch, let yourself feel whether the air is warm and balmy, as on a summer day, or cool and crisp like New England in the fall. Let yourself smell the scent of flowers, the dampness of the earth after a rain, or the pungent salty smell of waves rolling in from the open ocean. With your ears hear the birds singing, leaves rustling, waves crashing, or the cascading rhythm of a waterfall. There might even be a sweet taste in your mouth from fruit trees, or the tingling you get on your tongue after a thunderstorm in the desert or the high mountains. Wherever you choose to be, allow that place to become as real as possible through as many senses as possible. Take a few minutes and just enjoy being in this place where you feel perfectly safe and undistracted.

• Now look out in front of you about ten feet, and you will notice that the air is shimmering like heat radiating off a highway, creating the illusion of water. As you watch, the shimmering becomes a solid screen. What you can do now is to ask for an image or symbol of anything you want to change to appear spontaneously on the screen. It can be an image or fragment of an image or an abstract symbol of a psychological problem, a physical disease or disability, or a skill you wish to improve upon, anything from perfecting your tennis serve to composing music with more fluidity. Simply ask for an image to appear and it will. If the image seems contrived, then let it change, or if it seems that you forced a particular image to appear, then let it transform. If it appears to be odd or not obvious, that is fine. Just look at the image without judgment or criticism and take a few minutes to examine the details of whatever you are seeing. Sometimes a headache appears as a jagged red line or evenly knotted ropes, as in a television commercial. Whatever you see is fine; there is no "right" image. Let your other senses also come into play. The image may be accompanied by discordant music, a sense of cold or heat, or even a particular smell. Simply observe what you are seeing for a few minutes and suspend analysis or judgment for the time being.

• After a few minutes ask that the image be transformed in a positive way. This change will not necessarily be immediate, but it will be a beginning. You might notice that the jagged red line representing a headache becomes a soft blue cloud or that discordant music becomes a familiar, favorite symphony. Whatever change takes place, simply observe the transformation for a few minutes without judgment or analysis. After two to three minutes allow the image to fade and then allow the screen to fade as well. Acknowledge to yourself that a positive change has been rehearsed, that other alternatives are possible, that the change is real, and that you can return at any time to rehearse other alternatives or to complete and enhance the outcome that has just occurred.

• Finally, find yourself back in the place where you began. You might look around and notice that colors or sounds are more intense than before. Someone or something might be present or absent from the first scene that you envisioned. Take note of such details, but primarily take a few moments to enjoy being back in this familiar place. How you conclude this visualization is as important as how you began it. Just as in the general relaxation exercise, take a deep breath, draw your arms up toward your chest, and as you exhale, stretch your arms out over your head and open your eyes. Again, you might want to stand up, stretch, or move around after sitting still for so long.

You may want to record this relaxation and visualization strategy on tape and listen to your own voice guiding you, or you may want to have a friend read it aloud. There are many similar techniques available in books and on audiotapes, and there is no one right approach. What is most important is that you choose a method that appeals to you, that you practice this method, and that you apply it in your everyday life. Don't worry about finding that perfect method or dogma. There is a virtually infinite number of ways to open your heart and mind through relaxation techniques, prayer, meditation, and selfless service to others, to animals, or to the environment. The point is to quiet the body and mind enough to be able to get in touch with your higher self. Although seemingly simple, these two strategies—one physical, the other mental—are a significant first step toward establishing an inner state of balance and mental equanimity. In that place of quiet, one can examine, experience, and choose from among many possible thoughts and behaviors. With this quiet contemplation and experimentation, we enable ourselves to create—and feel—a more profound integration with people and the world at large.

JOURNEY OF A THOUSAND MILES

Over twenty-five hundred years ago Buddha achieved enlightenment, or awakening. His name is actually derived from the Sanskrit root *budd*, which means "to awaken," literally, to become aware of what was previously not known. To the extent that we remain unaware of our beliefs, attitudes, and self-imposed limitations, we are unconscious of their influence and of our other options. Unexamined beliefs, attitudes, and choices, both positive and negative, become calcified as habits. When we are awakened, we become receptive to alternate views of a situation and are able to choose what is the optimal alternative. To attain optimal health, we must be aware of our many options and choose only those that make us feel genuinely good.

We already know enough to take the first step to begin the journey of a thousand miles. But to choose a path of fulfillment, we must first look at where we are and where we want to go. That means facing the troubling questions that have been posed throughout this chapter: Why do so many rational people with access to health care still engage in personal and environmental practices that are risky and even life-threatening? Why do many health care workers continue to smoke? Why does an obese person continue to overeat? Why do we not use seat belts every time we get into a car? Guns, too readily available, are a main cause of the alarming increase in violent deaths; why is legislation delayed even thirty years after the assassinations of President John F. Kennedy, Martin Luther King, Jr., and Robert Kennedy? Do motorcyclists and bike riders not know how vulnerable they are when not wearing helmets? Does anyone doubt the value of a low-fat diet or the malnutrition of junk food diets? Why do women not conduct breast self-exams or have appropriate mammographies? Is exercise so onerous that despite the overwhelming number of television exercise programs and local YMCAs, regular exercisers remain a minority in our population?

Questions such as these virtually defy explanation. Certainly one factor is the debate between self-interest and the common good. Our own United States Constitution, strengthened by the Bill of Rights, ensures the protection of individual rights against undue infringement in the name of the common good. How this vital balance or creative tension is resolved in daily life is infinitely complex. Courts are constantly called upon to settle such disputes, and the pendulum swings depending on the current political climate.

Health issues are profoundly influenced by our historical and cultural legacy of individualism versus the collective will. Misplaced fixation on the narcissistic aspects of health—trying to achieve the perfect body through unduly restricted diets and cosmetic surgeries—is an extreme of individualism. Even health is a means, not an end in itself. Every individual I interviewed subscribed to this view. The following guidelines represent a summary of common approaches they employ in their ongoing process of moving toward optimal health. These can be broken down into six steps:

• Choose a particular area of interest or a nagging problem you'd like to solve or a habit you'd like to change. It can be smoking, drinking, or being more attentive to someone you love, but choose a specific area and decide exactly what you want to try to do about it. It is best to pick an easy problem or challenge first and then build on your success. Stating a problem too generally, for instance, "I'd like to fix my marriage"—is not a good starting point. Be more specific: for example, "My wife and I argue about money," or "My husband watches too much television." Also, be sure the problem is something you really want to change. Ask yourself if the problem is easy enough to start with. One helpful strategy is to write down the problem and define specifically the details of the current situation. Remember that one of the common characteristics among individuals in my interviews was their ability to be blunt about their own shortcomings, problems, and challenges.

• Consider the challenge and how you currently behave or react, both psychologically and physically. When you are faced with this problem, do you react physically? Do you breathe faster, get sweaty palms, cold hands, muscle tension, stomach upset, or a general feeling of fatigue? How about psychologically? Do you find yourself thinking that you have tried this before and failed? You might experience self-defeating thoughts—"I'm so stupid," or "Why can't I get things right?" or "I must be crazy to do this," and even "I am never going to learn my lesson." Write down how you react to the problem you have chosen to resolve. Note both your body's reactions and those of your mind.

How do these reactions affect your behavior? One way to find out is to complete the phrase, "When I am faced with this problem, I . . . ," followed by "smoke more," "drink too much," "lose my temper," "become anxious," "use drugs," "become violent," or "go off to be by myself," or whatever it is that you do. Be as honest and specific as possible, because resolving the problem requires a clear acknowledgment of how you truly react.

At this point you have the critical opportunity of handling the situation by taking charge. This literally means identifying and accepting the problem as well as your own reactions and feelings to it and about it. You now have an opportunity to ask the vital question, "What can I really do about this situation or problem?" And then, "Is my current way of handling the situation making me feel better or worse?" followed by, "Is my present reaction improving the situation or not?" Once you have honestly asked and deeply pondered these questions, you will have reached the fulcrum point of resolution.

• Physically, it is important to suspend your usual, habitual, and perhaps negative responses. Such reactions as a headache, cold or sweaty palms, or pain can distract you from the behavior you are trying to change and can distract you from your commitment. At this point it is very useful to practice a physical relaxation strategy such as the one described earlier. Remember that although there are many techniques, there is no one right approach except the one that feels right to you. Through practice you will begin to notice that your automatic, habitual reactions to the problem will begin to diminish. You might notice that you do not immediately feel hungry when you experience intense stress, or that you do not feel sudden fatigue at the thought of exercising. These are indications that you are beginning to suspend your previous, unexamined, habitual responses, which may have been making your identified problem worse rather than better.

Practice the relaxation technique until you can enter into this state comfortably and relatively quickly and remain undistracted by annoying physical sensations, such as an itch or muscle spasm, for five to ten minutes. This ability is beneficial in and of itself because it prevents the occurrence of negative physical responses, but more importantly, it clears your inner being to be more sensitive to new influences and sensations. Overeating dulls the sense of what one particular food feels like in your stomach; reducing the compulsive urge to eat can allow you both to taste and to feel how a particular food affects your digestion, mood, or energy level.

• After mastering the physical relaxation, you can begin to rehearse different ways of reacting. Once you are free of the old, automatic physical and psychological responses, you will see more alternatives and possibly better solutions. Think about it: What could you say differently to prevent an argument with your spouse or someone at work? Rehearsing specific alternative behaviors is a safe means of practicing new skills. Such physical relaxation and visualization strategies are used by everyone from Olympic athletes to CEOs of major corporations. They are applicable to any problem, no matter how trivial or formidable.

When practicing the four-step visualization exercise outlined earlier, you will literally see yourself thinking and behaving differently. There is no audience, no panel of judges other than yourself, no questions asked and no explanations needed. Very often during such visualizations you will see the humor in a situation that had become deadly serious, or have a sudden insight into another person. You may even find yourself delightfully surprised by a creative and novel solution to a supposed impasse.

• Try out the new attitude or behavior and see how it works in real life. For example, go out and exercise even if you are a bit self-conscious. Talk honestly and openly with a colleague with whom you have had a problem. Try eating a bit less or drinking less but enjoying the taste more. Decide to organize neighbors into a street watch to reduce crime or start them on a recycling program. No matter what you have rehearsed, you will find that you will modify and refine your new, more positive attitude and behavior every day.

Perhaps most importantly, you will be engaged in life with a new physical and psychological sensitivity, freed of negative, habitual, unexamined responses and behaviors. You will be sensitive to precisely what allows you to choose among vying options; you will literally feel what is right for you, whether you're working on diet, interpersonal relations, or a commitment to a greater cause for humankind. Surely you will take much of your past with you, but you will do so with a new appreciation because your view of the past will have been released from negative beliefs, attitudes, and assumptions. You can use this process to address all of the problems or challenges you can identify, all the while continuing to build your own personal strategies for optimal health.

• Finally, move beyond the self and give to other people, to animals, and to the environment. As was expressed by every individual in my study, health is a means of feeling good personally, of course, but it also fills us with the desire and energy to give back to our families and our communities. Get involved with your children, family, friends. Volunteer with programs for youth, the disadvantaged, homeless, or elderly. Help restore the environment with a recycling program or by planting a tree or two.

It is out of this service to others that we must profoundly experience what Professor John W. Gardner of Stanford University has termed the "resilience of the human spirit." Writing in *The Recovery of Confidence*, he sagely observed, "I speak for . . . an optimism that does not assume it has found a cure for all of life's ills, that recognizes the deep, intrinsic difficulties of social change, that accepts life's often unfavorable odds—but will not stop hoping, or trying, or enjoying when it's possible to enjoy. . . . There is the resilience of the human spirit. Hope runs deeper than intellectual appraisal. We were designed for struggle, for survival. Only fatal and final injuries neutralize that irrepressible striving toward the light. Our conscious processes—the part of us that is saturated with words and ideas—may arrive at exceedingly gloomy appraisals, but an older, more deeply rooted, biologically and spiritually stubborn part of us continues to say yes to hoping, yes to striving, yes to life." That is, ultimately, the essence of optimal health.

CHAPTER SEVEN

Doing Well by Doing Good

Love Is Feeding Everyone (LIFE) was started by the actors Dennis Weaver and Valerie Harper with several concerned Los Angeles community leaders in 1983. Initially the program provided food directly to four hundred people on a daily basis; now it feeds over sixty thousand people every day. Community action and empowerment is the basis for this food recovery and distribution project, which gathers food from area supermarkets, produce outlets, food drives, and bakeries and distributes it to social service centers, churches, and organized neighborhood groups through centers in South Central and East Los Angeles. Even amidst the rioting and destruction following the Rodney King beating trial, the program remained a beacon of hope for the hungry and homeless. Beyond the immediate focus on the hungry of Los Angeles, the LIFE program has received national attention as a prototype for similar community programs throughout the United States; it offers a training film and manual for other organizations interested in duplicating its success. In 1986 Dennis Weaver received the Presidential End Hunger Award and remains highly active in virtually every phase of the organization's growth and service.

Why would a successful actor at the height of his career turn down several lucrative roles to dedicate himself to feeding homeless people? Surely it seems atypical for an actor to defy the notorious self-indulgent narcissism of the entertainment industry, which was depicted so well in *You'll Never Eat Lunch in This Town Again* by Julia Phillips. Counter to this all-too-accurate stereotype, Dennis Weaver's career has been characterized by his strong, outspoken commitment to supporting world peace, drug abuse prevention, global ecology, and the battle against homelessness and hunger. Reflecting on his charitable work, Weaver said, "I guess I have always been one of those people who was service-oriented. I believe it really is more blessed to give than to receive. . . . I've been involved in several other hunger projects in the past, but nothing that's been this satisfying. We know that there are people all over this city who need food, but we have to take it one step—and one meal—at a time. I don't get too overwhelmed by what this program might become because I'm primarily concerned with what it is that we are doing *now*. And the things that keep me going are the genuine thanks I see in people's eyes and the fullness I feel in my heart.

"I have made many career decisions based solely on my personal values. They may not have been in the best interest of my career development or my checkbook, but the decisions were right for me ethically. I turned down a lot of things that were overloaded, in my view, with sex for the sake of it, with no redeeming dramatic qualities or purpose. I feel the same about violence, and I have simply chosen not to do those types of projects. It wasn't always easy to make those decisions. At one point in my career, in the seventies, I had just started doing *McCloud* and it became really successful. I got a lot of offers to do big-screen films, but I just couldn't bring myself to do them. At the time I thought, Why should I? I'm making a good living at television, and television seems to have some standards that coincide with my values. I don't believe that my values were ever an impediment to success. . . . My values are at the core of who I am and what I feel my life is about. They have given me confidence, balance, and a kind of calmness, which allows a sharper, heightened creativity within me. Certainly this approach to life has contributed greatly to my health.

"To be able to be on television and to reach and communicate with people is a powerful thing which I never take for granted. Art in its various forms, whether in film, television, or radio, is a key factor in the shift in consciousness that I see coming. Right now I am forming a producers' unit with John Denver and three others. Of course our first priority is to create a project that entertains and satisfies people, but we also want to say something important without preaching. We want to create important pieces through the dramatic interplay of people and characters. For example, one of the scripts I'm working on takes place in a rain forest. . . . Our films will challenge the audience to examine their personal and spiritual beliefs and attitudes. They will communicate that until we change our attitude, until we change our priorities, until we change our feelings, we will not change our behavior. And they will invigorate the audience with a palpable sense of how satisfying and rewarding it can be to do good on a greater scale—beyond your individual circle of family and friends."

Altruism, the ability to value and pursue another person's well-being as an unselfish goal, is a hotly debated phenomenon. Both Freud's psychoanalysis and Skinner's behaviorism assumed that people were ultimately capable of caring only for themselves. Today many sociobiologists, including Dr. Edward O. Wilson of Harvard University and Dr. Richard Dawkins of Oxford University in England, assume that people are genetically predisposed to be "selfish" in order to ensure their survival. However, even with this deterministic model, the sociobiologists concede that although genetic encoding may instruct people toward selfishness, they are not compelled to obey such directives. Given the complexity of the debate, it is impossible here to thoroughly outline, much less resolve, the conflicting positions. What is relevant to this chapter is the increasing evidence that altruistic behavior is an inherent trait of humans and other animals, even insects. There is an extensive body of research revealing that helping behavior toward others, sometimes at the cost of the helper's life, is found among insect colonies, birds, dolphins, porpoises, wild horses, African elephants, and virtually every animal species. Both anecdotal evidence and research have documented selfless concern for the welfare of others as predominant among humankind as well. Although we have a history of barbarism, cruelty, and unmitigated violence, there is no evidence that these behaviors are more prevalent than altruistic behavior.

As reported in *Science*, the compelling research on twins by Dr. Thomas J. Bouchard and his colleagues at the University of Minnesota indicates that behavioral factors ranging from "reaction time" to "religiosity" have a strong genetic basis. Among the many contemporary researchers refining the parameters of human altruism are Dr. C. Daniel Batson and his colleagues at the University of Kansas. Batson asserts that developing "empathy" for other people is at the heart of altruism and that such empathy can be learned and taught. He says that altruism appears to be an inherently powerful motivation that manifests itself in "our helpful acts, ranging from numerous small kindnesses and favors that we do for each other every day to the great acts of self-sacrifice of the Albert Schweitzers and Mother Teresas." It is in this sense of active empathy that the participants in the Sound Mind–Sound Body study exhibited an unequivocal and abiding commitment to altruism.

All of the participants in my study clearly attributed their success

and health to a higher or spiritual sense of inner values. Only three
expressed their spirituality in terms of adherence to an orthodox religious system, although all but one grew up within a traditional religion. One individual had a quotation from Pierre Teilhard de Chardin
on his desk that read: "Someday, after we have mastered the winds,
the waves, the tide and gravity, we shall harness for God the energies
of love. Then, for the second time in the history of the world, man
will have discovered fire." Every interview revealed some degree of
profound altruism or an abiding desire to be of direct service to other human beings. Building upon the compassion and forgiveness they
gave and received within their own personal social support systems,
these people moved beyond this network of immediate family and
friends to serve their fellow companions.

In San Francisco Dr. Meyer Friedman has concluded that by and
large the impatience, hostility, and all-consuming drive of some human beings result in a deadly absence of spirituality. According to
Friedman, spirituality does not mean having specific religious beliefs
but comprises "a basic concern for human relations and other interests that enrich life: As de Tocqueville stated in 1835, "Americans
want to get it all right now. And they start squeezing, getting greedy
for acquisitions, pretending that death doesn't exist. . . . as for getting spiritual sustenance from friendship—I don't believe they think
of that very often." To be of service to others may or may not be the
antidote to the isolation and anger leading to heart disease, but it is
certainly an inviting alternative. The desire to serve others is not a
mere belief or philosophical abstraction; it is a positive and sustaining drive toward a greater purpose in life.

Looking back at his two childhood years in a tuberculosis sanato-
rium, Norman Cousins articulated his sense of a greater purpose:
"There was never any doubt in my mind that I would survive. But
there was also the need to give thanks for my good fortune. At that
early age I discovered that philosophy was not just a matter of asking
where you came from, or what life means, but how you justified the
gift of life."

Surely such a sense of altruism and purpose is consistent with our
own highest self-interest, for it helps to free us from limitations, isolation, and loneliness to embrace greater challenges. This giving back
to others through service is a theme that pervaded the interviews in
a range of variations—the previously mentioned LIFE program of
Dennis Weaver, Walter Landor's Creative Arts Center, the anthropo-
logical research support of Gordon Getty, and John Tishman's educational fund. Each individual, in his or her own way, has moved

beyond the self to a fulfillment derived from genuinely humanitarian actions.

COMPASSION IN ACTION

Altruism is an expression of personal spiritual values, which have to do with finding the purpose and deepest meaning of life. This deeply personal, nonsectarian quest or spiritual journey is the underlying thrust of the world's great religions. It has also been a recurring theme in literature throughout the ages, as in the New Testament's powerful passage on "charity" from Paul's letter to the Corinthians, the epic of *Gilgamesh, The Canterbury Tales, Pilgrim's Progress, Don Quixote, Heart of Darkness* (and its film derivative, *Apocalypse Now*), and the classic *Siddhartha*, to name just a few. In our own era the release of films such as *Star Wars, Resurrection, Dances with Wolves, The Natural, The Milagro Beanfield War*, and, of course, *Field of Dreams* is a testament to the broad appeal of such powerful spiritual statements. Altruistic actions that arise from our quest for universal ethical principles constitute the sixth and highest stage of moral development as that development is formulated in the writings of Dr. Lawrence Kohlberg of Harvard University.

By asking people of different backgrounds and ages how they would respond to problems involving moral dilemmas, Dr. Kohlberg found that their answers fell into six systems of judgment, on which he based his six stages of moral development. All individuals begin with "concern about self" at stage one. But some individuals progress through increasingly higher levels of moral awareness until they reach the sixth stage, where universal ethical principles are addressed.

Kohlberg asserts that, for the most part, the "most important ethical principles deal with justice, equality, and dignity. These principles are higher than any given law." An ethical principle is different from a rule or law in that it is general, for example: All persons are created equal. By contrast, a rule is specific: Thou shalt not kill. One of the most famous statements of universal, spiritual ethics was formulated by Martin Luther King, Jr., in his "Letter from the Birmingham City Jail." In an often-quoted passage, King challenges the clergymen of the city:

> You express a great deal of anxiety over our willingness to break laws. This is certainly a legitimate concern. . . . One has not only a legal but a moral responsibility to obey just laws. Conversely, one has a moral obligation to disobey unjust laws. . . . To put it in

terms of St. Thomas of Aquinas: an unjust law is a human law that
is not rooted in eternal law and natural law. Any law that uplifts
human personality is just. Any law that degrades human personality is unjust.

Taking a moral stance requires deep introspection and honesty. It
can often require a willingness to challenge the status quo at great
personal sacrifice, although that is not always the case and is not a
requisite for the true expression of spiritual values and altruism.
Whether or not personal sacrifice comes into play, an abiding self-
knowledge, honesty, and the courage to engage in compassionate action are necessities.

Insights derived from spiritual quests are frequently experienced
in transient moments of intensity, termed "peak experiences" by the
late psychological pioneer Dr. Abraham Maslow. According to
Maslow, these peak experiences include many but usually not all of
the following characteristics: "an almost overwhelming sense of pleasure, euphoria or joy, a deep sense of wonder or awe, feeling in harmony or at one with the universe, altered perceptions of time and/or
space, a deep feeling of love, greater awareness of beauty or appreciation, and a sense that it would be difficult or impossible to describe
adequately in words." Such an experience transcends specific tem-
poral, cultural, geographic, or religious boundaries. Organized religion attempts to structure, rationalize, and claim exclusive ownership
over the spiritual experience by establishing a creed or set of beliefs,
a set of rituals and an authority, and often by intervening between the
individual and his or her direct experience of the spiritual.

One of the most scholarly yet engaging considerations of this ancient dilemma is *The Gnostic Gospels* by the Harvard University the-
ologian Dr. Elaine Pagels. With the clarity and precision of a
historian, Pagels describes the process by which the early Church
consolidated its doctrine, accepting some writings for inclusion in
what became the New Testament and declaring others heretical, including those that have become known as the Gnostic gospels. These
writings are a remarkable collection of thirteen leather-bound pa-
pyruses and loose papers that were eventually found in Nag Hammadi
in the upper Egyptian desert in 1945 when a farmer accidentally unearthed a large pottery jar that had lain buried for over sixteen hundred years. This discovery revealed manuscripts written at the time
of the New Testament gospels and then translated from Greek to Cop-
tic, which was the common Egyptian language of that time. Gnostics,
the authors of these manuscripts, viewed themselves as mainstream

Christians, not heretics. They differed from the Church in believing that spirituality was an inner experience, not an intellectual doctrine. However, their view did not lend itself to the hierarchical structure in which salvation could be achieved only through the authority of the Church bureaucrats, who demanded obedience and the tithing of increasing amounts of property and money to the Church, which in turn grew more and more powerful. Today this very emphasis upon the direct, transcendent spiritual experience has made Eastern philosophies appealing to many individuals who have become disillusioned by the hierarchies and bureaucracies of organized religion and the role it claims as an intermediary to the divine.

Considering organized religion's response to the AIDS epidemic, the Reverend Richard Dunphy, a Jesuit priest, has stated, "Organized religion can be even more susceptible than other human enterprises to a variety of abuses, because in religion one can be tempted to justify prejudices by appropriating the power of the holy. . . . When spiritual needs do surface, they may be dismissed as either irrelevant or oppressive, or they may be ignored out of fear of an anticipated rejection or inappropriate response by a representative of organized religion." Certainly the numerous scandals and abuses of the public trust by television evangelists have illustrated a compelling contrast between spiritual values and organized religion. The participants in my interviews clearly exhibited their values and altruism in spiritual rather than religious terms. However, this is not to assert that spiritual and religious values are inherently antagonistic, since the three individuals who do adhere to an organized religion found their personal spiritual values and those of their religion to be synonymous.

An ethical lifestyle does not protect us from pain and suffering. In the biographies of not only Martin Luther King, Jr., but also Mother Teresa of Calcutta, Gandhi, and Albert Schweitzer, the emotional pains and scars are evident. Indeed, they are a part of daily experience. Spiritually awakened individuals are not spared loneliness, emptiness, hopelessness. In her many interviews with reporters and visitors Mother Teresa has said that she felt like an empty vessel, a limp rag, alone, and even miserable. For many years Schweitzer also acknowledged that only at quite rare moments had he felt glad to be alive. He felt with a "sympathy full of regret" all the pain that he saw around him, not only that of humankind but of the whole of creation. However, it seems that what allows these modern saints to tolerate, perhaps even appreciate, the ordeals and sufferings they witness is their conviction that there are no higher or richer spiritual meanings to be detected in life than those found in the daily struggle to be of greater service to the world. In effect, the transformation of despair and emptiness into hope and meaning is the ultimate purpose in life, at least for them.

Perhaps it is such an action-oriented spirituality and altruism that will provide an antidote to the narcissistic fixation on the most superficial aspects of health. Empathy for—and assistance to—the more than 37 million people in the United States who have no health coverage is our most serious health challenge. These millions are predominantly women, children, and the elderly, with racial minorities disproportionately represented in all of these categories. A culture lacking empathy is one that slashes billions from essential programs for children, adolescents, and families while poverty rises and infant mortality and morbidity rates are among the highest of any modern nation. Homelessness and child abuse mount, mental and physical health suffer, chemical dependencies and AIDS continue their grim rise. Paralleling this social decay is the ongoing deterioration of the environment as the rain forests are destroyed, the park lands are deforested, tons of carcinogenic agents are pumped into soil and drinking water, and global warming becomes a reality. A willingness to rise to such challenges is one of the most striking characteristics shared by all the participants in my study.

Although politics, the environment, and spiritual values may seem like an unlikely fusion, their mix is what drives United States Congresswoman Claudine Schneider. As the youngest member of the United States Congress, Congresswoman Schneider is rapidly emerging as a moderate voice within the Republican party and an outspoken advocate of the environment. Growing up in a small town in Pennsylvania, she was raised as a Catholic but her parents "didn't talk about religion at home. We went through the motions of going to church on Sunday, but it was religion as opposed to spirituality. As a result, I was taught the basic aspects of the Catholic religion, such as Don't lie, Don't cheat, Don't hurt people. The Ten Commandments were all rote. Through the years I began to understand the real essence of the meaning behind those man-written words."

Her concern for environmental health arose out of her childhood experience. Reflecting back on her early surroundings, Congresswoman Schneider remembers, "In this small town, near Pittsburgh, where I lived, there was a cokeworks for coal processing. The sky was often orange at night, and the air was always sort of funny-smelling. As a young girl I used to think that everybody in the United States had to dust their house every day. That was my daily chore as a little girl. . . . It wasn't until I moved from Pittsburgh that I realized that the sun did actually shine and there was a pure and clean environment. When I developed cancer at age twenty-five, I wondered if there was any linkage to my childhood environment. It was quite clear that it had been detrimental to my health—the strange smells I was inhaling, and perhaps the water I was drinking. Who knows what? Eventually I started thinking about the linkages between my spiritual values, my health, and the environment. . . . In the seventies we talked about not killing the fish from a naturalist point of view. But in fact, we are killing ourselves. All parts of our ecosystem are interconnected. We have a responsibility, not only to other human beings, but also to the trees, the plants, the water, the animals, and everything else. My philosophy is like the sign in the National Parks—leave the park better than you found it. Now I feel that way about the whole earth. We have a responsibility here that we should leave this planet a little better than we found it."

This living philosophy of empathy and action has been reflected in the environmental protection policies sponsored by Schneider, who frequently stood alone among Republicans against first the policies of the Reagan administration that undermined environmental protection, and then against the hypocrisy of George Bush's refusal to sign virtually every major environmental policy statement at the 1992 Earth Summit in Rio de Janeiro. Difficulties that arose from Congresswoman Schneider's childhood gave her an empathic regard for others, which in turn generalized her concern to global issues.

In the majority of the interviews environmental issues were consistently cited as a critical area in which participants were either directly or indirectly involved. Compassion in action often means undertaking to look beyond individual needs and beyond the boundaries of nations and continents. Nobel Prize–winner Dr. Murray Gell-Mann, with his characteristic super-vision, has embodied this quest by leaping from his established field of expertise, the realm of subatomic particles, to the ecological diversity of the Brazilian rain forest. Throughout his illustrious career he has sought and discovered basic laws and general structures that describe and predict the behavior of subatomic particles. In 1952 he discovered the quality called *strangeness.* He has actually described his moment of discovery as occurring during a lecture at Princeton when a "slip of the tongue" in an equation he was presenting led him to a major insight about the "strange particles" he had been studying. Then in 1961 he proposed the *eight-fold way* classification scheme for organizing elementary particles. Later he proposed *quarks* and *colored gluons* as the fundamental constituents of strongly interacting particles such as the neutron and proton.

In describing his search for underlying order amidst complexity, he has observed, "We seek two basic principles that underlie all of physics and chemistry. One is the unified theory of all the elementary particles (the constituents of all matter in the universe) and of all the forces among them. . . . No matter how we try to describe the universe, through scientific research, through artistic recreation, or through appreciation of its beauties, it exhibits a wonderful interplay of simplicity and complexity." It is with this same outlook that Gell-Mann studies the interrelationships of biological diversity.

With a genuine humility and a notorious wit, Gell-Mann has pursued his lifelong interest in conservation and bird watching with the same passion as his brilliant career in physics. In addition to his position as professor of theoretical physics at Caltech, he is also a director of the John D. and Catherine T. MacArthur Foundation and chairman of its World Environment and Resources committee.

During my interview with him in his Caltech office, Gell-Mann reflected on the values underlying his passion for finding and preserving the "simplicity amidst the complexity" of global ecology. Looking back to his childhood, he noted, "I became a passionate conservationist at the age of five or six. My brother and I used to watch the disappearance of the wild areas around New York City. We were united by our hatred of [New York City Parks Commissioner Robert] Moses. Nowadays people write books about him in which they point out his flaws as well as his virtues, but at that time there were very few people who realized that paving the entirety of New York was not the best thing to do—that maybe leaving a swamp a swamp and not turning it into a playground might be a good idea. I was also sensitive to the problems of overpopulation; it seemed to me, even at that early age, that the world was getting filled up with too many people who were treading too heavily on the planet. I was a premature conservationist. . . . It was not until 1969 that I formalized the role. That year I was asked to be a member of the President's Science Advisory Committee, but unfortunately the president was Nixon. Regardless, it was a time when the environmental movement was really gathering a lot of political steam, and it seemed like a time when I could make a difference in this direction. I tried to set up a panel on environmental populations, but the political impositions of Nixon's henchmen on the members of the panel were a problem. After his first term he didn't want science advice anymore and finally dissolved the committee.

"Now I am the chairman of the Committee on World Environmental Resources, concerned with world environmental problems and also specifically with the conservation of biological diversity in the tropics and the associated problems of conservation science. A main focus is on sustainable economic development for the people who live in the vicinity of areas which contain precious biological diversity. Obviously these indigenous people must be brought into a position where they have a strong political and economic stake in the success of conservation. Today anybody who is smashing a road through some primitive area that shouldn't be disturbed claims to be doing "sustainable development," so a new concept—ecodevelopment—has been invented, the basis for which is that development activities bring local rural people into the game of conservation so they understand its value and have a real political and economic stake in its success."

On a recent bird-watching trip to the mountains of Mexico's southernmost state of Chiapas, Gell-Mann was pleased to see evidence of his basic philosophy in the form of an action-oriented and effective plan for preserving the ecosystem while enhancing the lives of the local population. Although he traveled to the region to observe its tropical birds, he left with greater hope about people and their interaction with their environment: "There are communal farms, or *ajillos*, around the base of the mountain range, and the people are learning about the value of protecting the watershed. Disputes arise about the altitudinal boundaries of the forest reserve, but apart from that, the people are enthusiastically in favor of it. Farmers have stopped killing the animals in the reserve and are limiting their coffee plantations to avoid encroaching on what they consider to be its boundaries. Now they are even supplying guides for people who come to see the wonderful animals, trees, and plants in the reserve. They will get some local funds from that. Also, they are supplying help to parties who want to go into the forest, as in the case of our party, which required twelve horses and several guides with assistants. Part of the effort is environmental education for the local people, but equally important is giving them a tangible economic stake in the outcome. These two goals are often synergistic. Thus, the people are helping themselves and the world at the same time."

ALTRUISM: BEYOND "SELFISH GENES"

Under the auspices of the Institute of Noetic Sciences in Sausalito, California, there are several ongoing research projects on altruism.

Predominantly funded by Laurance S. Rockefeller, they involve researchers at several major universities as well as innovative social organizations and representatives from Europe. To grasp fully the development and implications of compassion in action as an integral part of optimal health, it is important to understand this new and very promising area of research. In studying such complex and elusive phenomena as altruism, compassion, the health benefits of service to others, and similar positive emotions and behaviors, it is difficult if not impossible to confine them prematurely to the traditional research methods of control groups, longitudinal designs, and statistical analysis. As in any new domain of inquiry, these methods may prove to be appropriate at a later time. Despite their absence, there is a robust and insightful body of research that enriches and provides a context for a more complete understanding of the Sound Mind–Sound Body interviews.

Late in 1991 I was invited to attend a weekend-long meeting convened by the Institute of Noetic Sciences to exchange papers and ideas with other researchers in the area of altruism and its development. Among the first issues addressed by the group was the complexity of agreeing upon a working definition of altruism. There are essentially two schools of thought. One contends that true altruism entails no benefit to the individual, while the opposing view holds that the provider can and inevitably does benefit personally from his or her altruistic behavior. With virtual unanimity we discovered that all our independent research findings clearly supported the latter definition, and that is the basis from which we proceeded.

Among the most insightful findings were those presented by Dr. Anne Colby and Dr. William Damon of Brown University. Their studies focused on "moral exemplars," individuals whose beliefs and behavior exemplify the highest moral ideals of their day. These are individuals whose work and examples exert a profound influence upon others in their lifetimes and often beyond. As I did in my research, Colby and Damon attempted to determine how these individuals formed their patterns of moral beliefs and conduct over the course of their lives. The researchers hypothesized that a developmental approach would permit them to examine the dynamic interplay among altruistic issues they chose to address. Also parallel to my study, their research was based on clinical interviews, or case studies. They interviewed twenty-three men and women who were working in communities on a national level. Among the selection criteria for the participants were a sustained commitment to altruistic ideals, a disposition to act in a manner consistent with those ideals, a willingness to risk or sacrifice self-interest, an ability to inspire others, and a genuine humility. After formulating these initial criteria based on the limited previous research in this field, they depended upon expert referral to help them identify and select appropriate candidates for the interviews.

Probably the most important similarity between Colby and Damon's study and mine is that we made the same vital assumption: moral commitment to a lifestyle of compassion in action is normal in the sense that it is a basic drive inherent in people and able to be developed, though it is not usually exhibited to a great degree in most people. The only qualitative distinction between the study participants and other individuals is in the degree of expression of this basic drive. Furthermore, and perhaps more important, this commitment can be learned, elicited, and enhanced in the case of any individual, under even the most negative circumstances, as was illustrated in both their research and in my own.

Each of the researchers at the symposium had taken a slightly different approach to altruism, and therefore there were nuances of variation in selected populations, methodology, and outcome. Colby and Damon focused on people who had sacrificed personal gain and social position to serve their altruistic calling. My approach, in contrast, deliberately chose individuals who remained explicitly involved in their careers, in order to determine the extent to which their altruistic values determined and were impacted by the demands of their work. Despite this difference, the elements the Brown University researchers identified from their interviews and proceeded to analyze were remarkably similar to the pervasive themes that arose from my interviews with an entirely different group of people.

Conducting their study over three years, Colby and Damon found "striking similarities that cut across the very diverse group of people we studied. All of these similarities derive directly or indirectly from the phenomenon of unity between personal *moral goals* and the centrality of these goals to the individual's sense of self. . . . Among, the most striking cross-cutting themes are a certainty of belief, i.e., a lack of self-doubt or inner conflict in acting on their beliefs, a relative lack of concern for possible dangers or negative consequences, the absence of their having a sense of their own moral courage, *a positive attitude toward life* and *a deep enjoyment of one's work.*" All of these characteristics are consistently found among the individuals in my research as well. A number of findings were unanticipated. The researchers had expected to discover that the altruists had struggled with their own conscience or sense of social duty and that their consciences had finally won out, but that was not the case at all. In every instance those interviewed actually denied any sense of moral courage. It "*meant little to them*. It seemed that they did not see a 'choice' in the matter—that is, they wouldn't seriously consider doing otherwise. This was a striking finding, since many of these people had indeed placed themselves in danger by living out their values." There was a sense of certainty, not choice, in discovering their true purpose.

Consistent with my research, more than half of the participants in Colby and Damon's study were not religious in any traditional way but reported a sense of a spiritual mission in their charitable and altruistic work, a mission that transcended them and their immediate surroundings. Actually, Colby and Damon found that the hardest subject for their interviewees to discuss was their faith, spiritual beliefs, and motivations. Consistently they denied the significance of the particular form or denomination of their faith, even when they were involved in a traditional religious order. Instead they emphasized that the form of their spiritual values was simply the words, symbols, and rituals they used to communicate to a particular community of people. Spirituality was inherently not reducible to a particular organized religion. Taking both studies together, these are individuals who do not theorize about morals and a life mission; they act in ways that are not encumbered by excessive forethought, reflection, or hesitation. They deliberately engage other people and address the issues of the moment in a direct, hands-on manner. It is this real-life interaction that refines their beliefs and commitments, rather than an abstract ledger of checks and balances. These are individuals who are deeply involved in direct social engagement with other people.

Overall, Colby and Damon concluded that "in their explanation of their life decisions, moral exemplars . . . tend to offer justification based on actions, events, or circumstances rather than on generalizations or abstractions." This is quite different from the popular conception and theoretical literature, which assume that such individuals continually refine their internal beliefs before they arrive at a resolution and act. In the real world, that does not appear to be the case.

Research findings from Drs. Colby and Damon also reflected the Sound Mind–Sound Body themes of personal control, commitment, and an abiding sense of purpose. For the moral exemplars and others there is little if any discrepancy between their beliefs and their actions. In effect, there is a marked unity of self in thought, word, and deed, and a remarkable lack of denial, compartmentalization, or similar psychological defenses. Clearly these are individuals who embody the polar opposite of the disease- and mortality-inducing risk factors of isolation, hostility, and loneliness. According to the Brown University study, there is a "unity between personal and moral goals, a close relationship between one's moral convictions and one's sense of self, and a deep certainty and lack of conflict about one's moral beliefs. . . . It is as if they believe that their actions and situations speak for themselves, so there is no need to make explicit the values or principles underlying their moral choices." Throughout Colby and Damon's interviews there were many stories of how the moral exemplars drew their inspiration and guidance directly from other people, organizations, or specific causes. Very often they cited instances of significant mentors or role models, including parents, grandparents, teachers, or ministers, who provided support and inspiration during childhood traumas. Although the Brown University researchers did not elaborate upon this finding, these interactions appeared to be a vital formative experience for the moral exemplars. Paradoxically, these leaders portrayed themselves as followers!

Although the individuals in the Colby and Damon study were not nationally recognizable, there have recently been numerous examples of concerned individuals finding themselves so devoted to resolving major social issues that they were literally thrust into prominence. Andrei Sakharov, the Soviet dissident, was thirty-eight years old before his contact with dissidents awakened in him a deep sense of mission. His specific concerns over nuclear proliferation broadened into the greater humanitarian issues of freedom of speech, Jewish rights, and world peace, with which his name is now synonymous. During his acceptance of the Nobel Peace Prize he commented that he had been "pushed by others" to express his conscience. Similar statements are a matter of long-standing record for Sir Laurens Van Der Post with his concern for the Bushmen of the Kalahari; Lech Walesa in his dedication to the freedom of Poland and all of Eastern Europe; and Bishop Desmond Tutu, whose voice for peace was heard above the violence of apartheid. Clearly these are individuals whose conviction, moral commitment, and sense of purpose are consistent with their actions and extend far beyond the issues of personal fulfillment and even safety.

Finally, the interviews by Colby and Damon are consistent with the developmental aspect of my interviews in that they indicate an overall, long-term stability of the participants' inner values and commitments. The altruists' goals changed, under the influence of a few significant people, later growing to embrace even greater humanitarian issues. These individuals are unflinching self-critics who are unerringly truthful to themselves and those around them. It is this clarity that keeps their inner commitment alive. By acknowledging their own limits, shortcomings, and problems, they develop a quality of understanding and compassion that enables them to communicate with and inspire others in remarkable ways.

At the symposium Colby and Damon made one last observation. Although their study had not addressed any specific questions about mental or physical health, they did consistently note that the interviewees appeared to be in excellent health. This was particularly striking, as these men and women ranged in age from their early sixties to mid-nineties and were living in less than optimal circumstances. Together our independent research projects lend support to the premise that doing good for others is beneficial to the giver.

FOR LOVE AND PROFIT

Commitment to altruistic values and compassion in action is not only *not* antithetical to success, it may in fact *determine* that success. We need not journey to an underdeveloped country to express and behave in a manner consistent with our deepest convictions. In fact, it was in the domain of business enterprise that many of the individuals in the Sound Mind–Sound Body study translated their spiritual values into social action. Although altruistic behavior is all too frequently lacking in the quarterly earnings myopia of most businesses, there are notable exceptions.

At the time of his interview James E. Burke served as chairman of the board and chief executive officer of Johnson & Johnson, the world's most diversified health care company. During his leadership the company's worldwide sales grew from $2.5 billion to over $9 billion annually. Above and beyond his management responsibilities Burke issued a challenge to his company in 1977 to "become the healthiest employee population in the world." As a result of that challenge Johnson & Johnson developed an internal health promotion and disease prevention program called Live for Life. This successful program became the core of yet another company in the Johnson & Johnson family; it now markets its program to other companies under the name Johnson & Johnson Health Management, Incorporated. Today Burke continues his leadership on a national level as chairman of the board of the Partnership for a Drug-Free America. One of the best-known and most dramatic media messages from the Partnership was the image of an egg ("This is your brain"), which was then dropped into a heated frying pan ("This is your brain on drugs"). He also serves on the board of directors of IBM and the Prudential Insurance Company and is a member of the Trilateral Commission.

Known as an intensely private man with strong family ties, Burke eschews the label of "visionary" and focuses on the expression of simple, traditional values. When as a young man he first considered entering the business world, he was reluctant because he was not sure that he could retain his personal values and still do well in business. Looking back at his early decisions, he stated, "Actually, I went through a period in my life when I wasn't sure I wanted to be in business. My brother-in-law talked me into going to Harvard Business School, and that was a very big turning point in my life. Ironically, business school reaffirmed a lot of my own values. I realized that my values wouldn't get in the way of being in business, rather that they would affirm my success. Like many people I had this idea that you really cannot be honest and be in business. Where this belief came from I have no idea, and I am mystified by the fact that I carried it with me. One of the great interests in my life has been to try to reaffirm the importance of basic values to success. I am lucky that I came to Johnson & Johnson, because even though I found a lot of those same values at other companies, it was not to the same degree that I found them here.

"As I began to think about health, it seemed to me that television was an extraordinary opportunity to change the way in which the health care system would function. So I went to the president of the general executive committee and said to him, 'Why don't you buy a television station?' I suggested we then hire health managers, just like we have product managers: one would be in charge of diabetes, and so forth, and they would bid for the unused, unsold time available on a station, of which there was a great deal in those days. We would use the station to try to maintain wellness, to keep people from getting sick, or to promote early intervention. This was a long time ago, so while it was not really an original idea, no one had yet conceptualized it quite this way.

"Now while I was doing that, I was also thinking about the company and its future, and it seemed to me that Johnson & Johnson was going to change and grow for two reasons. One was that the public was now going to be getting more information about their own health and, as a result, take greater charge of it. And technology was about to explode, and the marriage of the two would provide the right syn-

ergy for a totally different Johnson & Johnson company. I then draft-
ed a document setting a goal for Johnson & Johnson to be the healthiest company in the world." Reframing the mission statement of a
major international corporation is not only unusual, it has proven essential in the "managed health care decade" of the nineties.

Building upon his experience with that first television station and
his growing interest in community involvement, Burke carefully
tracked and evaluated the initial programs for impact and cultural
change. Among his first targets was smoking: "I don't know at what
point I really got interested in preventing drug abuse, but I was interested in smoking cessation from the very beginning. Remember in
the early seventies, when many people stopped smoking because of
the anticigarette advertising? I had a five-year-old child who would
tug at my jacket after watching those commercials. So finally I gave
up smoking!" Burke then became convinced that drug usage in America was out of control when someone close to him became addicted
to prescription drugs.

"When we began the program, nobody was doing anything about
drug abuse and nothing was happening in the way of advertising."
Following a bitter dispute with the national Advertising Council,
Burke and several colleagues decided to form the Media Advertising
Partnership for a Drug-Free America. "In the midst of all of this my
brother, who is now a president of ABC, called me and said, 'We just
bought ABC, and somebody at work yesterday overdosed and
dropped dead. What do we do?' I told him about our internal program
at Johnson & Johnson, since by now it was considered a highly sophisticated approach. I was astounded by how little people in business knew about the problem, how epidemic it was, and how serious
it became. Finally we gave a big presentation to the Business Council, and I remember the chairman of Philip Morris politely suggesting he was going to sue me because I said that cigarettes were as
addictive as heroin."

Those challenges only spurred Burke to fulfill his mission of service to others—a mission far beyond the necessity of ensuring high
stock earnings for his Fortune 500 company. Just before my interview
with Burke, he had presented to then-President-elect George Bush
the results of his media campaign, which showed that the Partnership
for a Drug-Free America had been an integral part of preventing drug
abuse, as it still is today.

Burke's efforts continue to focus on helping communities organize
to prevent drug abuse and enhance overall health. In his extensive me-

dia campaigns, as well as his work with students, parents, community leaders, and the police, he emphasizes restoring healthy community values and creating jobs. Among the many influences upon Burke's thinking about communities and work sites are the Stanford Three-Community Study and Five-City Project conducted by Dr. John W. Farquhar and his colleagues at the Stanford Center for Research in Disease Prevention at the Stanford University School of Medicine, which will be detailed in chapter 8. In yet another in the series of convergences in Burke's foray into altruistic domains, both he and Farquhar received the Dana Foundation Award in 1991 for extraordinary achievement in public health.

Another notable altruist who is addressing society's crises through his business is the publishing executive, author, and poet James A. Autry. Acting from his firm belief that business should be socially responsible, he is in the process of implementing a national program for the homeless to be sponsored by his magazine *Better Homes and Gardens*. With his typical, inspiring enthusiasm, Autry exclaimed, "It is an abiding conviction that I have that the good companies, the companies which are going to succeed in the nineties, are the companies that realize they've got to provide an environment in which people feel fulfilled spiritually and personally, as well as financially. I mean companies where people can grow, where they're empowered to do their work. Selfishness is not congruent with the new workplace. People can overcome selfishness through interpersonal, relational activities, and altruistic programs. We all need to support programs for people who are outside a workplace, like the homeless program I have envisioned.

"Picture this: all over the country, the great middle and upper-middle class of home-owning American families helping the homeless. Families with homes helping families without homes. It can be terrific! There are thirty-seven million readers of *Better Homes and Gardens*. They have their own church campaigns, their own programs and charities, so why should they send money to us? Subscribers to *Better Homes* are not a club or a family, although we like to think of them that way. . . . They are our customers: we supply a service, they pay for it. Why should they sign on to help the homeless? Well, there's some mystical one-to-one connection between editors and the readers. I know that. My belief in that relationship leads me to believe they will respond.

"We should all be asking each other what we *really* care about. Business has taken a bum rap; I am very sincere in this conviction.

Business has taken a terrible rap, because in reality, business has done a lot of good things. Businesses seldom display it, because most are afraid that the stockholders will say, 'What the hell are you spending my money like that for?' So we're reluctant to blow our own horns and consequently have been attacked by the press, politicians, and consumer groups for being socially irresponsible. Obviously there are plenty of businesses which are not responsible. But if there's a quid pro quo, I want someday, maybe five years or seven years from now, for someone to get a subscription solicitation in their mailbox and say, 'Oh, *Better Homes and Gardens*. They're the people who do that wonderful homeless program.' Will I ever be able to measure that? No. But if we succeed in building transitional housing and funneling this money to the homeless by having these intervention programs, then my belief is that everybody associated with the company, everybody, is going to be so proud, they won't care how to measure it. They'll measure it by the way they feel."

That same motivation was also expressed by David Rockefeller. Although most recognized for his role as chairman of the board and chief executive officer of the Chase Manhattan Bank from 1969 to 1980, the story of his involvement with the business community, the arts, international politics, and urban renewal could fill volumes. Just to show the span of his interests, in international affairs he helped found the highly influential Trilateral Commission in 1973 to promote understanding and cooperation among the nations of North America, Western Europe, and Japan. On the domestic side he founded the New York City Housing Partnership, which is engaged in the large-scale construction and rehabilitation of affordable housing for moderate-income families. In the balance between his business and governmental activities is a deeply ingrained commitment to philanthropy through his work with many foundations, including the Rockefeller Brothers Fund, founded in 1940.

From a purely historical perspective it is astounding to realize that he worked with and knew on a personal basis such influential leaders as Nikita Khrushchev, Anwar Sadat, King Juan Carlos of Spain, Pope John Paul II, Helmut Schmidt, as well as United States Presidents Kennedy, Johnson, Nixon, Carter, Reagan, Bush, and Clinton. During the eighties, his youngest daughter, Eileen Rockefeller Growald, founded the Institute for the Advancement of Health, which focused serious attention on the field of mind-body interactions in health and disease. From the founding of the Institute, I served on her board of directors. At one of the board meetings at their family estate in Tarrytown, New York, a most insightful toast was offered by Norman Cousins, also a longtime personal friend of the Rockefeller family. Cousins said that perhaps there were families in the world with greater wealth and influence, but that no one family other than Rockefeller was known for great wealth used with such responsibility and compassion.

David Rockefeller is particularly clear about attributing his values to the examples set by his parents from the time he was very young. His father, John D. Rockefeller, Jr., had devoted his life to philanthropy in direct opposition to the ruthless business practices of the eldest Rockefeller, John D., Sr., the founder of Standard Oil, who himself turned to philanthropy in later life. David recounted his personal philosophy: "Basically, I was influenced by my parents, who stressed by implication that with opportunity goes responsibility. They always taught us that we should give ten percent of what we had away and save ten percent. So my brothers and I all established little savings accounts. We kept track of what we spent and gave at least ten percent of our allowance to church or other charities.

"Now, I have no doubt that one derives more satisfaction from doing things that are beneficial to others than from just doing things to promote one's own hedonistic pleasures. Not that I don't enjoy doing things for myself. But I think if it were a principal part of my life, I would soon tire of it. Doing something that is beneficial in some sense to mankind or to a cause gives you a greater sense of satisfaction."

During a luncheon address in New York City in 1988, David Rockefeller reflected on the health benefits of altruism and the hazards of its absence: "We have all experienced the good feeling that accompanies a gift of charity or public service or participation in a cause that assists our communities in some way. Do we experience something akin to the release of beta endorphins when we act in philanthropic ways? Is this part of nature's way of ensuring that we help our fellow man and also keep ourselves healthy? I do not know the answer to these questions, but I do think that the evidence that we have, mostly intuitive, tends toward a positive response. I have known a great number of people with large fortunes who have not used their resources very constructively. Almost without exception they have been extremely unhappy. On the other hand, there are many people who have much less in the way of financial resources, but who give of themselves generously and are both happy and healthy. I believe that this is much more than chance or coincidence."

NOT EVERYONE IS FAMOUS FOR FIFTEEN MINUTES

Not all those who live lives of compassion in action are well known or ever become known because of their efforts. Achieving recognition should be neither the goal of the individual nor a criterion for altruism. However, it is increasingly clear that a vital and overlooked aspect of optimal health is our capacity to care about others and to act on their behalf. An often-cited definition of this expression of altruism is "a regard for the interest of others without concern for one's self-interest." That definition is often interpreted as precluding the individual from receiving any benefit from the benevolent actions, and is sometimes even seen as including such great sacrifice as dying for another. These latter cases may be considered instances of altruism, although there are arguments that attribute what appears to be a purely self-sacrificial act to self-destructive behavior, guilt, miscalculation of risk, and suicide. What is most unfortunate about equating altruistic behavior with extremes of self-sacrifice is that it does a disservice to the individuals and organizations that may derive considerable benefit from their service to others. Such service is clearly compassion in action.

To date there has only been one matched group study of altruistic individuals. Over the course of several years the anthropologist Dr. Christie W. Kiefer has studied a group of altruists in the Human Development and Aging Program of the University of California School of Medicine in San Francisco. To select his participants, Kiefer stated two criteria: "(1) consistent unselfish concern for the well-being of strangers or for humanity at large, over a long period of time, and at considerable cost or effort; and (2) no obvious or serious character flaws, such as extreme vanity, self-destructiveness, poor reality orientation, or social unreliability." He then sought the names of individuals who were recognized to fit these specific criteria within their community, state, or, possibly, nation. Names were gathered through expert referral, as in the Colby and Damon study and my own. Through this process Kiefer identified twenty people whom he termed "natural altruists." In a unique dimension to his study, he then searched through the life histories of 216 people who had been interviewed for a life stages study at the University of California. After reading through these cases, he selected twenty individuals who matched the twenty natural altruists in age, religion, personal beliefs, values, social activities, ethnic background, education, and everyday behavior. Such a matching group is obviously not a true control group, nor is this approach a true experimental design, but its quasi-experimental approach did yield a basis of comparison between altruists and less prosocial people.

Surprises that occurred in the interviews add an even more subtle and intriguing dimension to the phenomenon of compassion in action. For instance, the accepted sociocultural theory proposes that individuals develop altruistic behavior out of a stable nuclear family. That was certainly not the case in my interviews, and Kiefer found that at least seven, approximately 30 percent, of his "natural altruists" reported significant childhood trauma, including sexual abuse, automobile accidents, or death of a parent. Both studies found, however, that the occurrence of a traumatic event is *not* as important as how the individual responded to it. This observation was confirmed by Kiefer's finding that six of the sixteen controls he was able to follow for the entire length of the study, or 40 percent, came from families that had been disrupted by divorce, death, mental illness, alcoholism, or other serious problems. Consistent with my research Kiefer found that the traumatic event was "transformed" into a positive experience through the help of an early childhood mentor. Eleven of the twenty altruists reported having parents or surrogate parents who "could be described as idealistic, and the young altruists absorbed a strong social conscience from them." By contrast, only five out of the control group reported such role models. Parents clearly played a role in the development of the early antecedents of compassion, but the individual's own response to trauma or challenge within such a social support system appears to play the more decisive role.

Teaching compassionate values to children is undoubtedly positive, but it need not be the parents who do the teaching. Providing a warm and supportive emotional atmosphere for the growing child is actually more important, and a combination of the two is most beneficial. However, it is extremely important to reiterate that the absence of one or even both of these influences does not doom an individual to isolation and impaired personal growth. In fact, during my interviews slightly over 75 percent, and in Kiefer's interviews over 60 percent, had successfully managed to transform their childhood trauma without external guidance or support.

Delving into early childhood experiences, Kiefer found, as I had, that the father played a major role, whether his influence was positive or negative and whether the altruist was male or female. Kiefer elaborated on this unusual finding in noting, "A remarkably high proportion of altruists—40 percent—had unusually close relationships with warm fathers, although only one described her mother in positive terms." Their fathers were not necessarily strong or powerful figures but were often described as warm or supportive. Several individuals in both studies suffered the death of their influential fathers at an early age, but the positive influence remained intact. In fact, Kiefer concluded, "Having no father appears to be better than having a cold, distant, noncommunicative, domineering, fear-inducing father." In contrast to the altruists, eight of the sixteen controls, or 50 percent, described their fathers in such negative terms as "cold," "angry," and "strict." This finding concerning fear is unique to the Kiefer study, which found that the altruists exhibited an unusual lack of fearfulness of or sense of threat from other people, both as children and adults, despite significant trauma caused directly or indirectly by others.

Perhaps it is this lack of fear uncovered in Kiefer's study, or in more proactive terms, the deep sense of purpose, commitment, and control that was evident in my interviews, that permitted the individuals studied to be open to new ideas, accept challenges, and enter into novel and demanding circumstances, both as children and adults. Interpreting his findings, Kiefer stated one conclusion that is completely consistent with my own observations: "All of the outstanding altruists were deeply curious about their environment, and questioning of things they did not understand. They seemed to have the uninhibited curiosity of healthy children and their thinking tended toward the highly unconventional. The non-altruists, by contrast, seem much more concerned with controlling their economic and social destinies—with winning approval from their parents, families and/or peers, or with steering clear of people and beliefs whose influence might lead to a loss of security and comfort. . . . The most important finding is that altruists are somehow able to integrate the emotional and the intellectual sides of their personalities, so that their behavior is not only *realistic*, that is, effective and socially admirable, but also *autonomous*, that is, coming from deeply felt convictions." This abiding and unshakable sense of purpose in life in general and in their lives in particular is a compelling dimension to optimal health.

At the developmental level the optimally healthy individuals in my study literally do not recall a sustained period of time in their lives when they were particularly confused, angry, resentful, isolated, or lacking in a strong sense of purpose or an inner strength and conviction. Through the transformed trauma of their childhood or adolescence, these individuals "discovered" a sense of their "true mission," "real vocation," or "destiny" usually in their mid- to late twenties. Often this discovery was accompanied by a sense of inevitability and a renewed, deeper commitment to the altruistic purpose they had sensed more vaguely as a child or young adult. Occasionally the discovery occurred during a period of crisis, or through a powerful but transient period of alienation, or within a spontaneous internal moment of insight or "enlightenment." The youngest participant in my research articulated this reinstatement of purpose most succinctly.

Surely the death of both parents during childhood is the most traumatic event possible in a child's development. At the time of our interview twenty-eight-year-old Michael S. Currier was the youngest member of the Forbes 400. The great-grandson of Andrew W. Mellon, Currier was six in 1967 when both of his parents died in a private airplane crash. Yet he has clearly attained a profound equanimity about his loss and transformed that tragedy into a sense of a higher purpose to his life. By anyone's appraisal Currier is an unusually modest, thoughtful, and honest individual. He recalled, "Sometimes an unhappy childhood gives you a lot of anger. I guess I had anger. Yet even without my parents, I seem to have discovered my own ideas and vision of ethical behavior through the people who raised me. As a child I had an uncanny sense of truth and integrity. From a very early age I had a serious code of ethics that I wouldn't breach.

"Sometimes from a negative experience you can become cynical, pessimistic, or bitter, but I chose a different path. Honestly, I don't know how I came out of that traumatic experience intact, and I do not take credit for it. It seems it was just meant to work out that way. That is my faith—that God or the universe said, 'Michael, you're gonna have your karma, bad karma, early on. We are giving you a big dose of it early. Then at about twenty or twenty-two you are going to learn about money, because you have a responsibility to use the money that has been given to you. That is your purpose.' " Through his philanthropy and by directing major investments into socially responsible and environmentally protective companies, Currier remains true to his convictions.

A fifty-two-year-old concert pianist in the Kiefer study went through a similar progression of early life difficulties followed by an altruistic adulthood. He had undergone a period of negative but transient alienation, which led him to study occult religions at age fifteen. It was not until he was an accomplished pianist at age thirty that he rediscovered the sense of vocation that he had previously, only dimly perceived. When he was asked to give a concert at a psychiatric hospital, he experienced, in Maslow's phrase, a peak experience. Suddenly he saw all of the parts of his life up to that time fit together in an intelligible pattern, accompanied by a sense of truly rediscovering the altruistic purpose to his life. Immediately and without reservation he passionately threw himself into developing a program of free concerts and plays for social outcasts, prisoners, psychiatric patients, and other shut-ins. When asked by Kiefer if his altruistic behavior required discipline, he responded, "Not so much a discipline, but a belief system that one is here for a reason—to achieve a certain amount of perfection before one can progress out of the world to a higher perfection. It's not seeking sainthood; it's more like a Buddhist concept—how you go about your business, what your karma is, and how you come to grips with it."

In analyzing his study and considering such statements, Kiefer developed a classification system to describe varying degrees of altruistic behavior. At one extreme were people who deceptively, both to themselves and others, portrayed themselves as having such values in order to win approval and respect. At the other, positive extreme he noted that individuals like the concert pianist were "rebels." For him such people were "in many ways, the most interesting group. . . . The rebels underwent powerful transformative experiences in latency or adolescence, which alienated them from their families and communities. All went through a period of more or less severe maladjustment, out of which they emerged in their twenties, having discovered their altruistic avocations in further transformations. The most intense personalities in the study were some of the most successful altruists."

Perhaps because one of the criteria for selecting my participants was prominence or achievement in their field, it appears that the vast majority of these individuals share many of the developmental characteristics of Kiefer's "rebels." I point out this similarity not to classify or categorize prematurely these individuals, but to note a significant developmental pattern of transformative experiences. This preliminary observation supports the findings of other case studies of altruism and optimal health, especially those of Dr. Abraham Maslow. Maslow believed that full moral maturity is achieved following the integration of a person's needs for security, intimacy, and social approval. It appears that the positive transformation evident in the individuals from my research was accomplished by liberating the emotional energy that had been previously bound up in a childhood trauma or challenge. During that process a sense of life's purpose, destiny, and altruism appears to be indistinctly perceived by the child or young adult. In the mid- to late twenties, the individual experiences an event—either positive or negative—that rekindles and reinstates the altruistic sense into a deeper and more profound adult expression of compassion in action.

Throughout the literature on moral development there is a hypothesis that the integration of an individual's intellectual and emotional life leads to a sense of self-confidence. Dr. Lawrence Kohlberg's pioneering work in identifying the six stages of moral development stresses the importance of such an integration in order for a person to attain the highest levels of moral achievement and expression. That hypothesis is clearly confirmed by the living examples of individuals in the altruism studies conducted to date. At the conclusion of his study Kiefer stated, "It is as though the achievement of awareness of one's internal states allows one to recognize those beliefs and actions that truly enhance life in the long run. Perhaps the most interesting fact about this is that such an awareness *always* leads to more altruistic behavior. I have yet to find an instance where personal transformation led to a *less* altruistic personality." What is ironic, though perhaps consistent with this sense of internal purpose, is that the actual expression of altruism may often be innovative, unconventional, and even controversial. Clearly the individuals in my research lacked the kind of lockstep inhibition and need for conformity that appears to bind the majority of people into conventional ways of thinking and living. By being less dependent upon the approval and direction of others, optimally healthy individuals hear and abide by their inner directives, not necessarily by the rules and mores of the collective society. One participant decried the excessive restraint of conventional thinking as typifying a "gray flannel brain" and defined his role as "challenging the conventional myopia and local customs" to provoke creative new insights and solutions. Such individuals are more willing to experiment with emerging values and new ideas, and to take considerable personal risks to enrich the lives of others.

"WHO ARE YOU GOING TO BELIEVE, ME OR YOUR OWN EYES?"

This quip from Groucho Marx perfectly encapsulates the fact that one need not take the reputed health benefits of altruism as a matter of abstract research data or even testimonials, but rather as personal experience. Although the vast majority of studies on altruism have not focused on specific health benefits, they have all parenthetically noted that the participants, although not absolutely free of disease or disability, were unusually vigorous or in unusually good health. The observation points to the possibility that altruistic behavior is directly related to optimal health. At the very least, having such an orientation surely demonstrates that there is a healthy way to have a disease and even a healthy way to die.

One of the best books to address the direct effects of altruism on health was written by a colleague and friend, Allan Luks, who is currently executive director of Big Brothers/Big Sisters in New York. With coauthor Peggy Payne he reported the results of a national survey on volunteers in his 1992 book, *The Healing Power of Doing Good*. The book formulated the concept of the "helper's high," which volunteers describe as a mental and physical sensation of well-being that they experience when helping others. The sensation was reported by over 95 percent of the survey respondents, equally by men and women. Volunteers who reported the sensation were more likely than other volunteers (and much more likely than nonvolunteers) to view their health as better than that of others of comparable age. It is interesting to note that nearly eight out of ten volunteers reported that these positive feelings returned, though with diminished intensity, when they remembered their helping activities. Luks also found that direct contact with people was the most satisfying form of volunteer work, and that helping complete strangers, rather than family and friends, appeared to be most conducive to the helper's high. Finally, there was a clear indication that commitment to serving a community and a personal expression of higher values through that service was of major importance to their health.

To be sure, there is little if any scientific research to demonstrate a causal link between altruistic beliefs and behavior and enhanced mental and physical health. Such a definitive role for compassion in action in optimal health remains unproven, but indirect findings from my research provide compelling preliminary support. In no way do I mean to rationalize or advocate such behavior for whatever personal health benefits might accrue. None of the individuals in my study, or in any other research, indicated that health was even a remote rationale for their behavior. In fact, none cited material security, wealth, conventional success, personal comfort, or desire for power or recognition as motivations. As I have noted, my study participants appear to live their lives in a manner consistent with the generic doctrines of the world's great religions, although the vast majority do not express their beliefs in terms of the tenets of any organized religion. That emphasized, let us make a brief foray into the growing body of research that points to both direct and indirect benefits of spiritual values and altruistic behaviors as an integral aspect of optimal health.

Baby boomers, entering middle age in the mid-eighties, entered into new positions of prominence and power. One dimension of their lives that has undergone profound transformation is the spiritual. In the first large-scale study of boomers' spiritual values, Dr. Wade Clark of the University of California at Santa Barbara surveyed four-teen hundred people by random polling in Ohio, Massachusetts, North Carolina, and California. Writing in *A Generation of Seekers*, he found that two thirds had dropped out of their orthodox faiths dur-ing long periods of alienation due to Vietnam, political assassinations, the civil rights struggle, and Watergate. However, he found that these individuals were returning to more unorthodox, hybrid, spiritual ori-entations to life not necessarily expressed through traditional reli-gions. He found that the individuals fell into five groups: loyalists, returnees, believers-but-not-belongers, agnostics, and seekers. Two of his groups, the believers-but-not-belongers and the seekers, are most similar to individuals from my interviews. More than 28 percent were believers-but-not-belongers, who indicated that they were spir-itual but not involved with organized religion. Nine percent were seekers, who asserted that their spiritual life flowed from their own direct experience of the spiritual. These people tended to be older, politically liberal, in more nontraditional marriages, morally liberal in tolerating different lifestyles, as well as more situational than rigid in their ethics and more concerned with self-fulfillment. Seekers are disproportionately inclined to practice various forms of meditation as well as to espouse beliefs in psychic phenomena and reincarnation. Although they may participate in groups for support, they follow their own unique path to spiritual fulfillment. Overall, Dr. Clark conclud-ed that boomers are not as secular and materialistic as is often as-sumed. Although many are antireligious, they are deeply spiritual and committed to a rediscovery of deeper values and altruistic service.

Consistent with the concern to redefine the aphorism of "healthy, wealthy, and wise" is a book entitled *The Pursuit of Happiness* by the social psychologist Dr. David Myers. Based on his research, Myers concluded that happiness is not related to wealth, not specific to any age or gender, and not even dependent on physical wellness. While good physical health was associated to some degree with greater sat-isfaction, he found that students disabled by illness were as happy as their physically able peers and that a health crisis could be emotionally transcended, leaving a deeper sense of fulfillment. Even the most tragic of physical injuries or illnesses did not necessarily inhibit a sense of personal happiness or delight in living. Myers concluded that personal happiness depended on more than physical health and defined optimal health in terms of a life fully lived. From his review of research studies and other sources, he concluded that a happy person is likely to have many friends, be married, and have a spiritual orientation to his or her life. He also found that happy people seem to spend as much time focusing on the well-being of others as on themselves. Concluding his book, Myers noted, "Well-being is found in the renewal of disciplined lifestyles, committed relationships, and receiving and giving of acceptance. To experience deep well-being is to be self-confident yet unself-conscious, self-giving yet self-respecting, realistic yet hope-filled." From many perspectives there is a growing movement toward a more profound definition of health and personal fulfillment that looks beyond such physical deficits as debilitating illness or the declines of advancing age. For health professionals and others alike there is an imperative to incorporate the intangible values of spiritual life and altruism as well as biology into the new model of health.

Surely any consideration of such a complex and powerful issue as the relationship between altruism, spiritual orientation, and the health of individuals and social systems inevitably leads to a sense of awe and respect for what remains unknown and undiscovered. To illustrate the expanse of the frontiers yet to be explored, there is a definitive bibliography of over thirty-six hundred cases of spontaneous remissions from cancer and other disease documented in the world's medical literature, which provides evidence that individuals' beliefs play a pivotal role in the status of their health. This annotated bibliography was prepared by the late Brendan O'Regan and his colleagues at the Institute of Noetic Sciences in Sausalito, California, and can be ordered from that organization.

Ever since 1883, when Francis Galton asked, "Do sick persons who pray or are prayed for, recover on the average more rapidly than others?" there have been attempts to address this elusive phenomenon. A triple-blind study by the physician Dr. Platon J. Collipp, who was chairman of pediatrics at the Meadowbrook Hospital in New York, indicated that prayers on behalf of children with leukemia appeared to reduce mortality. By contrast, a double-blind study by two researchers from the London Hospital Medical College concluded that prayers offered on behalf of forty-eight patients with chronic rheumatic disease had no effect at all. Then there are the meticulous procedures and records of the International Medical Commission at Lourdes, France, which is charged with stringently evaluating supposed miracle cures. Twenty-five medical specialists from throughout Europe make up this commission, which has determined that only sixty-four of six thousand cases recorded since the 1860s actually constitute "miraculous" cures. Considering the strict criteria and evaluation procedure, it is surprising that there are any cases at all that are considered miraculous.

Interest in the relationship between spiritual values, altruism, and health is not limited to a few researchers or investigators of miraculous remissions. In the widely read journal *Medical Economics* one of the editors reported on the Christian Medical Foundation, founded by the surgeon Dr. William Standish Reed. This organization predominantly of clinical practitioners claims a membership of over thirty-five hundred individuals who consider prayer for their patients to be an integral part of their practice. For too many decades such practices as these have been overlooked, ignored, or even ridiculed. Given the consistently cited role of spiritual values and altruism in the health and well-being of so many individuals and groups, they are in need of further serious exploration.

YOUR SECOND FIFTY YEARS

For most of the Sound Mind–Sound Body participants altruism required many years to develop and reached full expression only in their middle years. Perhaps it is in mid- and later life, when the demands of career, child rearing, and economic security are resolved, that altruism begins to flourish and become even more important for individual health. Research by Dr. Ellen L. Idler of Rutgers University and Dr. Stanislav V. Kasl of Yale University has found that public practice of spiritual or altruistic beliefs, such as church attendance or involvement in community service, had positive health benefits among adults over age sixty-five. From 1982 to 1989 the two researchers studied a group of over twenty-eight hundred residents of New Haven, Connecticut, who were actively practicing Catholics, Protestants, or Jews. Overall, the actively involved people had a lower incidence of physical disability and depression, and the Christians and Jews had a lower mortality rate before their religious holidays compared to state averages. The researchers concluded that active involvement in religious practice and the community provides social contacts, optimism, participation in group rituals, and a sense of meaning in daily life as well as during crisis. Given the consistency of such findings, it is clear that altruistic behavior benefits the individual donor as well as the recipient throughout life.

Below is an outline of several recommendations, derived from my interviews as well as related research, for eliciting and sustaining an altruistic orientation. Surely the actual recommendations are deceptively simple: simple in that the steps are explicit and clear, but deceptive in the sense that understanding them is not the solution. The challenge is in taking action. Compassion in action is at the root of altruism. All of these actions take place in a community context, whether they concern a friend, an animal, a plant, family, geographic area, or the greater family of all humankind.

• Identify any cause that strikes you as important. It can be visiting an ill or disabled family member, developing a recycling program at your work site or in your neighborhood, or tackling a major social problem, such as hunger or homelessness. Know that you can make a difference. Speak your mind and get involved.

• Spend more time with people you care about and who care for you. Loving, unselfish dedication to one person is as great an expression of altruism as the attempt to resolve a major global crisis. Devote time to being of service to particular groups of people, such as children, the disabled, or the elderly. Very often altruistic individuals find their greatest satisfaction in working with those who need help the most.

• Volunteer in your children's school, local political campaigns, or fund-raising events for charitable organizations in any way that allows you to join together with like-minded individuals committed to a common cause. Best of all, try to find an activity in which your entire family can be involved.

• Join an environmental or animal protection organization. Consistently, the altruistic individuals studied cited their dedication to the environment and animals, as much as to other people, as eliciting and sustaining their sense of devotion to a greater purpose. Just consider the fact that the United States covers 1.5 percent of the earth's surface, has only 5 percent of the world's population, and produces 70 percent of the planet's trash and pollutants. Think about the beauty and wonder of the complex interrelationships between the earth, plants, and animals; then look at that delicate balance in the context of environmental pollution and the wanton killing of wild horses, dolphins, elephants, and other highly evolved species. This kind of awareness will inevitably lead to a personal vision beyond immediate and physical gratifications.

• Develop a self-care group for others who wish to work together on a common problem—alcoholism or child care, for example—or to share the enjoyment of a common interest like bird watching or walking. Sharing a common interest with others is an excellent way to gain a perspective on your own life as well as to relate to and understand the way other people see and respond to the world around them.

If there is any single compelling lesson to be derived from the altruistic orientation expressed in the interviews, it is to take any one step toward compassion in action. That one action, no matter what it is, will provide the most direct experience of the benefits of altruism. In 1990 the Dalai Lama received the Nobel Peace Prize in recognition of his lifelong advocacy of peace, even when confronted by the continuing cultural genocide perpetrated for decades by China on the people of Tibet. Perhaps no other world leader embodies compassion in action more than the Dalai Lama. Addressing a symposium on the relationship between compassion and health, he said, "Love and kindness cannot be regarded as a luxury. Even without religion we can manage, but without these it is difficult to find happiness and tranquility. . . . Sincere motivation based on compassion and love not only brings happiness and calmness to an individual but also affects the social environment. . . . Moreover, I think the reality of the modern economic structure is telling us that human beings need a genuine sense of cooperation and universal responsibility. The natural environment, the mother planet itself, is now telling us, her children to be careful. These indications are now very clear. So now the reality, the actual situation itself, is showing us the proper way to act and think. Much depends on the eradication of narrow-mindedness and self-centered thinking and action. Otherwise there will be long-term disaster. Lastly, I think we can develop a sense of universal responsibility provided we use the proper education of love and kindness." As the living voice of a two-thousand-year-old tradition of compassion in action, the Dalai Lama's exhortation might remain a matter of idle philosophizing if our survival as a species did not depend upon the answer.

CHAPTER EIGHT

Where There Is No Vision,

the People Perish

Alice in Wonderland queried the Cheshire Cat: "Would you tell me, please, which way I ought to go from here?" To which the cat responded with a smile, "That depends a good deal on where you want to go." Lewis Carroll's classic tale, a disguised treatise on formal logic, is brought to mind as the question of direction becomes a fundamental issue for both individuals and institutions as they confront the current crises in medical care. One unequivocal finding from the Sound Mind–Sound Body project is that optimal health is not attainable by plugging into a formula, nor is it an end in itself. Rather it is an inner attitude or lifestyle orientation that can be present in anyone at any age. In this new model, health may persist during periods of crisis and illness; a paraplegic may be healthy, while a superb athlete may be very unhealthy. This revision in our current model of health will have profound consequences on how we restructure medical care for the future, how we provide access for the uninsured, and how we care for the exploding number of the elderly. We cannot solve these problems under the "patch 'em up when sick" model. We need a new model of health that does not entail more medicine, more doctors, more hospitals, more drugs, or more money. We need an approach that involves us and empowers us, as individuals and institutions, to be integral and responsible participants in our own health, to help others who are less fortunate, and to help the nation as a whole.

Why do we even need to examine something so abstract as a "model" of health? Because our fundamental assumptions set our direction, as individuals and as a nation. Our beliefs establish our conscious and unconscious goals and are the basis for our day-to-day choices. These individual choices aggregate into group behaviors, which in turn result in this country's horrifying statistics on heart attacks, automobile accidents, AIDS, rape, violence, and the never-ending litany of disaster and death. Writing in the *Journal of the American Medical Association*, the physician Dr. Roger J. Bulger of the Association of Academic Health Centers in Washington, D.C., described the outmoded approach to health as a "Newtonian, reductionist, biomedical model, which emphasizes the understanding of disease and therapeutics at the molecular level. One gene, one enzyme, one protein, one disease fairly describes the overarching gestalt of modern medicine." Behind the heated debate on financing health care, the emotional confrontations concerning its rationing, and the political rhetoric, which usually protects the same staid and vested interests, is a fundamental lack of direction and vision. Before specific choices can be made, it is necessary to commit to a goal of health, rather than to the management of disease. By overcoming personal crises and becoming committed to health as a means to resolve the larger issues of our time, the actions of individuals in my research serve as prototypes of a health-oriented direction, one that can be adopted at both the personal and the national policy level.

Surely when the American medical system is good, it is very good. In August 1992 the noted health economist Victor R. Fuchs of Stanford University wrote an article in the *Journal of the American Medical Association* entitled, "The Best Health Care System in the World?" In addressing this question, he noted, "Americans enjoy the best health care system in the world. So says former President Bush, and many physicians agree with this claim. But frequent repetition doesn't make it true. What kind of evidence would an objective observer examine to evaluate different systems of health care? . . . the 'best' health care system may be like the 'best' spouse—it all depends on what you are looking for." Fuchs added that the United States is where the "super-rich from Third World countries go when they want high-tech medical care." Genetic engineering and biotechnology have literally revolutionized the practice of medicine and eliminated such diseases as septic shock, once the country's thirteenth leading cause of death. High technology imaging devices permit noninvasive diagnoses with unprecedented precision by providing clear, moving images of the brain and other internal organs. Advances in orthopedic surgery have yielded artificial joint replacements and new prosthetic limbs, improving the quality of life for millions of people. Pharmaceutical companies have developed new generations of drugs to enhance the immune system. Coronary bypass surgery has saved and extended the lives of many. These are indisputable achievements, and nothing that has been discussed in this book is intended to lessen or denigrate these triumphs.

Medicine bashing may be in fashion and is often justified, but there is no inherent contradiction between an emphasis on health promotion (as an individual and national priority) and appropriate medical care. Allopathic or conventional Western medicine is very good at managing trauma, acute bacterial infections, medical and surgical emergencies, and other crises. It is very bad at managing viral infections, chronic degenerative disease, allergy and autoimmunity, many of the most serious kinds of cancer, mental illness, functional illness (a disturbance in the function of an organ in the absence of major physical or chemical changes), and those conditions in which the mind plays an active role in creating susceptibility to disease. It is not wise to seek allopathic care for a disease that conventional medicine cannot treat. It is also not wise to resort to alternative practitioners when you have a disease that conventional medicine can treat very well. Determining what is or is not appropriate care and how we can strike a new balance between prevention and intervention is a hotly contested issue.

Before a direction can be determined and solutions implemented, it is essential to unearth the roots of the current crisis. From the results of my interviews and a growing body of other research, it is clear that health cannot be relegated to biological reductionism and that individual adaptation, as in the case of early life trauma, must be taken into account. Individuals, not statistics and technology, need to be restored to the forefront of our emerging model of health. We need to encourage people to adhere to guidelines for disease prevention while also making clear that there is no lifestyle, no matter how hedonistic, that assures disease. Conversely, there is no lifestyle, no matter how austere or virtuous, that assures optimal health and longevity. Winston Churchill's often-quoted quip, "Perfectionism spells paralysis," is applicable to any fixation upon personal health practices. By restoring a more balanced view of health, and by learning from healthy and highly functional individuals who share the traumas and diseases common to us all, we can move beyond mere biology toward psychological, emotional, and social responsibility.

This call for change presents enormous implications for the way that medicine is practiced in the United States today. America's disease management industry, which is huge and growing, would be substantially affected. More than 14% of the total Gross Domestic Product goes to support this "health care system," yet it is one of the least effective and least satisfying in the world, in terms of its ability to elicit and sustain health. There is deep dissatisfaction with the quality of the relationship between health practitioners and patients, as all too often patients are seen as a cluster of symptoms, not as human beings with complex psychological, social, and spiritual dimensions. Prevention guidance is negligible, and medical care costs continue to escalate out of control. More than 37 million uninsured Americans have little access to health services, particularly high-cost and high-technology interventions, such as heart bypasses, which are readily available only to the well insured or the wealthy. Stop for a moment and consider that number: 37 million people. It may be difficult to grasp the scope of that figure, which translates into one out of every seven Americans. According to a 1992 report of the U.S. Senate Democratic Policy Committee, this number is equivalent to the entire population of twenty-three states (including Oregon, Nevada, Arizona, Nebraska, South Carolina, Maine, New Hampshire, and Alaska, to cite but a few examples!). At the present time the only other modern nation that does not provide access to medical care for all its people is South Africa.

As costs continue to skyrocket, assuring more equitable access to health care has become an overwhelming problem. Changes in behavioral and lifestyle approaches would make the pursuit of health less expensive and more accessible, while promoting a way of life that is healthier for the individual and less damaging to the environment. At a time when the number of elderly people is rising dramatically, both in absolute terms and as a percentage of the total population, and chronic long-term illness is rising proportionally, health promotion holds the promise of improving the quality of life for the chronically ill and even providing effective treatment for a wide range of major disorders.

Health promotion and disease prevention also include nontraditional techniques ranging from meditation to environmental protection. These inexpensive and readily available practices return a great deal of power to the individual, who is no longer solely a passive recipient. In this respect such an approach to health care is very compelling. However, the threat it poses to vested interests within the medical, insurance, pharmaceutical, and hospital industries cannot be underestimated. A reorientation toward disease prevention runs against the grain of conventional medical thinking, and it will not be warmly received by many in the industry. Many medical practitioners are confident in their conventional physical treatments for illness. Moreover, the economic considerations will be of great significance to everyone.

Existing institutions have a stake in existing treatment strategies. A major industry, earning over $7 billion annually, has grown up around heart bypass operations. Another huge industry—pharmaceuticals—is oriented entirely to the medication of diseases. Some powerful insurers and licensing boards with important interests in the medical area would be inclined to resist health promotion intervention as they would be less able to limit the kinds of practitioners whose services would be reimbursable. They may also, however, offer some incentives for the wider use of practices that might reduce the number of days a patient spends in the hospital. These issues need to be carefully considered, and an effort should be made to encourage cooperation in making health the priority—a viable and acceptable one—in the medical care system overall.

Health promotion has grown up in the shadow of standard, allopathic medicine and has been erroneously associated with countercultural institutions and lifestyles. As health promotion succeeds in establishing mainstream legitimacy, a new set of strategies will have to be developed to assure that its fundamental character is not lost. There will be significant questions about how established organizations will adapt to it; certainly some of them will try to co-opt it. Rules and roles in the medical arena, which are now geared to disease-dominated medicine, will also have to be reconsidered. In addition the responsibilities of individuals and their freedom to make choices should be emphasized, as corporations, professional societies, and insurance companies look to create incentives for healthy lifestyles.

FROM THE INDIVIDUAL TO THE COLLECTIVE . . . AND BACK AGAIN

Why should an individual be concerned about a model of health or issues of national policy? What can be learned from studying the personal health strategies of fifty-one healthy, prominent individuals? And how can this knowledge begin to resolve the current health care crisis? Make no mistake, the crisis cannot be resolved by individuals, no matter how perfect their individual health practices might be. Reg-

ular exercise and a good diet are necessary to health but are ultimately insufficient by themselves. Influences far beyond individual
control—the environment, socioeconomic status, race, ethnicity, and
even sex—determine so much of what we see as health that they may
ultimately prove to be of greater influence than today's commonly
accepted health determinants such as weight and cholesterol levels.

Clarifying this point most eloquently is a study by Dr. Richard Poll
of Oxford University, reported in the *American Journal of Public
Health* in July 1992. Poll examined the differences in life expectancy in the United States over time, between males and females and between whites and nonwhites, as well as worldwide between the
"market" or postindustrial nations and the emerging Third World
countries. He wanted to determine the relative importance of factors
contributing to the life expectancy differences among these groups.
Among the influences he examined were personal behavior, medical
care, psychosocial factors, and changes in the physical environment.
After analyzing these factors, he concluded that personal behavior
was not the most important influence but that "the principal environmental hazards world-wide are those associated with poverty of
individuals within the market economies and of communities in the
developing countries and that in the future, they will be the effects of
overpopulation and the production of greenhouse gases." In contrast
to the older reductionist and molecular model, a new model of health
must encompass the overarching influences on public health—the environment, economics, and policy decisions—that affect each and
every one of us day in and day out.

This orientation toward larger issues is clearly reflected in the lives
of the Sound Mind–Sound Body participants, all of whom have
moved outward toward addressing the crises of the world at large. All
of them have experienced a marked benefit in their personal health
and well-being through their altruistic dedication to resolving the
pressing crises of our modern times. They have literally journeyed
beyond their personal health strategies to embrace the collective or
common good.

Surely the best solution to the current crisis in medical care needs
to follow this same pattern: individual health practices within a community must be maximized and supported by state and national policies, which in the long run will return substantial benefits to the
individual. Consider how this might affect an individual's choice to
quit smoking. This choice obviously requires individual willpower,
but the availability of behavioral and pharmacological programs, the

support of the person's family and friends, clean air, no-smoking policies in all public areas as well as in all work sites, and further limitations on cigarette advertising could very well make the difference between success and failure. Smoking cessation is one of the many issues of disease prevention pointedly addressed by Dr. William H. Foege, an internationally prominent physician with the Carter Center of Emory University who has been a long-standing, articulate, and highly regarded advocate of a new model of health. In his article entitled "The Growing Brown Plague" in the *Journal of the American Medical Association* he noted, "Executives in the tobacco industry . . . daily make the decision to kill for money, to become 'hit men' on a colossal scale . . . the annual global toll of tobacco will equal the total death toll of the Holocaust of Nazi Germany. . . . Tobacco advertising is held to different standards, where seemingly any deception is tolerated, and implying benefits of health, vigor, and attractiveness is condoned. To explain this will be the burden of future historians. It would be similar to learning that merchants of old were responsible for deliberately spreading the Black Plague, simply to increase their wealth. We would reject the possibility that *people of honor* could behave that way." Foege and many others advocate a model of health that enhances individual choice within a supportive environment. In essence, this is the "systems" model—moving from the level of individual choice, to the molecular level of nicotine addiction, to the public policy level of laws and regulations, and back again to reinforce and sustain the initial individual choice.

We as individuals may not be able to change laws, regulations, policies, or cultural values directly, but we do need to know more specifically what the problems are in order to seize every opportunity to exert whatever influence for good is possible, no matter how large or small. Now is not the time to sit on the sidelines or expect someone else to make the right decisions for us.

Within the confines of this book it is not possible to weave through the complexity of the legal, political, and financial labyrinth of public policy, nor is it desirable, since it is a bewildering maze of acronyms, vested interests, political lobbying, and legal maneuvering. Many excellent books have been written that detail the positive clinical and policy approaches necessary for a true health care system, including *America's Health Care Revolution* by Joseph A. Califano, Jr., *The Nation's Health* by the U.S. Assistant Secretary of Health, Dr. Philip R. Lee and his colleague Dr. Carroll L. Estes at the University of California School of Medicine in San Francisco, the

United States Government Printing Office document entitled *Healthy People 2000*, and the highly influential *Guide to Clinical Preventive Services*, edited by the well-respected physician Dr. Robert S. Lawrence of the Rockefeller Foundation.

Obviously the issues behind the health crisis are not new. What *is* new is that the problems are becoming much more specific; it is now absolutely imperative that the medical crisis be solved before it results in an economic as well as a human disaster. Despite the overwhelming magnitude of the crisis, there is reason for considerable optimism; later in this chapter I will detail some of the positive steps individuals and institutions are taking to create a true health care system.

Today the United States spends more money per person per year than any other medical system on earth, with a 1993 total of over $900 billion, or more than $2 billion per day. According to a report in *The Nation's Health*, published by the American Public Health Association, the medical expenditures in 1991 "rose 10.5 percent, twice as fast as the 5.1 percent increase in the gross national product." There were some years during the eighties when medical inflation ran three to four times higher than the overall rate of inflation. In releasing these figures, Health and Human Services Secretary Louis W. Sullivan said, "Rapid spending growth places a severe strain on the resources of families, business, and government alike." He noted that none of the reforms proposed in Congress include meaningful cost containment measures and that health promotion and disease prevention programs are absent from these proposals. If uncontrolled costs continue, an expert panel from the national Health Care Financing Administration reported in *Health Affairs* in 1992, medical spending could account for upward of "40 percent of the nation's gross national product by the year 2030." Consider the implications of this projection, specifically the other programs that will be cut back or eliminated to sustain that staggering expenditure.

Comparative statistics on medical expenditures for the United States and other nations are most revealing. In 1990 medical costs stood at 12.3 percent of the Gross National Product for the United States, compared to 8.8 percent for Sweden and 8.7 percent each for Canada and France. Since 1990 not only have our costs escalated even more disproportionately, but countries that spend less—Sweden, Canada, France, Germany, Japan, and every other developed nation—rank higher than the United States in every internationally accepted index of the health of a nation, including heart disease, cancer incidence, homicides, infant mortality, and average life expectancy.

In short, we spend more money than every other nation on the globe and simply aren't getting the "health" we're paying for. A special 1990 issue of the widely respected journal *Health Affairs* contained an article written by a major spokesman for public health, Dr. Lester Breslow, formerly dean of the School of Public Health at the UCLA School of Medicine. Breslow reported the results of a study comparing both the costs of and subjective levels of satisfaction with the medical care systems in ten developed nations, including the United States and Japan. He found that Canadians were the most satisfied with their system, contrary to what many Washington political lobbying groups now contend, and that the United States ranked ninth in satisfaction, followed only by Italy. An overwhelming 89 percent of people in the United States indicated dissatisfaction: 60 percent said the system needed "fundamental change," while 29 percent wanted to "completely rebuild the system." The highest annual cost per person for health care was $2,051 in the United States, followed by Canada at $1,483, and Italy at $841.

As human beings, we share the same basic body, but among comparable nations there are profound differences in the way we're treated medically, as the journalist Lynn Payer of the *International Herald Tribune* reports in the book *Medicine and Culture*. Offering a detailed analysis of the varying practices in the United States, England, Germany, and France, Payer notes the following significant differences between Americans and their European counterparts: American women have two to three times as many hysterectomies as European women; prostate surgery is more frequently performed on both older and younger men in America; European women have fewer radical operations (for example, they would be more likely to have a lumpectomy rather than a mastectomy). These observations have been underscored recently by the Stanford University medical economist Victor R. Fuchs, who found that the most cost-effective medical care was that of England: "Although high-tech medicine is severely rationed, England's level of public health is about the same as America's and it manages to provide a considerable amount of service while spending only $1 per capita for every $3 spent in the United States." To be sure, there are many complex cultural factors that affect the provision of medical care in any country, and these cannot be overlooked in accounting for such wide variation in practices and costs. However, given that these other countries provide universal access to care at much lower costs, and boast a comparable health status for most citizens, longer average life expectancies, and much

higher levels of subjective satisfaction, there is obviously a great deal
to learn from them about creating a true health care system.

Studies have been conducted to determine how necessary, appropriate, or effective many diagnostic and intervention strategies really are, and the results are astonishing. Writing in the *Journal of the
American Medical Association* in September 1990, Dr. Mark B. Wenneker and his colleagues at the Harvard School of Public Health compared hospital care for insured versus uninsured people admitted to
Massachusetts hospitals in 1985. Among those suffering from cardiovascular disease, insurance coverage was strongly associated with
the use of certain cardiac procedures. Researchers compared the situations of private, paying patients versus uninsured patients undergoing three expensive heart procedures: angiography, bypass surgery,
and angioplasty. Based on the researchers' analysis, the privately insured patients were at least twice as likely to undergo these procedures as the uninsured or Medicaid patients. After accounting for
other variables, the odds of procedure use for privately insured patients relative to those with no insurance were 80 percent greater for
angiography, 40 percent greater for bypass grafts, and 28 percent
greater for angioplasty. Medicaid patients also underwent all three
procedures significantly less often than private patients.

These results could indicate that Medicare and uninsured patients
are receiving undertreatment simply because they do not have the
means to pay for adequate treatment. However, they could also mean
that privately insured patients are receiving excessive or inappropriate treatment simply because they have the means to pay. Or they
could indicate both. Beyond the cost involved in performing excessive or unnecessary procedures, there is the issue that many of them
are risky and can cause death.

Using a similar methodology, a later study of insured versus uninsured care was performed by Dr. Jack Hadley and his colleagues
from the Georgetown University School of Medicine. For this study,
reported in the January 1991 issue of the *Journal of the American
Medical Association*, the researchers selected the discharge records
of 592,598 patients who were admitted in 1987 to hospitals throughout the nation. Again there were systematic and marked differences
in the care provided to insured versus uninsured people. Uninsured
patients were 29 to 75 percent less likely to undergo each of five
high-cost or high-discretion procedures, yet there was an indication
that the uninsured patients were actually more ill, as they were 50
percent less likely to have tissue biopsies that were normal. In addition, death rates for uninsured people were 1.2 to 3.2 times higher in

eleven out of sixteen groups of patients in the study.

In addition to these findings there is ample and persuasive evidence of inappropriate variations in practice patterns, of unnecessary and sometimes dangerous testing, and of self-serving decision making by medical providers. Pioneering work by Dr. John Wennberg of the Dartmouth School of Medicine has repeatedly demonstrated that the rate at which physicians use a particular treatment can vary by a factor of four or five times between one hospital and another. Overuse of medical practices has nothing to do with the quality of care or clinical necessity. In fact, inappropriate care may actually cause more harm than good! Among the recent evidence of this phenomenon are the following findings: 1) A study by the public Citizen Health Research Group found that use of cesarean sections in birth deliveries varies enormously from city to city, topping 50 percent in some (the estimated appropriate rate is 12 percent). Cesarean sections increase the risk of maternal death two to four times and cost about 1 billion dollars more per year (in 1987 dollars) than appropriate vaginal deliveries; 2) A 1988 Rand Corporation study found that 32 percent of carotid endarterectomies (removal of fatty deposits from neck veins) are unnecessary and that 10 percent of patients undergoing the procedure died or suffered a stroke as a direct result; and 3) Approximately 15 percent of physicians have a financial interest in medical testing laboratories. A recent study of Medicare physicians showed that those who an interest in such laboratories ordered 45 percent more tests than those that did not have such interests. These are common situations and indicative of a system that is increasingly mismanaged and out of control.

In the February 1991 issue of the *New England Journal of Medicine* a pair of articles were published on two studies that looked into the frequency of medical negligence in hospitals. In the first study an interdisciplinary team led by Dr. Troyen A. Brennan from the Harvard Medical School reviewed the medical records of more than thirty thousand hospitalizations in New York State during 1984. The findings are sobering. The team estimates that of the 2.7 million hospitalizations in New York during 1984, there were twenty-seven thousand adverse events due to medical negligence, and that 25 percent of these negligence problems led to death. The main reasons for the medical negligence were drug complications and injuries secondary to improper or delayed diagnosis. These adverse events were markedly more frequent among the elderly. The latter finding was not explained by differences in the severity of illness.

In the second study a research team headed by Dr. Lucian L. Leape of the Harvard School of Public Health looked at a sample of 30,195 randomly selected hospital records and identified 1,133 patients (3.7 percent) with disabling injuries caused by the medical treatment itself. These adverse events were correlated to error, negligence, and disability due to medical mismanagement. Two physician reviewers independently identified the adverse events and evaluated them with respect to negligence, errors in management, and extent of disability suffered by the patient. The adverse event most commonly found was drug complications, followed by wound infections and technical complications. Nearly half (48 percent) were associated with an operation. Although the prevention of many of these negative events must await improvements in medical knowledge, the high proportion due to management errors suggests that many others are potentially preventable right now.

Compounding the inability of a disease-focused system appropriately to manage existing chronic and acute diseases is the rise of what have been termed the "new plagues." In August 1992 a series of articles in *Science* documented that viruses and bacteria that were thought to be under control or eliminated are again emerging, in new forms as well as old, to cause new disease epidemics. Changes in living patterns are one of the prime causes of this resurgence; lifestyle changes themselves may hold the key as well to containing these diseases. Among the new or reemerging plagues are AIDS; toxic shock syndrome; outbreaks of tuberculosis, especially among the poor and homeless; Lyme disease; increased streptococcal infections; and numerous strains of influenza that are particularly life-threatening for the elderly. Overuse of antibiotics has actually fueled the new plagues. Writing in *Science,* Dr. Harold C. Nev of Columbia University has indicated that a range of diseases that impact the skin, lungs, intestines, and urinary tract are "now resistant to virtually all of the older antibiotics. The extensive use of antibiotics in the community and hospitals has fueled the crisis." This crisis cannot be resolved by new drugs. It will require more effective public health measures for disease detection, changes in personal and group lifestyles, better hygiene, more efforts to improve the environment, and a great deal of attention to the conditions of poverty and homelessness that have given rise to the new plagues and have allowed the old plagues to take hold once again.

Consumer Reports published a series of three articles beginning in July 1992 that illustrated how pervasive the medical crisis really is. In the first paragraph of the first article *Consumer Reports* stated, "Of the $817 billion that we will spend this year on health care, we will throw away at least $200 billion on over-priced, useless, even harmful treatments and on a bloated bureaucracy. We are no healthier than the citizens of comparable developed countries that spend half of what we do and provide health care for everybody. In fact, by important measures such as life expectancy and infant mortality, we are far down the list." Underlying causes of this $200 billion waste include excessive litigation by ambulance-chasing attorneys, unduly high insurance company overhead and profits, lobbying by disease management PACs (political action committees) to maintain the status quo, out-and-out billing frauds (estimated to stand at 10 percent of all costs by the U.S. General Accounting Office), and, of course, the unnecessary, inappropriate, expensive, and deadly overuse of medical interventions. *Consumer Reports* concludes that "our $200 billion figure is truly a minimum estimate."

In its April 25, 1992, issue, *The New York Times* published an op-ed piece entitled "Making a Living Off the Dying," written by Dr. Norman Paradis, a physician and director of emergency medicine at New York University's Bellevue Hospital. His father, also a physician, was diagnosed at age 75 with terminal pancreatic cancer. When he arrived at his father's bedside, Paradis found that he was being subjected to a barrage of diagnostic testing. The son made his family's wishes clear to the attending doctors. Paradis remarked, "It's an old story of inflated fees charged by subspecialists with procedure-based practices." He again stated his family's requests, and when his directives continued to be ignored, he was joined by his brother, an attorney. Together they protested to the hospital that procedures were being performed without consent, but to no avail. For two weeks their father remained in the hospital subjected to "unnecessary 'billable' high-tech therapy that could not possibly cure him or relieve his pain." Finally the brothers invoked the power of attorney to the hospital administrator and chief of staff to stop all unnecessary procedures. That night their father underwent yet another surgery. Angered and desperate, the brothers tried to transfer their father to another hospital but were repeatedly assured that he was in "the best of hands." Each time they arranged for him to be moved home or to a hospice, "a test or procedure would be performed, making him temporarily too unstable to be transported." After finding his father sitting alone in a hallway after yet another examination, Dr. Paradis was finally able to move him to a New York hospice. He died the next morning.

For months afterward Dr. Paradis agonized over the question, "If

my brother and I—a lawyer and a doctor—could not get decent care
for our father, also a doctor, what chance does the general public
have?" This tragedy demonstrates precisely why it is necessary to
move far beyond limited individual efforts into areas where personal strategies and choices, whether in health or in crisis, are sustained
by the health care system, not destroyed. To add insult to tragedy,
Medicare paid the bill of over $150,000 for a patient who "needed
only a bed and some morphine." When Dr. Paradis contacted the
Medicare inspector general's office to file a complaint against the
hospital for billing for unauthorized procedures, there were so many
pending cases of fraud for over a million dollars that a case involving
a mere $150,000 would not even be investigated. Trying to salvage
some benefit from his personal anguish, Dr. Paradis concluded, "Our
health care system is structured to meet reimbursement rather than
patients' needs. Tremendous amounts of money are spent prolonging
death, not life. If the story of my father's suffering can help improve
our medical system it will have been worth telling. Though I was unable to get him the care he deserved, I believe he would forgive me."
Dr. Paradis's dramatic account of an all-too-frequent tragedy has re-
inforced the concern of every responsible clinician, hospital, government agency, and professional society to redirect the resources of
a system that places profits first and people last.

One obvious conclusion from this brief and gloomy foray into the
current crisis of the so-called health care system is that the dangerous practices, the inequitable access to care, and the policies of greed
must be corrected. However, we must remember that treating appropriately or even curing a disease does not result in health. Resolving
the larger health crisis requires a fundamental redirection of our individual and collective resources toward the evolution of a true health
care system.

LIGHT AT THE END OF THE TUNNEL

A crisis of the magnitude inherent in the present disease management
industry is surely overwhelming to the individual, yet it is necessary
for us all to be aware of the factors causing the crisis, even though
they may be beyond our control, because they directly influence our
options, choices, and day-to-day health. In facing up to this reality,
we can learn from the experiences and choices of and the paths tak-
en by the participants in the Sound Mind–Sound Body study. These
optimally healthy individuals, and a growing number like them, rep-

resent a direction and an end point—a destination or goal for the development of a true health care system. Once you know your destination, the journey may be demanding but you at least have a direction and a means for gauging your progress. All too often the proposed solutions to the current crisis get bogged down in elaborate managed care mechanisms, legal or economic barriers keeping people from getting access to appropriate care, or an endless litany of government acronyms for competing alternatives. To a degree this is a necessary process, but it is meaningless and will get us nowhere without an appropriate model of health for both individuals and institutions.

What is this abstraction—a model of health—and why is it so important? One of the most articulate answers to this question has been given by Dr. Harry Sultz of the School of Medicine at the State University of New York at Buffalo. Writing in the April 1991 issue of the *American Journal of Public Health*, he said, "Neither a society nor a health care system can survive without virtue or a cause that supersedes individual interests. Our health care cannot progress without an articulated purpose, a common vision expressed as policy that eliminates ambiguity of purpose, ambivalence towards performance standards, conflicts or principles, and contradictions of goals." Such a model or shared vision needs to be flexible and adaptable to meet the demands of a rapidly evolving society, but there must be an initial direction. Billions of dollars are spent and other billions wasted in treating diseases and emergency-room traumas resulting from underlying social pathologies, which only remain unaddressed. Chronic unemployment, the breakdown of the family structure, increasing domestic violence ranging from rape to handgun deaths, poverty, homelessness, drug abuse, and environmental contamination are the base causes of the vast majority of conditions that we attempt to treat by increasingly expensive and ineffective medical interventions. These social pathologies become real medical problems, but they are not inherently biological diseases. They end up in emergency rooms, intensive care units, and morgues—not at all appropriate to where they begin and where it is possible to make a difference.

Expectations that tinkering with the anachronistic disease management industry will resolve the crisis are misplaced at best, because they overlook fundamental questions. As early as 1976 noted social analyst Ivan Illich descried the inadequacy of a medical-model approach to health. Prophetically, he warned in *Medical Nemesis: The Expropriation of Health* that "health care is turned into a standard-

ized item; when all suffering is 'hospitalized' and hopes become in-
hospitable to birth, sickness, and death." Now, nearly two decades
later, even the most mundane aspects of ordinary life and pleasure,
from birth to grandparenting, are being medicalized and hospitalized.
Illich's apparently extremist alarm in 1976 turns out to have been an
understatement. In a country rife with teenage pregnancy and sexu-
ally transmitted diseases, troubled youths have been fatuously ad-
vised to "just say no." Looking back at the decade of the eighties with
its simplistic add-ons to an inherently ineffective system, Dr. Harry
Sultz observed, "Equating the pressure to take drugs with being offered a scone at a tea party, this national campaign typified the flight
from reality that gripped all of society in that era." For the nineties
and beyond, effective solutions will necessitate a profound individual and organizational introspection, accompanied by fundamental
reorganization, rather than sound-bite solutions.

Addressing the real challenge ahead is Dr. Myron Allukian, the immediate past president of the American Public Health Association
(APHA). While applauding the *Healthy People 2000* goals for achieving health for the nation, he is sharply critical of its shortcomings and
outlines the more positive additional steps that need to be taken. In
the October 1990 issue of *Nation's Health*, an official publication of
the APHA, he observed that the health crisis in America is widening
the gulf between the haves and the have-nots, the insured and the
uninsured, and whites and minorities, and that the closure of these
gulfs is long overdue. Allukian noted that approximately forty thousand babies died in the United States before their first birthday. This
figure ranks the United States twenty-second in infant mortality after Japan, France, Canada, Hong Kong, and every other postindustrial nation. He also observed that over one hundred thousand
Americans die or are disabled from unintentional injuries that involve
automobiles and/or alcohol. He pointed out that the *Healthy People
2000* report unfortunately omits any objectives for the nation on
handgun control, family planning, school-based clinics, and tobacco
and cigarette taxes. Although such objectives are supported by thousands of experts, agencies, and institutions, the political administration has yet to upset the powerful alcohol, tobacco, and gun lobbies,
or the "religious zealots who refuse to address human sexuality." Resulting from this dismaying compromise is a prescription for health
that cannot be filled.

In another major criticism of *Healthy People 2000* Allukian noted
that it blames victims for their health problems. Throughout its pages
the document asks the elderly, poor, and minorities to accept re-

sponsibility for their ill health, ignoring the fact that many health problems are rooted in poverty and that improved living standards result in improved health. No one chooses to live in drug- and rat-infested neighborhoods or on the street. Some of the most significant health improvements in the last hundred years occurred as a result of societal or governmental action. Cleaning up the water supply, instituting pure food laws, providing nutritional fortification, better housing, improved nutrition, and fluoridation of water all require national social policies rather than specific individual responsibilities. It is true that to a large degree individuals are responsible for their own health, but to achieve fully and in an equitable manner the objects of *Healthy People 2000*, a true community partnership is required. Individuals, families, businesses, health organizations, and civic groups must join with government in providing leadership and resources to resolve the growing crisis.

As Allukian pointed out, there is a trend toward emphasizing individual responsibility, but placing responsibility on individuals is not an adequate solution to an overwhelming problem. Additionally, there is evidence that the focus on individual health behaviors as a means of dealing with the present disease-model crisis is being oversold. Prevention costs money. Changing behaviors is difficult, and not all prevention efforts are effective. One argument against the health model is that successful prevention may just mean that people live longer, eventually succumbing to chronic conditions that are expensive to treat. However, it may not be more expensive to treat diseases in late life. In reality, the most dollars are spent during lingering chronic illnesses that result in long periods of decline. The longer a healthy individual lives, the more likely it is that he or she will experience what Dr. James F. Fries of the Stanford University School of Medicine refers to as "the compression of morbidity and mortality," meaning that a healthy older person afflicted with a fatal disease will die more quickly than an unhealthy person, and therefore cost less. Some believe that medical care for the elderly should be rationed, but we cannot salvage our medical system, cure our social ills, or reduce medical costs by exacting revenge on our elderly. We need to address the reasons why we want or need to ration medical care for a particular group, whether it's the poor or the chief executive officers of Fortune 500 companies. Before we target any groups for rationing, we need to set priorities, find the type of medical care that is needed for a long and healthy life, and decide how we are going to pay for it. We also need to pay a great deal more attention to defining the kinds of procedures that are necessary to good medical care and identifying those that are unnecessary, gratuitous, or indeed life-threatening.

In a September 1990 editorial in the *New England Journal of Medicine*, then editor-in-chief Dr. Arnold S. Relman faced the question of rationing medical care for the elderly: "Rationing is not likely to be successful in controlling costs unless we deal with that basic problem. Given the huge sums we are now committing to medical care as compared with other developed countries, we should be able to afford all the services we really need, provide we use our resources wisely." Not a single serious analyst has demonstrated that cost containment has come anywhere near reaching its goal. If we could only eliminate unnecessary, untested, or wasteful diagnostic services in medical treatments, do away with excessive malpractice claims, and tear away expensive bureaucracy, we might well be able to provide equitable care. Indeed, it would be a mistake, not to mention morally objectionable, to ration health care before we have exhausted all means of achieving cost containment and making care more efficient.

In considering solutions to the rationing problem, Relman observed that the current medical care system has a "built-in incentive for waste and inflation" in the way that medicine is organized and delivered. To avoid rationing, what is needed most is not more money but the will to change those aspects of the present system that are responsible for the present financial crisis. Any new model of health needs medical and ethical, not simply economic, justification. Addressing the needs of the aging population requires a vital balance between individual responsibility and collective changes in current policies. Neither solution alone is adequate to the challenge.

An aging and growing population, rising public expectations, and the continual introduction of new and expensive forms of technology generate a virtually unlimited demand upon medical services. Inevitably this unchecked demand will exhaust the resources we are willing and able to devote to medical care. Sooner or later we will be forced to limit expenditures by restricting service, even those that are beneficial. This crisis and the limitations on access resulting from high costs stem from an inherently inflationary and wasteful medical care system.

Redirecting the largest and fastest-growing industry in the world to place an increasing emphasis on a model of health rather than of disease, or health promotion and disease prevention, requires both the vision and the courage to implement the difficult decisions that lie ahead. What will this revolution require? Writing in the *Washington Post* in 1990, Dr. Uwe Reinhardt, professor of political economy at Princeton University and a highly respected expert on health policy and economics, stated, "First, we will really have some dark days. Our medical system now is like a sick man who knows he is sick but doesn't want to go to the doctor because he fears what he might find out. We all know the system is failing. But almost nobody wants to sit down and figure out what we need to do to make it work." In the September 1992 issue of the *Journal of the American Medical Association* there was a long follow-up interview with the outspoken Reinhardt, who raised himself out of poverty in West Germany, where he and his family lived "in a toolshed," to become one of the most articulate and respected analysts of the medical crisis. During the interview he chided, "Imagine . . . a group of colleagues . . . all of you too impaired to drive home. Instead you play 'Building America's Health Insurance System.' Would you, even while dead drunk, construct a system that does this?" From that point on he elaborated on every inequity considered above, and more, to describe a system that simply does not work. Yet no matter how clear the need for change is, few special interests are willing to give up what they hold dear. Doctors want freedom from bureaucracy. They want to be able to make decisions without insurance companies or hospital boards second-guessing them on an economic basis. State governments do·not want to take the unpopular step of raising taxes, even though their state medical plans sag under the load of hospital inflation. Perhaps the most positive sign is that the American people, according to polls, constantly indicate that they want more and better health services and also want more people to have access to more services.

In response to these observations Dr. James Todd, executive vice president of the American Medical Association, has stated, "The first thing that is going to have to happen is that the level of expectation about what people can expect from health care will have to be reduced. Americans want all the access in the world. They want their choice of doctors, they want fancy technology, and they want more people to have a fair shot at the system. There is just no way to grant all those wishes to everyone." Limitations are inevitable, and determining those limits requires defining our collective direction. We need to set priorities, allocate resources, and establish which services are best provided to which people at what cost.

TOWARD A NEW MODEL OF HEALTH

From the comments of the Sound Mind–Sound Body interviewees to those of participants in numerous national surveys, it is evident that we know what to do to attain optimal health. In previous chapters we delved into the psychological, developmental, behavioral, and spiritual dimensions of optimal health. We saw that successful personal strategies in those areas are moderate, widely known, and attainable by virtually anyone who is at least assured of basic economic, social, and environmental security. We know what to do, both as individuals and as a nation. The time for implementation is now.

Developing a true health care system is an acknowledged individual and national priority, according to an article in the *Journal of the American Medical Association* by Dr. Robert A. Hahn of the Division of Surveillance and Epidemiologic Studies at the National Centers for Disease Control and Prevention in Atlanta. Dr. Hahn led a study in which a team of researchers assessed the mortality from the nine major chronic diseases in the United States for the year 1986. They found that the reduction of mortality from these nine diseases would mean an average increased life expectancy of four years. While an additional four years of life might not be enough to motivate people to change their behavior, they would not only be extending their length of life but enjoying an enhanced day-to-day quality of life. Dr. Hahn concluded, "Though there are nonpreventable (for example, genetic) contributors to mortality for many diseases, our understanding of what must be changed in the population to achieve lowered mortality levels from the nine diseases and to increase longevity is reasonably well-established. Preventable exposures include cigarette smoking, hypertension, obesity, high cholesterol, lack of exercise, heavy consumption of alcohol, and failure to use screening techniques such as mammography and pap smears. Both reduction of exposures to known risk factors and increased utilization of known screening measures are important means in the control of chronic disease, particularly in disadvantaged populations. The critical challenges remain to implement established knowledge, to increase awareness and motivation for healthy living, and to provide resources for equitable access to appropriate care." By supporting and reinforcing individual choices with innovations in policy and programs, we *can* achieve health.

Emphasis in the last part of this chapter will be on elaborating the new programs and policies necessary to support individual efforts. These ongoing and future programs are designed to help individuals sustain their own optimal health in order to achieve the goal of health for every family, every community, and the nation as a whole. Such individual and collective efforts combined will lead to the creation of a true health care system.

. . .

Health promotion—and establishing health as a goal—needs to be the first step. Surely the most widely accepted statement of this viewpoint was written in 1987 in the Ottawa Charter for Health Promotion, which proposes the integration of individual and community efforts as a means to achieve optimal health.:

> Health promotion is the process of enabling people to increase control over, and to improve, their health. To reach a state of complete physical, mental and social well-being, an individual or group must be able to identify and to realize aspirations, to satisfy needs, and to change or cope with the environment. Health is, therefore, seen as a resource for everyday life, not the objective of living. Health is a positive concept emphasizing social and personal resources, as well as physical capabilities. Therefore, health promotion is not just the responsibility of the health sector, but goes beyond healthy lifestyles to well-being.

This orientation toward health is a potent challenge to the status quo, and yet its goals are attainable. However, a new health system depends on our making a commitment to resolving our social and environmental crises before they become medical emergencies. At the present time there is no complete picture of how to resolve them all, but some pieces of the jigsaw puzzle are falling into place.

One of the most fundamental issues to be addressed is the fact that 10 percent of our population, people with catastrophic or chronic disease, actually account for as much as 70 to 80 percent of all annual medical expenditures. There are several promising approaches to this issue, foremost among them the use of behavioral changes and drug treatment instead of expensive surgeries to reverse heart disease.

Cardiovascular disease is still the leading cause of death, followed by cancer and injuries, of those under age seventy-five. Today 1.7 million adults suffer heart attacks each year and over five hundred thousand of them die! Angioplasty, thrombolytic therapy, coronary bypass surgery, heart transplantation, and many new heart medications buy time and alleviate symptoms. But none of these interventions do anything to treat the underlying arterial disease that is the cause of heart attacks. Looking at this situation, the eminent physician Dr. Alexander Leaf, chairman emeritus of Preventive Medicine at the Harvard Medical School, posed this rhetorical question in a *New England Journal of Medicine* editorial: "Are we developing ingenious, technologically sophisticated, and expensive treatments for established disease and ignoring the fact that the malady is potentially preventable and reversible? . . . It would seem that a health care system that improved the health of the patient and of the public would be preferred to one that focused only on extending life. This is what preventive measures should accomplish, especially with coronary heart disease." Significant regression of coronary artery blockages has been achieved by a reduction of risk factors, through medications, or with a combination of the two. This news generates a new and more optimistic perspective on heart disease, the number-one killer of people under age seventy-five. Three research studies have demonstrated that drug intervention with advanced heart disease can slow the progression of the disease, and four studies have shown that lifestyle change can even reverse the disease. One of the latter, a purely behavioral study conducted by Dr. Dean Ornish and his colleagues, was popularized in his 1992 book, *Dr. Dean Ornish's Program for Reversing Heart Disease*. Given the small number of people in his study, the extremely intensive and expensive intervention—the preparation of virtually all of the meals for the participants, intensive psychotherapy and yoga classes, and other unique aspects of the program—it remains to be demonstrated that such a program is practical for large numbers of people.

One study is of particular significance not only because it demonstrated a 50 percent slowing in the rate of progression of heart disease, but because it represents a practical model that could in fact be implemented today. That project is the Stanford Coronary Risk Intervention Program (SCRIP), led by Dr. William L. Haskell and his colleagues at the Stanford University School of Medicine. For the vast majority of participants the combination of lifestyle change plus appropriate use of medications was much easier to maintain than a program that required stringent lifestyle modification only. SCRIP is the first study to evaluate this combined impact of comprehensive lifestyle changes—diet, exercise, weight loss, smoking cessation, and counseling—together with medications. For the study a total of 259 men and 41 women were randomly assigned, 145 to the SCRIP program and 155 to usual care at another medical school. After the initial examination, the SCRIP intervention was delivered by trained nurses over the telephone.

At the conclusion of the four-year study, the people in the SCRIP group showed major improvements beyond the people receiving usual care. Significant reductions occurred in the form of 40 percent lower cholesterol consumption, a 23 percent reduction in the low-density lipoproteins ("bad" cholesterol), along with a 12 percent rise in high-density lipoproteins ("good" cholesterol), and a 20 percent increase in exercise. There were three deaths in each group, but there were only twenty-five hospitalizations in the SCRIP group versus forty-four under usual care. Both groups showed some progression or worsening of the disease, but the SCRIP patients demonstrated 47 percent less narrowing of their arteries. Furthermore, a small number of patients in SCRIP experienced actual reversal of blockages. Beyond the clinical findings this study is unique in that it was the largest, longest study to use inexpensive nurse-delivered telephone intervention, yet it still had a major positive impact. Because it required no special facilities and combined basic lifestyle changes plus medications, it represents a model that can be used by any hospital, clinic, or individual practice.

Building on that research, Dr. Haskell and his colleagues, including Dr. John W. Farquhar and me, are currently developing the Stanford Coronary Atherosclerosis Management Program (SCAMP) clinical research project in conjunction with Blue Shield of California. This is a major clinical and policy coup because Blue Shield, along with the states where Blue Shield and Blue Cross are integrated plans, constitutes the largest insurance company in the world. For the first time medical practitioners will be reimbursed for providing a lifestyle-plus-medication program on an equal footing with invasive surgeries. Insurance companies have long known that for every unnecessary coronary bypass surgery, they can save a minimum of thirty thousand dollars per person. Now some forward-looking insurers are taking the prudent steps necessary to make that savings in dollars and human suffering a reality. More and more patients will find that their individual choices will be supported and reimbursed by at least one major insurance company, and others will follow this innovative lead.

While heart disease has declined over the last ten years, cancer has actually increased. It is the second major cause of death today. After twenty years of the "War on Cancer" and the quest for a "magic bullet" to kill various forms of the disease, this quasi-military assault has failed. According to the National Cancer Institute, the number of women dying from breast cancer is increasing despite a $1 billion expenditure during the last ten years. Writing in *Science* in December 1991, Dr. Eliot Marshall cited a report of the Government Accounting Office that "in many respects, what's happening with breast cancer is an extreme example of the way the War on Cancer is going in general. After spending $22 billion in the past two decades . . . overall death rates from many common cancers remain stubbornly unchanged—or even higher than when the war began. . . . Nowhere in the pipeline is there any drug that is going to transform the situation dramatically." With mounting evidence of this failure, there is a clear mandate to move away from reactive treatment to proactive prevention. Compounding this deficiency in the old model is the fact that socioeconomic factors play a major role in cancer survival. One recent study of 2,089 patients suffering from six different common cancers looked at predictors of the person's survival. Overall, the best indicators of whether or not the person died were type of cancer, severity of illness, income level, and education level. Poorer patients with lower education levels were at highest risk, partially because they delayed consulting or did not have access to doctors. The study concluded that educational programs about cancer treatment aimed at poorer people would improve their survival rates and actually prevent some cancers as well.

In contrast to heart disease, the treatment of cancer has not yet shifted toward a greater focus on prevention, despite the fact that socioeconomic, educational, dietary, and environmental factors are increasingly documented as causes of common cancers. Using breast cancer as an example, two very recent studies, one from Vermont and another from Israel, indicate that women who develop breast cancer may have been exposed more often to toxic chemicals than women who remain cancer-free. Future funding and programs in a health model will need to focus on reaching the poor and the less educated, on eliminating all tobacco products, on creating and implementing dietary guidelines that include the elimination of carcinogenic additives in all foods, and on removing carcinogenic chemicals from the earth and the air. Clearly these are efforts far beyond individual control, but they represent areas in which people can both act individually and act and speak out in larger public forums.

Pogo's wonderful quip, "We have met the enemy and he is us," is particularly appropriate to the issue of environmental quality, perhaps the single most potent element in a true health care system. Environmental deterioration and pollution have direct negative effects upon health globally. Writing in the *New England Journal of Medicine*, Dr. Alexander Leaf pointedly links environmental degradation to its devastating effects on health. He enumerates in no uncertain terms the catastrophic consequences that will result from the greenhouse effect, explaining that not only could it cause 50 million people in coastal areas to become environmental refugees, forced to abandon their homes to rising oceans, but the depletion of the protective ozone layer in the earth's atmosphere will also increase cancer incidence, kill the phytoplankton photosynthesis in our oceans, and make land less fertile, compounding global hunger. There will be increased mortality from heat stress, atmospheric pollutants will cause even more lung cancer and asthma, skin cancer will result from the continued thinning of the ozone layer, increased rainfall will cause proliferation of insect-borne diseases, deterioration of water quality will create sanitation-related diseases, and increased ultraviolet radiation will suppress the human and animal immune systems. Leaf also observes that the oceans have been increasingly overfished and "desecrated with garbage, sewage and toxic substances, many of which are not biodegradable."

Concluding his article, Leaf cites the positive efforts of the Worldwatch Institute and the United Nations Environment Program as steps toward a healthy solution. Summing up, he observes, "The effects of environmental change may be analogous to those of nuclear war, which although it basically involves political, economic, and military issues, has the potential to harm human health to an unprecedented and intolerable degree. . . . Only an educated and aroused public is likely to force antiquated nationalistic political systems to cooperate in promoting family planning, energy conservation, and the protection of the global environment in time to prevent the direst possibilities from occurring." Efforts at the level of the individual, such as recycling, using nonaerosol sprays, buying "cruelty-free" products that are not tested on animals, are all necessary first steps. But our efforts must progress to the next level: social and political action.

Concurring with these observations is Dr. Joyce L. Lashoff, chairman of the School of Public Health at the University of California at Berkeley and immediate past president of the American Public Health Association. A long-standing and highly prominent spokeswoman for prevention, she dedicated an editorial column in *Public Health Reports* to issues of environmental quality. Among the issues she cites for collective action are preventing climate changes due to global warming and increased carbon dioxide levels from burning fossil fuels, preserving biodiversity, controlling unchecked population growth, protecting the world's forests (both domestic parks and tropical rain forests), and saving the oceans from rampant pollution. She also mentions the noted Toronto Conference on the Changing Atmosphere, which warned in 1988, "Humanity is conducting an unintended, uncontrolled, globally pervasive experiment whose ultimate consequences could be second only to a global nuclear war." Leaf and Lashoff, as well as many other individuals and environmental organizations, are critical of the Republican administrations of the eighties for failing to support domestic and international environmental protection programs while reducing available money for the treatment of the resulting increases in diseases and deaths.

On the positive side there are a growing number of companies that remain profitable and successful while actively cleaning up the environment and/or engaging in nonpolluting industry. Such investment mutual funds as the Calvert-Ariel Growth and Calvert Managed Growth, Dreyfus Third Century, Pax World, New Alternatives, and Parnassus funds, as well as such investment managers as Winslow Management of Boston, have demonstrated that it is possible to be socially and environmentally responsible *and* profitable. Among the many environmental organizations worldwide, Peter Seligman's Conservation International in Washington, D.C., pioneered the "debt for equity" exchange strategy of allowing underdeveloped countries to write off some of their national debts in exchange for preserving rain forests and animal habitats.

What if the talented professional men and women who have been employed in the defense industry were to apply their genius to the problems of cleaning the oceans, enhancing the quality of drinking water, recycling automobile tires into building materials (as used in Dennis Weaver's Colorado home), developing efficient solar and wind power as alternatives to fossil and nuclear fuels and their disposal problems, and developing a whole range of positive, life-affirming industries that would be both health-enhancing and profitable? According to an April 1992 article in *Science*, the highly respected National Research Council released a report indicating that "environmental pollutants are having a deleterious effect on immune systems." As one example, pollutants have been shown to increase asthma, which has risen 58 percent since 1970. Increasing environmental pollution may underlie the diagnosis of "multiple chemical sensitivity," a condition in which pollutants may increase "arthritis, hay fever, depression, even hallucinations or a combination thereof." We need not wait for further research to begin taking steps toward stricter control of indoor air pollutants to alleviate the increasingly common sick-building syndrome. Together we will solve this crisis of human health, or together we will perish.

One major public figure who has been a consistent proponent of positive practical approaches to the environment is Vice President Al Gore, who while serving in the U.S. Senate wrote the sweeping, pragmatic book *Earth in the Balance*. Reflecting on the current status of the environment and the choices that are before us, Gore wrote, "Humankind has suddenly entered into a brand new relationship with the planet Earth. The world's forests are being destroyed; an enormous hole is opening in the ozone layer. Living species are dying at an unprecedented rate. Chemical wastes, in growing volumes, are seeping down to poison groundwater while huge quantities of carbon dioxide, methane and chlorofluorocarbons are trapping heat in the atmosphere and raising global temperatures. How much information is needed to recognize a pattern? How much more is needed by the body politic to justify action in response? . . . The environment is becoming a matter of national security—an issue that directly and imminently menaces the interests of the state or welfare of the people. . . . In the not too distant future, policies . . . will join, or perhaps even supplant, our concern with preventing nuclear war as the principal test of statecraft." Today it is necessary for every individual to take a stand—to give a voice to our hopes and aspirations for ourselves, our children, and for the Earth.

In order to provide a healthy environment in which to pursue optimal personal health, communities must become healthy cities. During the mid-1970s Dr. John W. Farquhar and his colleagues at the Stanford Center for Research in Disease Prevention of the Stanford University School of Medicine developed the first intervention and evaluation models for working with entire communities to enhance health. That initial project was the well-regarded Three-Community Study, which focused on an inexpensive, community-wide intervention to reduce cardiovascular risk in three small cities in California. Its comprehensive approach used local regulations (such as no-smoking laws), environmental factors, and changes in personal behavior to elicit and sustain healthy lifestyles in an atmosphere of social support. Drawing upon the success of this initial study, Dr. Farquhar and his colleagues launched the even more ambitious Five-City Project, the results of which were reported in the July 1990 issue of the *Journal of the American Medical Association*. This study, fourteen years in duration, compared the effects of community intervention promoting cardiovascular risk reduction in two cities of approximately 122,800 people versus three control cities of approximately 197,500 where there was no intervention. Interventions consisted of education about the risk of heart disease (four to five education programs per year focused on specific risks, such as smoking and cholesterol), community classes and contests, one-on-one counseling, special programs in Spanish, and school-based programs for grades four, five, seven, and ten. Following the first five years of intervention, the researchers reported reductions in cholesterol, blood pressure, heart rate, smoking, and heart disease risk scores, as well as a 15 percent reduction in total mortality risk scores. Data from this innovative intervention is still being collected by Dr. Stephen P. Fortmann and his colleagues of the Stanford University School of Medicine. Although the decreases in risk were acknowledged as significant but relatively small, and the focus was specifically on heart disease prevention, the Stanford Five-City Project has generated an invaluable model that has been and can continue to be replicated in other communities to elicit and sustain individual efforts to achieve optimal health.

Two other complex and equally well tested programs have also been conducted, with similar results. The Minnesota Heart Health Project studied six cities with a combined population of 356,000, and the Pawtucket Heart Health Project looked at two Rhode Island cities with a total of 173,000 people. These studies and the Stanford studies together included a total of thirteen cities and over 890,000 people. Their combined results are indeed significant, given the number of people, the diversity of geographic location, and the demonstrated effectiveness of the interventions. With such large numbers of people involved, these community-based programs create an essential foundation for the low-cost implementation of a true health care system. Although these programs are all within the United States, community programs are equally applicable internationally. Among the best known are projects in Finland, South Africa, Switzerland, and Australia.

Given the positive results of all of these studies, Dr. Farquhar and his colleagues have concluded that "the cost of such national programs is moderate, but the cost of *not* launching such programs is to accept the notion that the energies of communities cannot be harnessed for planned social change for health benefit." Today that challenge forms the basis of a model Healthy Cities program in Chico, California, led by Dr. Walt Schafer, chairman of sociology at the California State University campus in that town of eighty-five thousand. In 1993 Dr. Schafer and the entire community of Chico launched Healthy Chico 2000, a project based on the studies described above to provide a practical and replicable model of what a motivated community can achieve. Beyond the specific health promotion programs, the Chico project plans to include the construction of "healthy homes" incorporating the most up-to-date environmentally friendly materials, an innovative telecommunications link between these homes and community health care providers and hospitals, as well as new insurance plans. As an example of how the power of communities can be harnessed to increase optimal health, the results of the Chico program can serve as a pragmatic model for the nation.

Another innovative model for community health action is a unique program in Birmingham, Alabama led by R. William Whitmer, president of Wellness South. Somewhat different from the previous studies, this program is primarily focused on the work-site rather than on the community. It is quite expansive, though, including all of the approximately four thousand employees of the city of Birmingham. That city, like every city and employer in the United States, has had to respond to unchecked escalations in medical costs by paying higher premiums, cutting back on coverages, or dropping medical insurance altogether. In September 1985 the city of Birmingham received and matched a $1.5 million grant from the National Institutes of Health. With that total of $3 million the city implemented an integrated system of health promotion programs for active employees and their dependents. What is most remarkable about the plan is that participation was required in order to be eligible for medical benefits: those employees who declined to participate did not get access to the medical insurance screening that launched the five-year program. Conducting the actual interventions was Whitner and his team of psychologists, physicians, and nurses. During the five years of the program there were major reductions in all risk factors, in the occurrence of illness, and in mortality. Beyond these clinical outcomes were the very impressive indications of cost effectiveness. In 1985 the medical cost per employee was $2,050, or $300 above the national average. By the end of the demonstration phase of the program in early 1991 Whitner and his colleagues reported, "The city had no increase in the per employee cost of medical benefits." Considering the out-of-control escalation of medical costs during the same time period, this was indeed good news for Birmingham.

There are four important aspects of the Birmingham project that are unique: 1) All employees were prescreened as a prerequisite for medical coverage. Of course, employees also had the option of not participating and seeking their own medical care independently. Any mandatory participation is inevitably controversial, but it is certain that future programs will include some form of required participation, with individuals having the option to find their own coverage or pay a higher premium for coverage. 2) Aggressive physician referral was necessary for 13 percent of employees found to be at high risk, mostly for heart disease. 3) Assistance was provided in establishing a strong patient-clinician relationship. All too often it is assumed that people understand their medical plan and have a sound relationship with their physician and other providers. In Birmingham over 40 percent of the employees did not have an active relationship with their doctors. 4) Regular medical office visits were encouraged. This practice was directly opposed to the unfortunate tactic many employers have adopted of discouraging utilization of their medical plans. In Birmingham the philosophy now is that "employees should be educated and encouraged to see their primary-care physician regularly. The correction and monitoring of illnesses or premature death is an important part of cost effective health promotion." Perhaps one of the best aspects of the Birmingham project is that the providers are not perceived by the insurer as the enemy.

Work site–based health promotion and disease prevention programs are my greatest professional interest. More significant and effective innovations have taken place in work sites, from small to large, in the last five years than in the entire period since the Industrial Revolution. Programs to address lifestyle and environmental risks parallel earlier efforts in child labor laws, shorter work hours, fire codes, and health and safety regulations. Work environments are a mainstay in the generation of a true health care system because at the workplace it is possible to reach the largest number of people and their dependents, for the most years of their adult life; at the workplace both the individual and the employer have a vested interest in that individual's health and well-being. According to the U.S. Health Care Financing Administration, companies are currently spending 48.3 percent of their after-tax profits on providing medical care for employees and their dependents. That figure is conservatively expected to increase to over 60 percent by the year 2000. Professor Regina Herzlinger, an influential medical economist at the Harvard Business School, has cited an even more startling fact, based upon a graph she designed by taking the average rate of profitability of all of the Fortune 500 companies and projecting it into the future. She then did the same with the rate of increase in their medical costs and discovered that in about 1997, these two lines cross, meaning that the medical costs of the Fortune 500 companies will be equal to their profits! After that time, Herzlinger reports, medical costs will continue to grow more rapidly than profits. Corporations, large and small, represent the single largest segment of the United States that has a vested interest in health, if for no other reason than to eliminate the cost of employees on sick leave. Beyond the economic factors, the presence of health promotion programs at the work site has the added benefits of attracting and retaining key personnel, decreasing absenteeism, enhancing productivity, improving the company's public image, and encouraging employees' loyalty.

Actually, the verb *to incorporate* is derived from the Latin word *incorpore*, which means "to take on a body." A corporation literally takes on a body that has a life and rights of its own, and within that body are the cells—employees—that animate it and are integral to its health. Increasingly, the fact that healthy people equal a healthy business is being recognized as a fundamental underpinning for the successful company of the twenty-first century. Dr. Robert H. Rosen, author of the insightful book *The Healthy Company*, has observed, "Healthy people make healthy companies. And healthy companies are more likely, more often, and over a longer period of time, to make healthy profits and to have healthy returns on their investments. So healthy people and healthy relationships are at the very core of success in business, but for too long the old fear-based hierarchical paradigms of management and of management-employee relationships have driven the way business is done in America. I might add that those old paradigms also have just about driven business into the ground." The new model for business is one of healthy individuals within a healthy organization making contributions to a healthy community and environment. This requires not unbridled altruism but a recognition of the inextricable interdependence of a company's health and those people who work in that organization.

To address these issues, I founded a program in 1984 that has evolved into the Stanford Corporate Health Program in the Stanford Center for Research in Disease Prevention of the Stanford University School of Medicine. The program is a collaborative research effort between the university and twenty-two major corporations, including Aetna, American Airlines, AT&T, Bank of America, Blue Shield, Healthnet, IBM, Amdahl, Chevron, Hewlett-Packard, ARCO, Johnson & Johnson, Levi-Strauss, Lockheed, Shaklee, Syntex, and Xerox. Medical and personnel directors of these companies meet with Stanford University faculty on a regular basis to develop and evaluate innovative health and medical programs. Over the last ten years we have worked together on small projects, such as bringing mobile mammography vans to the work site, as well as highly complex endeavors like the five-year study of an innovative managed care plan for over eighty thousand employees of a major telecommunications company. Together we have created a database of knowledge for companies to use in making better decisions about allocating their annual medical budgets between treatment and prevention. Drawing on my work with the program, I wrote an article in 1991 and an updated

version in 1993 for the *American Journal of Health Promotion*, sum-
marizing the results of the forty-eight studies conducted since 1980
that have evaluated the health and cost effectiveness of comprehensive work site–based disease prevention and health promotion programs. This cumulative research clearly indicates that every program
demonstrated improvements in health. Additionally, for those programs that undertook cost-effectiveness or cost-benefit analyses, the
studies all indicated that the results were positive and saved money
as well as lives. Since my 1991 and 1993 reviews there have been additional studies, which have added further evidence to the observation that healthy people create healthy companies.

Yet there are still two missing partners in this collaboration. Together with the corporations and universities, we need the participation of insurance carriers and medical providers in these health
promotion projects. This point may seem obvious, but indeed, many
efforts in health promotion and in managed care are wasted on legal
and financial strategies. All too often the providers of care are treated as the enemy by managed care reviewers while the clinicians see
the managed care experts as interfering with their clinical practices.
This is an artificial, time-wasting, adversarial relationship that serves
no productive purpose. Happily, some former adversaries are forming new alliances to create truly innovative solutions, rather than ar-
guing over preserving the status quo or tinkering with an obsolete
system. One such project was reported in an article in the September
1992 issue of the *New England Journal of Medicine* citing a new consortium in Minneapolis, long a center of innovation in managed care,
of employers and health providers working together to resolve their
mutual problems. Among the companies in the project are Dayton
Hudson and General Mills, and the medical care providers range from
the Mayo Clinic to local health maintenance organizations. These
corporations and providers of care will work together to improve the
health of their more than 125,000 employees and dependents. Their
plan includes a "newly established institute [that] will develop guidelines for practice aimed at reducing variation in practice patterns and
eliminating unneeded care." If all goes as planned, the health and cost
effectiveness of health promotion programs will be an integral part
of this institute.

Currently the Stanford Corporate Health Program is also moving
toward a working alliance of companies, universities, and providers
of medical care. During the first years of the program, all care
providers were excluded to prevent any marketing or sales activities
that would cloud our research objectives. However, it seems certain

that the next stages in creating healthy work sites for healthy people will result from collaboration, not competition or antagonism. To that end Blue Shield of California (representing a national consortium of Blue Cross and Blue Shield Plans), the Kaiser Permanente Hospital System, Aetna Health Plans, and Johnson & Johnson are increasingly working together toward common solutions. This exciting new direction will lead to the development of innovative programs across the health care spectrum. For example, some will use nurses and computer interventions for advanced heart disease, while others will be oriented specifically to women or retirees. These collaborative efforts will create a symbiotic relationship between working people, their companies, and health care providers.

Women's health will be a major focus in the nineties and beyond. It is not coincidental that this long-overdue emphasis was made an important policy commitment by Dr. Bernadine Healy, who served as the first woman director of the National Institutes of Health prior to her resignation. Within a week of her confirmation as director she announced that she had a dramatic plan to redress what she called the years of neglect of women's health issues. In early 1993 she launched a ten-year program involving 140,000 women and an expenditure of over $500 million. Her proposal for the project was reviewed in *Science*, which summarized it as "a three-part study of postmenopausal women: one part would involve some 70,000 women in a set of clinical trials to measure the effectiveness of hormone replacement therapy, dietary modification, and vitamin supplements to combat heart disease, cancer, and osteoporosis; a second would seek effective ways to promote healthy behavior within local communities; and a third would be an observational study involving a minimum of 70,000 women over age 50 who would be screened for signs of progressive diseases and predictors of future illnesses." Healy's study will emphasize interventions—behavioral combined with pharmacological— to reduce heart disease, cancer, and osteoporosis in women between fifty and seventy-four, and it will pay particular attention to minority women.

Heart disease is the most common cause of mortality in older women: approximately 500,000 women die from it annually, accounting for 29 to 48 percent of all deaths in the age range of fifty to seventy-nine. This is greater than the mortality figure for men—approximately 470,000—yet virtually all of the research to date has focused on men.

Drops in the level of the hormone estrogen after menopause poses a major risk of heart disease for older women. It is thought that when women are premenopausal, estrogen protects them from heart disease, and ironically, it may very well be this protective effect that permits women to develop risky lifestyle habits, such as smoking, weight gain, and high-fat and cholesterol diets, for longer periods of time than men without the negative consequences becoming evident. Published studies have found that women taking estrogen replacement have a reduced risk of developing coronary heart disease. These reductions were observed for nonfatal as well as fatal coronary heart disease and cardiovascular disease. In several of the studies risk reduction appeared to be even more substantial in women with existing vascular disease. However, it is not clear from these observational data whether the apparent benefits of estrogen replacement might not be largely due to self-selection (perhaps healthier individuals are prescribed estrogen replacement), to other selection biases in the inclusion of subjects, or to the reporting of study results. Biases may not only exaggerate the apparent benefits but might also underestimate the magnitude of adverse effects. To clarify this complex question, the interventions in Healy's study will consist of single interventions and various combinations of hormone replacement therapy, low-fat diets, and supplementation of calcium and vitamin D, all within a behavioral program to help women make healthy choices and stay with them.

Using similar interventions, the study will also seek to reduce cancer, including breast cancer and colorectal cancer. In the United States breast cancer among women is the cancer with the highest incidence and has, after lung cancer, the second highest mortality rate. In 1991 an estimated 175,000 cases of breast cancer were diagnosed, and 44,500 deaths occurred. Breast cancer incidence has increased about 1 percent per year since the early 1970s, and international studies show a strong association between fat consumption on one hand and breast cancer incidence and mortality rates on the other. It seems that breast cancer is more common in countries with a high average consumption of total and saturated fat, animal protein, and total calories. Breast cancer incidence rates are more than five times higher in the United States than in Japan, and people migrating from areas with low rates of fat consumption to areas with high rates do indeed acquire the higher cancer and heart disease rates of their adopted country. For example, Japanese migrants to Hawaii and Italian migrants to Australia experience higher rates of breast cancer, suggesting that environmental and lifestyle factors may be of great importance.

Colorectal cancer is the third leading cause of cancer deaths in women. An estimated 78,500 new cases were diagnosed in 1991, and approximately 31,000 deaths occurred. Both human and animal studies conducted over the past few decades have established a strong link between dietary factors and colorectal cancer, and various dietary constituents have been implicated, including total fat consumption, excess calories, and low dietary fiber. As with breast cancer, studies of migrants from areas with diets low in animal fat and protein to areas with a more typical Western diet show an increase in the incidence of colorectal cancer when compared with the incidence in the country of origin. In case control studies the link between dietary fat and colorectal cancer is not readily demonstrable. Several international correlation and case control studies have shown that risk of colorectal cancer decreases with an increased intake of high-fiber foods, just as a high intake of fruits and vegetables has been consistently related to a lower risk of colon cancer.

Finally, the broad-based study of women will attempt to decrease osteoporosis, or loss of bone density, which leads to increased bone fractures for women, especially at older ages. Although fractures are not a major overall cause of death, those women who are hospitalized for hip fractures have a mortality rate as high as 30 percent from such complications as thromboembolism, fat embolism, pneumonia, and surgical problems. Fractures are common at older ages and are a major cause of the loss of mobility. Fracture rates, which increase markedly with age, are negligible at ages below fifty-five. At any age the rates in women are twice as high as those in men. Risk factors relating to bone loss include female gender, increasing age, Caucasian race, oophorectomy (removal of the ovaries), early menopause, prolonged immobility, and insufficient dietary calcium. Protective factors include estrogen replacement therapy, weight loss, and physical activity.

Conducting this exceedingly large and complex series of studies throughout the United States over the next decade will be a major challenge, but it will provide a wealth of information. It should be remembered that this study marks a historical point in medical research, not only because it is a clear commitment to learning more about women's health, but because it emphasizes prevention as well as behavioral and pharmacological methods to enhance optimal health.

At the same time that women are approaching equal access to employment opportunities, they are also gaining equal exposure to a variety of health hazards, ranging from the stress of white-collar work to toxic substances in the workplace. As a result some observers have detected evidence of a decline in women's health. At present an American woman's life expectancy is some eight years longer than a man's, but according to Dr. Nancy Milio of the University of North Carolina's School of Public Health, if current trends continue, the gap is likely to narrow by the end of this century. Milio predicts, "In the future women will die of cirrhosis of the liver at a rate almost equal to men, and their rate of death from circulatory and digestive diseases will not improve as rapidly as that for men." Just as their lifestyle patterns are changing, women's behavioral patterns are also changing. More women today are smoking, and the consequence is an increase in lung cancer. Also, the incidence of alcoholism, depression, sleep disorders, and chronic illnesses is on the rise. Collectively, the new research efforts will benefit women and their families by addressing a long-overdue need to understand the unique circumstances of women.

New technologies and new uses of existing technologies will be invaluable tools in helping individuals attain optimal health. Within medicine itself some major advances in high technology include the introduction of such imaging technologies as the magnetic resonance imaging (MRI) and position emission tomography (PET), the use of laser and laproscopic surgeries, and the use of sound waves for viewing the intrauterine fetus (ultrasound) and dissolving kidney stones (lithotripsy). Within a health care system that emphasizes health promotion and seeks to reduce medical costs, while preserving the quality of care, the telephone and computer are also achieving many sophisticated applications.

Use of the telephone has been linked to medical issues since its inception. In fact, the first transmission over Alexander Graham Bell's new "voice line" was a medical call. On March 10, 1876, Bell called his assistant, Thomas Watson, to help him after he had spilled acid on his skin! Now, more than a century later, the telephone is assuming a role of increasing importance in health care delivery. I mentioned earlier how the SCRIP program at the Stanford Center for Research in Disease Prevention is introducing the use of telephones in conjunction with computer guidelines so that nurses can intervene in advanced coronary heart disease. Similar projects are under way to work with smokers and arthritis sufferers. The telephone "house call" is an effective means of extending health care beyond the office, clinic, hospital, or work site. In the *Journal of the American Medical Association* of April 1992 there is an article concerning the work Dr. John Watson and his colleagues at the Dartmouth Medical School did with 497 men (fifty-four years or older) using clinician-initiated telephone calls. Approximately half of the men were randomly assigned to a group that received three telephone contacts per year plus more frequent face-to-face contact, while the other half followed the usual care recommended by their doctors. After two years the men receiving follow-up phone calls on their care had fewer clinic visits, used less medication, had fewer admissions and shorter stays in the hospital, and fewer days of intensive care. Expenses for these patients were 28 percent less over the two years, leading researchers to conclude that it is cost-effective to substitute telephone care for some limited aspects of care. Similarly, there is a burgeoning number of ways in which telephones, computers, and nurses and other health care providers can work together to provide "electronic house calls."

Other technological innovations in medicine are highly significant. Computer-assisted psychotherapy in the form of a Therapeutic Learning Program or TLP has been developed by the psychiatrist and author Dr. Roger Gould in Santa Monica, California. Preliminary data from this approach indicate that patients improve more rapidly and actually reveal more to the computer-interactive system than they do in face-to-face therapy. In the September 1992 issue of the *Journal of the American Medical Association*, Dr. Steven E. Locke of the Harvard Medical School, author of *The Healer Within*, published an innovative study using computer-based interviews to screen blood donors for the HIV virus, which causes AIDS. Interviews took only eight minutes and were more effective than standard questionnaires and interviews. Clearly such an application would offer even greater safety for the national blood banks. In San Francisco Dr. Albert R. Martin and his colleagues at the Interpractice Systems Company have worked together with the Harvard Community Health Plan and EDS, the company formerly run by Ross Perot, to develop a computer system linking a patient's home to a central clinic. Based on preliminary studies, these patients required fewer actual clinic visits, cost the Harvard Community Health Plan less to provide care, and themselves experienced a greater sense of satisfaction with what they perceived as a higher quality of care. Another innovative application of telecommunications has been used with patients after a heart attack, stroke, or coronary bypass surgery to help them return to work. Research by Dr. Robert F. DeBusk, professor of medicine and director of the Cardiac Rehabilitation Program at the Stanford University School of Medicine, has focused on contacting the person in the hospital as soon as possible during recovery and having nurses follow up with the patient by telephone after discharge from the hospital. To date his research indicates that it is possible for people to return to work sooner, at a higher level of activity, with fewer subsequent problems, and at a much lower cost than has previously been the case. Surely such an intervention is of great benefit to both employers and their employees, who most often do want to return to their careers and occupations.

Finally, a very interesting innovation in the use of telecommunications for house calls is part of the community-based health program in the Northern California town of Chico, mentioned earlier in the chapter. The Healthy Chico 2000 project is one of the first comprehensive programs to apply the principles of creating a healthy community and thereby achieve the goals set out in the United States government document *Healthy People 2000*. If this were the extent of the Chico project, the program would be unique, but it is actually more innovative than it appears. Working with local health and medical care providers, the project has proposed to develop the Video HouseCall. In the 145 environmentally healthy single-family homes to be built for the project, a special feature will be the linking of the homes to clinics and hospitals. Borrowing from the innovations of Interpractice Systems, the demonstration project will add the dimension of visual images by using the AT&T VideoPhone. It will then be possible to establish visual contact between patients and their physicians, greatly enhancing the quality of information provided by the telephone interaction. It is anticipated that Video HouseCall will allow many problems to be solved and many conditions to be treated without requiring a visit to the physician's office. This innovation should result in great savings in medical costs while enhancing the ability of limited numbers of primary care physicians to provide high-quality medical care to more patients. In addition to connecting patients' homes and physicians' offices, this demonstration project will link multiple work sites with a hospital emergency department and occupational health center. Through combining a community-based intervention, including health and medical providers, with creative applications of the new AT&T VideoPhone technology, the project represents a major innovation in helping individuals to elicit and sustain optimal health.

Mind-body interventions, including relaxation techniques, hypnosis, meditation, biofeedback, and visualization, are being given new credibility thanks to more sophisticated research and clinical applications. Mind and body are inextricably linked, and their second-by-second interaction exerts a profound influence upon health and illness, life and death. Attitudes, beliefs, and emotional states ranging from love and compassion to fear and anger can trigger chain reactions of every

cell and organ system in the body—from the stomach and gastrointestinal tract to the immune system. All that is now indisputable fact.
However, there is still great debate over the extent to which the mind
can influence the body and the precise mechanism of the influence.
There is even greater debate over whether, and how, the mind-body
connection can be harnessed to help people stay well or recover from
illness.

Yet despite the uncertainties, effective, responsible mind-body approaches are beginning to be used widely in university and private
clinics, in hospitals, and as an integral part of health promotion programs offered by such Fortune 500 corporate giants as AT&T, Johnson & Johnson, IBM, Du Pont, Bank of America, Coors, and General
Motors. These programs are gaining support because they empower
individuals, teach them skills for self-management, and give them the
knowledge to make informed choices that can promote better health.

Today the medical research community is also taking mind-body
interactions more seriously. One recent sign of this shift in attitudes
was found in a report by the Institute of Medicine, a branch of the National Academy of Sciences, which conducted an inquiry into behavioral influences on the relationship between hormones and
immunity and found a positive link. Similarly, researchers at the National Institutes of Health noted the role of stress in a wide array of
psychiatric problems, autoimmune diseases, coronary heart disease,
functional disorders of the intestinal tract, chronic pain, and a range
of other medical and psychological disorders. On the more public
side of such issues is an article by Charles R. Halpern in the
March/April 1992 issue of the *American Journal of Health Promotion*. After a distinguished career in public law, Halpern is now the
president of the Nathan Cummings Foundation in New York City. Re-
viewing the mind-body field from the political, economic, and public policy standpoint, he concludes, "In short, mind-body approaches
can be seen as posing a challenge, a threat, and an opportunity to a
major American industry—the medical care industry." Never content
to philosophize, Charles Halpern and the Cummings Foundation together with the MacArthur Foundation have funded the new Center
for the Advancement of Health in Washington, D.C., to provide a national clearinghouse for exerting quality control within this burgeoning area.

Early in 1993 Consumers Union, publishers of *Consumer Reports*,
published the first major popular book in this area under the title
Mind/Body Medicine. The book was funded by the Fetzer Institute,
endowed by the late John E. Fetzer, and accompanied the highly vis-

ible Bill Moyers's series *Healing and the Mind*. As I noted in the overview chapter I wrote for *Mind/Body Medicine*, it is clear that the most significant challenge faced by mind-body clinicians is to find ways to maximize the functioning of the immune system to enhance health. That research is likely to lead to two types of treatment: new uses of behavioral approaches and new drugs used with or without behavioral interventions. Meditation, visualization, hypnosis, biofeedback, and various relaxation techniques already show promise in helping prevent and treat a variety of illnesses, including coronary heart disease, autoimmune disorders, chronic lung disease, headaches, and gastrointestinal problems, as well as panic attacks, depression, and other psychological disorders.

Researchers are now trying, with some encouraging results, to demonstrate that such mind-body approaches can also directly affect the immune system. In one study conducted by Dr. Janice Kiecolt-Glaser and her colleagues at the Ohio State University College of Medicine, geriatric nursing home residents who were taught relaxation and guided imagery showed both increased activity of certain immune system cells and better resistance to the herpes virus. Other studies have suggested that humor, positive emotions, and hypnotic suggestion may also affect the immune response. Under hypnosis some subjects are able to increase the number of white blood cells in their bloodstream. Although these findings are not definitive, they do suggest that the mind may be able to control and perhaps optimize the immune system.

In one innovative study, reported in the *Archives of Internal Medicine*, researchers at the University of Arkansas College of Medicine worked with a thirty-nine-year-old woman who was an experienced meditator. After her normal immunological responses were measured, the woman was able voluntarily to reduce her immunological reaction to a skin test for a period of three weeks. At the request of the researchers, she was then able to bring it back up to her normal level voluntarily. While other similar volunteers failed to produce this effect, this study shows that it is possible, in principle, for a practiced individual voluntarily to regulate a specific immune response through meditation and visualization. I conducted a similar series of studies with the researchers Joe Kamiya and Erik Peper at the University of California in San Francisco back in the early 1970s. We found clear evidence that experienced meditators could control pain, bleeding, electrical activity in the brain, muscle tension, and infection.

Given the current crisis in medical care, it would serve us well to pay greater attention to health promotion and disease prevention, including the role of psychological factors and mind-body interventions. Research is also needed to clarify the role of such hard-to-measure factors as beliefs, positive emotions, and even spiritual values. Although these subjects might seem to be grist for idle philosophical speculation, studying them is crucial to our understanding of psychological well-being and physical health and will undoubtedly help us to develop a true health care system.

Higher or spiritual values are becoming an integral part of optimal health for individuals and institutions alike. Our values determine what is most important to us every day, and our values influence the most important choices we make. A major finding from the Sound Mind–Sound Body research was that literally all the participants said that their spiritual beliefs and values guided their personal and professional lives. Increasingly, the advances in medicine are engaging the most profound questions of human existence and values. Many of us have struggled with the question of when or if to end life support and terminate a life. Pro-life versus pro-choice debates have been unfortunately raised to a political totem, with the government overstepping its boundaries and intruding into the realm of personal choice. Whose rights prevail? Genetic testing can detect evidence of inherited diseases for which we have no cure. So what does the doctor reveal to the patient? These matters are on a continuum with moral questions that have been pondered for millennia in the great religions of the world and in literature throughout recorded history. They are issues that reach far beyond the domain of health and medical care into law, ethics, philosophy, issues of culture and ethnicity, religion in its broadest and narrowest sense. These questions can never have one right answer. Because of their changing and unique circumstances, we must look at their many dimensions and answer them, finally, with the voice of our higher selves.

While organized religion has eroded over time, modern Western medicine has begun to encroach on the infinite complexities of the spiritual domain. Dr. Wade Davis, an anthropologist and the author of the controversial book *The Serpent and the Rainbow*, wrote in *Newsweek*, "Western medicine tends to dismiss the ideas that lie at the heart of traditional healing—ideas concerning the spiritual realm, mind-body interactions, the interplay among humanity, the environment and the cosmos—for they don't fit readily into its scientific model. Yet there is a growing recognition that the mysteries of health and healing cannot be separated from the totality of the human experience." Every individual in my study was engaged in seeking this higher level of meaning in his or her life. For them, I found, health was a means to that end, not an end unto itself. This process deeply challenges personal identity in that people lose the widely accepted and shared definitions of the "consensus reality." In their pioneering work William James, Carl G. Jung, Abraham Maslow, Stanislav Grof, and the author Ken Wilber have spoken of the positive aspects of this search for meaning using terms such as *self-actualization, spiritual emergencies*, or *peak experiences*. Whatever the terminology, they all speak of the deeply felt experience that irrevocably confirms for the individual the existence of a realm of human experience beyond the rational mind and physical experience.

Dr. Larry L. Fahlberg and his colleagues at the University of Wyoming are delving into this complex realm. Writing in the "Spiritual Health" section of the *American Journal of Health Promotion*, Fahlberg recognized the increasing intersection of optimal health and spiritual issues. Addressing both the issue of health care providers and the evolution of a true health care system, Fahlberg concluded, "There is much evidence lending itself to the suggestion that spiritual awakening, peak experiences, self-transcendence, and spiritual emergence are valid, beneficial, necessary experiences. Today, a growing minority of people are beginning and continuing their growth into the transpersonal realms. The path of such transformation is often fraught with great difficulties and peril, and the ego often has to suffer crisis before it opens to self-transcendence. For the health promotion profession, which incorporates health enhancement and wellness, it may be necessary to recognize, facilitate, and support spiritual growth." Every individual in the Sound Mind–Sound Body study spoke of having such an experience, whether they entered into it involuntarily in a crisis or voluntarily in the search for a deeper meaning and purpose to their lives. Whether in crisis or in quest, whether in childhood or at the moment of death, the issue of spiritual health cannot be denied. It resides in the vital balance between the tangible and intangible, between biology and the human spirit that underlies the optimal health of individuals and society as a whole.

Individually and collectively these newly emerging areas constitute the foundation of a true health care system. As there are so many other positive instances that could be cited, these are intended to be representative, not definitive. Only recently the National Institutes of

Health created the Office of Complementary Medicine in Bethesda, Maryland, under the direction of Dr. Joseph Jacobs. For the first time this important governmental institution is examining nonorthodox approaches to medicine and health by supporting serious, unbiased clinical research into the validity and efficacy of such approaches. Among the areas under consideration are acupuncture, the psychological support treatment for cancer patients espoused by Dr. Bernie Siegel in *Love, Medicine, and Miracles*, the ayurvedic or Indian medicine popularized by Dr. Deepak Chopra in *Quantum Healing*, homeopathy research of the caliber of the work published in *Lancet* by Dr. Jacques Benveniste of Paris, and the study of the documented instances of spontaneous remission from terminal diseases abstracted from the world's medical journals by the late Brendan O'Regan of the Institute of Noetic Sciences. At the present time, the National Cancer Institute is supporting a study of twenty-five patients to determine if shrinkage of an established tumor can be documented following treatment with only psychotherapy and visualization. Inquiry at such a high level of government is an indication of how far and rapidly the frontiers of health are evolving. For the vast majority of individuals in the Sound Mind–Sound Body study these interventions were both familiar and frequently used. Given their educational and economic freedom, they have had access to the best that could be offered from conventional Western allopathic medicine but often found it insufficient. Creating a true health care system will require the careful, selective incorporation of the best from these nonconventional approaches to health and the treatment of disease—a formidable challenge for the decades ahead.

CONCLUSION

There are many well-known, moderate, and effective strategies that virtually all individuals can use to attain optimal health. It is certain that many more will be learned and disseminated. That is all to the good. However, as commendable and necessary as these personal strategies are, they are not sufficient conditions for achieving optimal health. That challenge is far, far greater. Individuals do not live just at home or spend all their time at work or at local recreation facilities or shopping centers. Individuals live in communities. The community as a whole is where truly effective health promotion strategies must be implemented. Having presented the personal experiences of the prominent individuals in the Sound Mind–Sound

Body study, together with some of the most promising innovations in health promotion and disease prevention, I have attempted to frame what is the most formidable challenge before us now. That challenge is to reach beyond ourselves and beyond personal gratification to create a true health care system that elicits, sustains, and enhances these individual efforts for the collective good. Whether the efforts are in economics, political policy, helping the poor and homeless, curtailing the rising incidence of handgun violence, working in the environmental area to prevent poisoning of our planet while simultaneously protecting other animal life, or preserving the oceans of the world and their marine inhabitants, the imperative for each of us is to do whatever we can, whenever we can, no matter how much or how little.

Most importantly, we need to restore individual and social well-being as the focus of our health care system, rather than allowing the perpetuation of a system mired in procedures and economics. When we focus on what an individual needs rather than on what economic priorities dictate, then those artificial limitations are without merit. Often the fate of one individual can lead to an epiphany for a physician; such an experience was articulated in a brief article in *Newsweek* by Dr. Sam Brody. Seeing a terminally ill, eighty-three-year-old woman with Alzheimer's disease elicited deep introspection for the gastroenterologist. Reflecting on the moment when the woman died in the anonymity of the hospital, Dr. Brody wrote,

> I realize that if DNR meant 'Do Not Reimburse' instead of 'Do Not Resuscitate' far fewer of the terminally and hopelessly ill would receive pointless treatment. . . . Have I come to see them as human loaves of bread in the health-care supermarket? The anonymity of life in a nation of mass convenience seems even more appalling in these very human terms. . . . In coming so far it seems we have left some very important things behind. . . . Faxes, car phones, beepers, scanners, specialists skilled in the latest technology are wonderful. They save time and lives. And we can bill the government for them because they are easier to quantify than judgment, compassion, and kindness. As I drive home I imagine I am standing on a podium before the entire nation. My speech contains the answers to all the problems that face health care in America. In my Utopia, doctors will make enough money but not too much, striving always for what is best for their patients while keeping a vigilant eye on waste. The public will not only take on greater

responsibility for their own health but will also come to understand the complexity and limitations of medical technology. The audience roars its approval for this sweeping vision.

It is in these moments of insight, when the fate of one person touches us all, that the seeming contradiction between the personal and political vanishes.

We know what is conducive to optimal health. According to Dr. J. Michael McGinnis, Deputy Assistant Secretary for Health in the U.S. Department of Health and Human Services, better control of fewer than ten well-known risk factors could "prevent 40 percent to 70 percent of all premature deaths, 33 percent of all cases of acute disability, and 67 percent of all cases of chronic disability. In contrast, technologically oriented medical treatment promises to reduce premature morbidity and mortality by no more than perhaps 10 percent to 15 percent." We know how to identify and eliminate risk factors. Means to enhance health are also becoming increasingly known, as demonstrated by the interviews throughout this book. Reaching a satisfactory solution is largely beyond the realm of individual action: it requires the active, informed, and empowered involvement of all individuals—together.

A new model of health is essential for setting personal as well as political priorities and goals that stretch beyond ourselves and into future generations. Models are not abstractions; they have a very real impact. They are paradigms or ways of viewing ourselves and the world. An old model crumbles when a new model, encompassing new data, takes on new challenges better. Even learning about a new model creates an irrevocable change. Once the world was discovered to be round, long before the voyage of Columbus in 1492, it became impossible to cling to the notion of its being flat. In 1543, Copernicus demonstrated that the earth was not at the center of the solar system, and we began the still-unfinished quest to discover our more humble position in the galactic hierarchy. Breakthroughs such as Rutherford's description of the structure of the atom and Niels Bohr's formulation of the foundations of quantum physics in 1913 erased physical matter into a blur of probabilities and energy fluctuations. Perhaps more than any other individual, Einstein with his theory of general relativity engendered shifts in our models of physical reality that scientists are still struggling to comprehend. Closer to the present time, the cosmological challenges posed by Dr. Stephen Hawking's book *A Brief History of Time* actually reached an even wider audience with the 1992 feature-length film of the same name. To some degree these momentous changes in our models of the universe are easier to digest than challenges to our model of health, because they do not necessarily engender profound individual, social, political, economic, and environmental transformation.

Today there are numerous political, social, religious, and economic gurus vying for dominance over the way we think and act. Perhaps at the root of the search for optimal health are individuals seeking the ideals missing from our petrified modern religions, seeking inner peace and harmony. Perhaps the achievement of optimal health frees an individual of all fears and all cages and offers a state of unconditional freedom based upon a profound inner equilibrium. Buddhism and Hinduism refer to this condition as *samadhi*, a state of consciousness characterized by a sense of unity with all animate and inanimate beings and an end to the fear of suffering and death. Toward that end there is no external road map. Among the great teachers of wisdom in this century, Krishnamurti has been one of the most outspoken in advocating that individuals attend to their own inner directives. In a 1928 lecture he stated, "The time has come when you must no longer subject yourself to anything. . . . I hope you will not listen to anyone, but will listen only to your own intuition, your own understanding, and give a public refusal to those who would be your interpreters. . . . Do not quote me afterwards as an authority. I refuse to be your crutch. I am not going to be brought into a cage for your worship."

Perhaps the most striking revelation of all in the many hours of talking with the participants in my research study was their abiding commitment to a deeper, altruistic spiritual purpose beyond ourselves. Surely it is the magnitude of what remains to be done for all of humankind that makes genuine humility and compassion so evident in their lives. Now that we are closer than ever to a deeper understanding of mind and body, it seems possible at last to bridge the gap between spiritual purpose and optimal health. Our direction is clear, for medical technology alone cannot provide the answer. Twentieth-century science has permitted humankind to peer with electron microscopes into intercellular space and chart the helical coils of the DNA molecule at the very heart of all life. Arcane Buddhist scriptures formulated thousands of years ago advocated the journey inward toward wisdom and enlightenment, the essence of the soul. Whether we are scientists or mystics, these perennial mysteries instill in us all an abiding sense of awe, humility, and compassion.

ACKNOWLEDGMENTS

Throughout the nearly five years of researching and writing this book there were many people who made the work possible through their encouragement, support, generosity, and shared vision. Writing this acknowledgment has given me the opportunity to reflect on how meaningful each person's contribution has been and to extend yet another heartfelt thank-you to many friends and colleagues.

First I would like to express my deep appreciation to Laurance S. Rockefeller, who generously funded this research over the five years it took to develop and complete the interviews. Clearly he is one individual who epitomizes optimal health, but his funding of this project and his well-known modesty precluded his inclusion in the research.

It was personally very insightful and inspiring for me to spend many hours with each of the participants. These interviews were a personal odyssey for me. Being a typical professional overachiever, I learned a great deal from talking with people who have created a vital balance between accomplishing and reflecting, doing and being, loving and being loved. My hope is that the reader will also get the feeling of sitting with, listening to, and talking with these remarkable men and women. Of course, I am most thankful to all the participants for taking hours out of their demanding schedules to provide extensive background materials, then to be interviewed, to proofread and correct the transcriptions, and to invite me into their homes for our most insightful discussions.

At the beginning it seemed almost impossible to gain access to these people, and I am most thankful to several friends and participants who had the patience and forbearance to work with me and refer me to others. Among these special people are my friend and longtime mentor Norman Cousins as well as close friends including John E. Fetzer, Michael S. Currier, Laurel Burch, and Walter Landor.

During the development and refinement of the interview structure and background, numerous friends and colleagues provided a great deal of insight, for which I am thankful, especially Dr. John W. Farquhar, Dr. Daniel Goleman, Mrs. Ellen Cousins, Dr. Philip R. Lee, Dr. Joel Elkes, Dr. James F. Fries, Dr. Rachel Naomi Remen, Dr. David Sobel, Dr. Michael Lerner, Dr. Jon Kabatt-Zinn, Dr. David Spiegel, Dr. Herbert Benson, Dr. Dean Ornish, Dr. Steve Locke, Drs. Joan and Myrin Borysenko, Dr. C. Barr Taylor, Dr. Jerry Jampolsky, Dr. Bernie Spiegel, Dr. Carl Thoresen, Dr. Steven A. Schroeder, Ronald P. Sturtz, and Drs. Anthony E. and Nitsa Elite. Also, a most heartfelt thank-you is extended to my greatly missed friend and colleague Brendan O'Regan for his gifts of encouragement, insight, and wit. A special note of thanks is due Dr. Jonas Salk, who provided many more hours of thought-provoking discussions than I ever thought possible.

During analysis of the research and preparation of the manuscript, Anne Weinberger, Marc Wilson, Rita Kary, Cheryl Chaffin, Cindy Watts, and Lauri Cardwell dedicated themselves to work of the highest quality. At several points in the research additional funding and assistance were provided that enabled us to explore questions and issues that we had not anticipated at the start. For that extra measure I must thank Tom Hurley and Wink Franklin of the Institute of Noetic Sciences, and grants from the American Health Association.

Finding the right agent and most appropriate publisher is often a formidable task, and I am most thankful for the sage guidance of my literary agents, Esther Newberg and Suzanne Gluck of International Creative Management. Through their willingness to listen to and counsel me, I am most fortunate to work with Frederic W. Hills and Laureen Connelly at Simon & Schuster. For many years I had admired the books shepherded by Fred Hills, and I feel very lucky to have had the opportunity to work with him and know firsthand how deserving he is of the praise from his authors.

For his inspiration I wish to express my deep appreciation for the opportunity to read the writings of and meet with His Holiness the Dalai Lama, who evoked so many of the thoughts that led to this book. Finally, yet the most heartfelt of all, I extend my love and deepest appreciation to my wife, Elizabeth, who always provided an unswerving course amidst times of doubt and inspired me with the purity of her heart and soul to express to others the hopes, aspirations, and love we have shared for these, our many lifetimes.

Just as I completed this book, my in-laws, Vincent Lawton Giantvalley and Virginia Halle Giantvalley, underwent a major trauma when Vincent was diagnosed with cancer. At sunset on a clear October evening and surrounded by his family, Vincent quietly shook off his mortal body and crossed over. Nature was his love in life and outside his hospital window one lone maple tree blossomed its full fall colors many weeks too early. During the ordeal of intensive care, he remained a man of dignity, compassion, humor, and courage. A courageous person is not without fear but is one who accepts the fear and proceeds against all odds. His final gift to our family was the time we spent together when three generations of two families came to understand, forgive, and know each other's hearts and minds with an unprecedented clarity and immediacy. We all miss you . . . and we all love you.

KENNETH R. PELLETIER
Diablo, California
January 1994

SELECTED BIBLIOGRAPHY

CHAPTER ONE

Allukian, Myron (1990). Healthy People 2000 and our domestic gulf crisis. *The Nation's Health*, October, 2.

———(1990). Presidential address: Something is wrong with our non-system. *The Nation's Health*, November, 9.

Angell, Marcia (1990). The interpretation of epidemiologic studies. *New England Journal of Medicine* 12:823–825.

Astin, A.; Green, K.; Korn, W.; and Schalit, M. (1987). *American freshmen: National norms for fall.* Los Angeles: Higher Education Research Institute, University of California.

Barsky, Arthur J. (1989). Fitness mania: The body as our temple. *Harvard Medical*, Spring 11–15.

Berkman, L., and Syme, S. (1985). Social networks host resistance and mortality: A nine-year follow-up of Alameda County residents. *American Journal of Epidemiology* 109 (2): 186–204.

Breslow, Lester (1990). A health promotion primer for the 1990s. *Health Affairs*, Summer, 6–21.

Business and Health (1992). Health care spending may reach 40% of GNP, analysts say. March, 24.

Chopra, Deepak (1993). *Ageless body, timeless mind.* New York: Harmony Books.

Consumer Reports (1992). Are HMOs the answer? August, 519–529.

———(1992). Wasted health care dollars. July, 435–448.

Doll, Richard (1992). Health and the environment in the 1990s. *American Journal of Public Health* 82(7): 933–940.

Fahlberg, Larry L.; Wolfer, John; and Fahlberg, Lauri A. (1992). Personal crisis: Growth or pathology? *Spiritual Health* 7(1): 45–52.

Folkman, S., and Lazarus, R. (1980). An analysis of coping in a middle-aged community sample. *Journal of Health and Social Behavior* 21:219–239.

Fuchs, Victor R. (1992). The best health care system in the world? *JAMA* 268(7): 916–917.

Goleman, Daniel, and Gurin, Joel (1993). *Mind body medicine: How to use your mind for better health.* New York: Consumer Reports Book.

Green, Richard (1987). *The "sissy boy syndrome" and the development of homosexuality.* New Haven: Yale University Press.

Hall, H. (1983). Hypnosis and the immune system: A review with implications for cancer and the psychology of healing. *American Journal of Clinical Hypnosis:* 25(2–3): 92–103.

Halpern, Charles R. (1992). The political economy of mind-body health. *American Journal of Health Promotion* 6(4): 288–289.

Hornig, Rohan M., and Locke, S. E., eds. (1985). *Psychological and behavorial treatments for medical disorders.* Vol. 1, *Psychological and behavorial treatment of disorders of the heart and blood vessels.* New York: Institute for the Advancement of Health. Includes annotated bibliography.

Horowitz, Mardi; Adler, Nancy; and Kegeles, Susan (1988). A scale for measuring the occurrence of positive states of mind: A preliminary report. *Psychosomatic Medicine* 50:477–483.

Idler, Ellen (1988). Healthy aging. *Social Forces* 66:226–238.

Keicolt-Glaser, J.; Fisher, L.; Ogrocki, P.; Stout, J.; Speicher, C.; and Glaser, R. (1987). Marital quality, marital disruption, and immune function. *Psychosomatic Medicine* 25(2–3): 92–103.

Kristein, M.; Arnold, C.; and Wynder E. (1977). Health economics and preventive care. *Science* 195:457–462.

Levenstein, Charles (1989). Worksite health promotion. *American Journal of Public Health* 79(1): 11.

Levitt, Theodore (1975). Marketing myopia. *Harvard Business Review,* September-October, 26–178.

Locke, S. E., and Colligan, D. (1990). *The healer within.* New York: E. P. Dutton, 1986. Reprint, New York: New American Library. Spanish, Italian, Japanese, German editions.

Mandell, Harvey, and Spiro, Howard (1987). *When doctors get sick.* New York: Plenum Press.

Marshall, Eliot (1990). Experts clash over cancer data. *Science* 250:900–902.

Morris, Jeff (1991). Through a glass, darkly. *Newsweek,* December 30, 5.

Moyers, Bill (1993). *Healing and the mind.* New York: Doubleday.

Norman, Colin (1988). Rethinking technology's role in economic change. *News and Comment,* May 20, 977.

Ornstein, Robert, and Sobel, David (1989). *Healthy pleasures.* Reading, Mass.: Addison-Wesley.

Oullette-Kobasa, S.; Maddi, S.; and Kahn, S. (1982). Hardiness and health: A prospective study. *Journal of Personality and Social Psychology* 42:168–177.

Pattishall, Evan G., M.D. (1989). The development of behavioral medicine: Historical models. *Journal of the Society of Behaviorial Medicine*, 43–48.

Payer, Lynn (1992). *Disease mongers: How doctors, drug companies, and insurers are making you sick.* New York: John Wiley.

Pelletier, Kenneth (1979). *Holistic medicine: From stress to optical health.* New York: Delacorte Press.

———(1981). *Longevity: Fulfilling our biological potential.* New York: Delacorte and Delta/Seymour Lawrence.

———(1984). *Healthy people in unhealthy places: Stress and fitness at work.* New York: Delacorte and Delta/Seymour Lawrence.

Pelletier, K., and Peper, E. (1976). Alpha EEG feedback as a means for pain control. *Journal of Clinical and Experimental Hypnosis* 25(41): 361–371.

Pilisuk, M., and Parks, K. (1985). Health and social support: Caring relationships and immunological protection. In *The healing web: Social networks and human survival,* edited by M. Pilisuk and S. Hiller. Boston: University of New England Press.

Pollack, Susan (1989). The return of the case study. *Psychology Today,* November, 74–75.

Reynolds, Kim D., and Slenker, Suzanne E. (1990). Fostering a broader understanding of health and health care: The health psychology model. Book review. *Annals of Behavioral Medicine* 12(3): 125–126.

Rowe, John W., and Kahn, Robert L. (1987). Human aging: Usual and successful. *Science,* July 10, 143–149.

Schrage, Michael (1992). Defining what is a disease is biggest health question. *San Jose Mercury News,* June 6.

Seeman, Julia (1989). Toward a model of positive health. *American Psychologist,* August, 1099–1109.

Skolnick, Andrew A. (1992). Manufacturer of "Death Cigarettes" says he's working to bring about the death of smoking. *JAMA* 267(2): 204–207.

Simon, Herbert A. (1990). A mechanism for social selection and successful altruism. *Articles,* December 21, 1665–1668.

Smith, G.; McKenzie, J.; Marmer, D.; and Steele R. (1985). Psychologic modulation of the human immune response to varicella zoster. *Archives of Internal Medicine* 145:2110–2112.

Strohman, Richard (1993). Ancient genomes, wise bodies, unhealthy people: Limits of a genetic paradigm in biology and medicine. *Perspectives in Biology and Medicine,* Autumn.

Sullivan, Louis W. (1990). Healthy people 2000. *New England Journal of Medicine* 323(15): 1065–1067.

Thomas, C.; Krush, A.; Brown, C.; Shaffer, J.; and Duszynski, K. (1982). Cancer in families of former medical students followed to mid-life— Prevalence in relatives of subjects with and without major cancer. *Johns Hopkins Medical* 151(5): 193–202.

Wallack, Lawrence, and Winkleby, Marilyn (1987). Primary prevention: A new look at basic concepts. *Social Science Medicine* 25(8): 923–930.

Wright, Robert (1992). Science, God, and man. *Time* (cover story), December 28, 37–43.

Wynder, E., and Bross, L. (1959). Factors in human cancer development. *Cancer* 12:1016

CHAPTER TWO

Adler, Tina (1991). Seeing double? *APA Monitor* 22(1): 1.

Barnett, Mark A., and McCoy, Sandra J. The relation of distressful childhood experiences and empathy in college undergraduates. *Journal of Genetic Psychology* 150(4): 417–426.

Barnett, Mark A. (1987). Empathy and related responses in children. *Cambridge University Press* 7:146–162.

Barsky, Arthur J. (1989). Fitness mania: The body as our temple. *Harvard Medical,* Spring, 11–15.

Bower, B. (1993). Some lasting memories emerge at age two. *Science News* 143 (June 12): 372.

Breslau, Naomi, et al. (1991). Traumatic events and postraumatic stress disorder in an urban population of young adults. *JAMA* 266(8): 1070.

Coles, Robert (1990). *The spiritual life of children.* New York: Houghton Mifflin.

Conger, John Janeway (1988). Hostages to fortune: Youth, values, and the public interest. *American Psychologist,* April, 291–299.

DeAngelis, Tori (1990). Should wellness model replace disease focus? *APA Monitor,* December, 30.

Drossman, D. A., et al. (1990). Sexual and physical abuse in women with functional or organic gastrointestinal disorders. *Ann. Intern. Med.* 113 (December 1): 828–833.

Ebersole, Peter, and Flores, Joan (1989). Positive impact of life crises. *Journal of Social Behavior and Personality* 4(5): 464–469.

Ebersole, Peter (1990). Life crisis often has positive effect, study shows. *Brain/Mind Bulletin* 15(2): 5.

Ferrucci, Piero (1990). *Inevitable grace: Breakthroughs in the lives of great men and women.* New York: Tarcher.

Gibbons, Ann (1993). Empathy and brain evolution. *Science* 259 (February 26): 1250–1251.

Goertzel, M. G.; Goertzel, V.; and Goertzel, T. G. (1978). *Three hundred eminent personalities.* San Francisco: Jossey-Bass.

Goertzel, V., and Goertzel, M. G. (1962). *Cradles of eminence.* Boston: Little, Brown.

Green, Richard (1987). *The "sissy boy syndrome" and the development of homosexuality.* New Haven: Yale University Press.

Hall, C. Margaret (1986). Crisis as opportunity for spiritual growth. *Journal of Religion and Health* 25(1): 8–17.

Harris, T. George (1987). The new individualism. *Fitness in Business,*

February, 141–144.

Howe, L. T. (1988). Crises and spiritual growth. *Pastoral Psychology* 3:230–238.

Kohlberg, L.; Ricks, D.; and Snarey, J. (1984). Childhood development as a predictor of adaptation in adulthood. *Genetic Psychology Monographs* 110(1): 91–172.

Leo, John (1990). The trouble with self-esteem. *U.S. News and World Report,* April 2, 16.

Locke, Steven E., M.D., and Gorman, James R. (1989). *The comprehensive textbook of psychiatry.* 5th ed. Baltimore: William and Wilkins.

Marantz, Paul., M.D. (1990). Blaming the victim: The negative consequences of preventive medicine. *American Journal of Public Health* 80(10): 1186–1187.

Ornstein, R., and Sobel, D. (1987). *The healing brain.* New York: Simon and Schuster.

Pelletier, K. R. (1977). Adjunctive biofeedback with cancer patients: A case presentation. *Proceedings of the Biofeedback Society of America.* Denver: Biofeedback Society of America.

———(1977). Biofeedback. *Collier's encyclopedia.*

———(1977). Mind as healer, mind as slayer. *Psychology Today,* February, 35–42.

Pelletier, K. R., and Peper, E. (1977). The chutzpah factor in altered states of consciousness. *Journal of Humanistic Psychology* 17(1): 83–73.

Pennebaker, James W.; Kiecolt-Glaser, Janice K.; and Glaser, Ronald (1988). Disclosure of traumas and immune function: Health implications for psychotherapy. *Journal of Consulting and Clinical Psychology* 56:239–245.

Richman, N., and Flaherty, T. (1988). Parent's emotional support predictive of kids' well-being. *J. Nerv. and Mental Dis.* 175:703–712.

Riegel, K. F. (1975). Toward a dialectial theory of development. *Human Development* 18(1–2): 50–64.

Rogers, Tony (1991). Why some people transcend their traumatic childhoods. *San Francisco Chronicle,* October 30, 1–2.

The Nation's Health (1990). Peak ages for developing mental illness are childhood, adolescence. November, 7.

Verhofstadt-Deneve, L. (1985). Crises in adolescence and psychosocial development from a dialectical viewpoint: A seven-year follow-up study with juvenile delinquents. *International Journal of Adolescent Medicine and Health* 1(3–4): 371–390.

Werner, E. E., and Smith, R. S. (1982). *Vulnerable, but invincible: A study of resilient children.* New York: McGraw-Hill.

CHAPTER THREE

Alfred, Kenneth D., and Smith, Timothy W. (1989). The hardy personality:

Cognitive and physiological response to evaluative threat. *Journal of Personality and Social Psychology* 56(2): 257–266.

Altruistic Spirit, The (1991). Sausalito,Calif.: Institute of Noetic Sciences. Report of a program of the institute, 1987–1990.

Bellingham, Richard (1990). Connectedness: Some skills for spiritual health. *Spiritual Health,* 18–23.

Colby, Benjamin N. (1987). Well-being: A theoretical program. *American Anthropologist* 89(4): 879–895.

Crandall, Manes E., and Rasmussen, Roger D. (1975). Purpose-in-life as related to specific values. *Journal of Clinical Psychology* 31(3): 483–485.

Crichton, Michael (1990). Greater expectations: The future of medicine lies not in treating illness but in preventing it. *Newsweek,* September 24, 58.

Drucker, Peter F. (1988). Leadership: More doing than dash. *McKinsey Quarterly,* spring, 67–70.

Emmons, Robert A., and King, Laura A (1988). Conflict among personal strivings: Immediate and long-term implications for psychological and psysical well-being. *Journal of Personality and Social Psychology* 54(6): 1040–1048.

Ferguson, Tom, M.D. (1989). The anatomy of empowerment. *The Last Word,* January/February, 72–75.

Frankl, V. E. (1969). *The will to meaning.* New York: New American Library.

———(1973). *Psychotherapy and existentialism: Selected papers on logotherapy.* Harmondsworth Eng.: Penguin Books.

———(1978). *The unheard cry for meaning: Psychotherapy and humanism.* New York: Simon and Schuster.

Ganellen, R. J., and Blaney, P. H. (1984). Hardiness and social support as moderators of the effects of life stress. *Journal of Personality and Social Psychology* 47:156–163.

Goleman, Daniel (1989). The mind: Healthy illusions. *Longevity,* April, 40–41.

Hiroto, D. S., and Seligman, M. E. P. (1975). Generality of learned helplessness in man. *Journal of Personality and Social Psychology* 31:311–327.

Hull, Jay G.; Van Treuren, Ronald R.; and Propsom, Pamela M. (1988). Attributional style and the components of hardiness. *Personality and Social Psychology Bulletin* 14(3): 505–513.

Hunt, Morton (1991). "Don't worry, be happy": There's something to it. *Longevity,* December, 80–83.

Jemmott, John B., III; Hellman, Caroline; McClelland, David C.; Locke, Steven E.; Kraus, Linda; Williams, R. Michael; and Valeri, C. Robert (1990). Motivational syndromes associated with natural killer cell activity. *Journal of Behavioral Medicine* 13(1): 53–72.

Kobasa, S. C. (1979). Stressful life events, personality, and health: An inquiry into hardiness. *Journal of Personality and Social Psychology* 37:1–11.

————(1982). Commitment and coping in stress resistance among lawyers. *Journal of Personality and Social Psychology* 42(4): 707–717.

————(1984). How much stress can you survive? The answer depends on your personality. *American Health,* September, 64–77.

Kobasa, S. C.; Hilker, Robert R.; and Maddi, Salvatore, R. (1979). Who stays healthy under stress? *Journal of Occupational Medicine* 21(9): 595–598.

Kobasa, S. C.; Maddi, S. R.; and Courington, S. (1981). Personality and constitution as mediators in the stress-illness relationship. *Journal of Health and Social Behavior* 22:368–378.

Kobasa, S. C.; Maddi, Salvatore R.; and Kahn, Stephen (1982). Hardiness and health: A prospective study. *Journal of Personality and Social Psychology* 42(1): 168–177.

Kobasa, S. C.; Maddi, S. R.; and Zola, M. A. (1983). Type A and hardiness, *Journal of Behavioral Medicine* 6:41–51.

Kobasa, S. C., and Puccetti, M. C. (1983). Personality and social resources in stress resistance. *Journal of Personality and Social Psychology* 45:839–850.

Locke, Steven E., M.D. (1982). Stress, adaption, and immunity: Studies in humans. *General Hospital Psychiatry* 4:49–58.

Locke, Steven E., and Colligan, Douglas (1986). Stressed for success. *New Age Journal,* June, 30–64.

Martin, Toni (1993). Review of *Disease-mongers: How doctors, drug companies and insurers make you feel sick. New England Journal of Medicine* 328(3): 218.

McClelland, David C. (1989). Motivational factors in health and disease. *American Psychologist* 44(4): 675–683.

Minkler, Meredith (1986). The social component of health. *Social Health,* Fall, 33–38.

Murphy, Michael (1986). The mysterious powers of body and mind. *Esquire,* May, 151–154.

Novak, Philip (1986). The Buddha and the computer: Meditation in an age of information. *Journal of Religion and Health* 25(3): 188–193.

Overmeier, J. B., and Seligman, M. E. P. (1967). Effects of inescapable shock upon subsequent escape and avoidance responding. *Journal of Comparative and Physiological Psychology* 63:28–33.

Payer, Lynn (1992). *Disease mongers: How doctors, drug companies, and insurers make you feel sick.* New York: John Wiley.

Pelletier, K. R. (1979). Holistic medicine: From pathology to prevention. *Western Journal of Medicine* 131(6): 481–483.

————(1979). Stress/unstress: A conversation with Kenneth R. Pelletier. *Medical Self-Care* 5:3–9.

————(1980). The mind in health and disease. In *Holistic medicine: An annotated bibliography,* edited by A. Hastings, J. Fadiman, and J. S. Gordon. Rockville, Md.: National Institute of Mental Health. Reprinted in

Health for the whole person, edited by A. Hastings, J. Fadiman, and J. S. Gordon. Boulder, Colo.: Westview Press, 1980.

———(1981). Psychosomatic approaches to healing. In *Folk healing and herbal medicine,* edited by K. Blum, J. Cull, and G. G. Meyer. Springfield, Ill.: Charles C. Thomas.

———(1983). A preventive approach to behavioral medicine: Biofeedback and beyond. In *Mind, body and health,* edited by D. E. Bresler, D. A. Jaffe, and J. S. Gordon. New York: Human Sciences Press.

———(1983). Stress: Etiology, assessment, and management in holistic medicine. In *Selye's guide to stress research,* edited by H. Selye. New York: Van Nostrand Reinhold Company. Reprinted in *Selected issues in drug abuse.* Community Epidemiology Work Group Proceedings. Washington, D.C.: U.S. Department of Health and Human Services, National Institute on Drug Abuse, 1983, Vol. 2, 16–51.

———(1983). Stress management: A positive approach to optimum health and longevity. *Generations: Journal of the Western Gerontological Society,* Spring, 26–30. Reprinted in *Wellness perspectives.* Lincoln: University of Nebraska Press, 1984.

Peterson, Christopher, and Seligman, Martin E. P. (1987). Explanatory style and illness. *Journal of Personality* 55(2): 237–265.

Peterson, C.; Seligman, M. E. P.; and Vallant, George, E. (1988). Pessimistic explanatory style is a risk factor for physical illness: A thirty-five year longitudinal study. *Journal of Personality and Social Psychology* 55(1): 23–27.

Pines, Maya (1980). Psychological hardiness: The role of challenge in health. *Psychology Today,* December, 34–98.

Reker, Gary T.; Peacock, Edward H.; and Wong, Paul T. P. (1987). Meaning and purpose in life and well-being: A life span perspective. *Journal of Gerontology* 42(1): 44–49.

Rhodewalt, Frederick, and Zone, Joan B. (1989). Appraisal of life change, depression, and illness in hardy and nonhardy women. *Journal of Personality and Social Psychology* 56(1): 81–88.

Rodin, Judith, and Langer, Ellen J. (1977). Long term effect of a control-relevant intervention with the institutionalized aged. *Journal of Personality and Social Psychology* 35: 897–902.

Rosener, Judy B. (1990). Ways women lead. *Harvard Business Review,* November/December, 119–125.

Ruffin, Julian E. (1985). The anxiety of meaninglessness. *Journal of Counseling and Development* 63:40–42.

Ryff, Carol D. (1989). Happiness is everything, or is it? Explorations on the meaning of psychological well-being. *Journal of Personality and Social Psychology,* 57(6): 1069–1081.

Schier, Michael F., and Carver, Charles S. (1985). Optimism, coping and health: Assessment and implications of generalized outcome expectancies. *Health Psychology* 4:219–247.

Schnall, Peter L., M.D.; Pieper, Carl; Schwartz, Joseph E.; Karasek, Robert A.; Schlussel, Yvette; Devereux, Richard B.; Ganau, Antonello, M.D.; Alderman, Michael, M.D.; Warren, Katherine; and Pickering, Thomas G., M.D. (1990). The relationship between "job strain," workplace diastolic blood pressure, and left ventricular mass index. *JAMA* 263(14): 1929–1935.

Seligman, M. E. P. (1975). *Helplessness: On depression, development, and death.* San Francisco: Freeman.

Seligman, M. E. P., and Maier, S. F. (1967). Failure to escape traumatic shock. *Journal of Experimental Psychology* 74:1–9.

Shafer, Walter E., and McKenna, John F. (1991). Perceived energy and stress resistance; A study of city managers. *Journal of Social Behavior and Personality* 6(2): 271–282.

Shapiro, Harold T. (1990). The willingness to risk failure. *Science* 250(4981): 609.

Shors, Tracey J.; Seib, Thomas B.; Levine, Seymour; and Thompson, Richard F. (1989). Inescapable versus escapable shock modulates longterm potentiation in the rat hippocampus. *Science* 244:224–226.

Soderstrom, Doug, and Wright, E. Wayne (1977). Religious orientation and meaning in life. *Journal of Clinical Psychology* 33:65–67.

Suls, J., and Mullen, B. (1981). Life events, perceived control, and illness: The role of uncertainty. *Journal of Human Stress* 7:30–34.

Syme, S. Leonard (1991). Control and health: A persona perspective. *Advances* 7(2): 16–26.

Tillich, P. (1952). *The courage to be.* New Haven: Yale University Press.

Trotter, Robert J. (1987). Stop blaming yourself. *Psychology Today,* February, 31–39.

Wallerstein, Nina (1992). Powerlessness, empowerment, and health: Implications for health promotion programs. *Behavior Change* 6(3): 197–205.

Weiner, Yoash; Muczyz, Jan P.; and Gable, Myron (1987). Relationships between work commitments and experience of personal well-being. *Psychological Reports* 60:459–466.

Wellness Letter (University of California at Berkeley) (1991). The middle of life: A good place to be. August, 4–5.

Wheeler, Robert J.; Munz, David C.; and Jain, Ashish (1990). Life goals and general well-being. *Psychological Reports* 66:307–312.

Wong, Paul T. P. (1989). Personal meaning and successful aging. *Canadian Psychology* 30(3): 516–525

Yarnell, T. D. (1971). Purpose-in-life test: Further correlates. *Journal of Individual Psychology* 21:76–79.

Zautra, Alex, and Hempel, Ann (1984). Subjective well-being and physical health: A narrative literature review with suggestions for future research. *International Journal of Aging and Human Development* 19(2): 95–110.

Zika, Sheryl, and Chamberlain, Kerry (1987). Relation of hassles and personality to subjective well-being. *Journal of Personality and Social Psychology* 53(1): 155–162.

CHAPTER FOUR

Ader, R. (1981). *Psychoneuroimmunology*. New York: Academic Press.

Barraclough, J., et al. (1992). Life events and breast cancer prognosis. *Behavioral Medicine Journal* 304 (April 25): 1078–1081.

Behavioral influences on the endocrine and immune systems. (1989). Division of Health Sciences Policy, Division of Mental Health and Behavioral Medicine, Institute of Medicine. Washington, D.C.: National Academy Press.

Borysenko, Myrin (1987). Area review: Psychoneuroimmunology. *Annals of Behavioral Medicine* 9:3–9.

Chrousos, George P., and Gold, Philip W. (1992). The concepts of stress and stress system disorders. *JAMA* 267(9): 1244–1252.

Cohen, Sheldon; Tyrrell, David A. J.; and Smith, Andrew P. (1991). Psychological stress and susceptibility to the common cold. *New England Journal of Medicine* 325(9): 606–612.

Cohen, Sheldon, and Williamson, Gail M. (1991). Stress and infectious disease in humans. *Psychological Bulletin* 109:5–24.

Davison, Gerald C.; Williams, Marian E.; Nezami, Elahe; Bice, Traci L.; and DeQuattro, Vincent L. (1991). Relaxation, reduction in angry articulated thoughts, and improvements in borderline hypertension and heart rate. *Journal of Behavioral Medicine* 14(5): 453–468.

Dohrenwend, B., and Dohrenwend, B. (1974). *Stressful life events: Their nature and effects*. New York: John Wiley.

Dorian, Barbara, M.D., and Taylor, C. Barr, M.D. (1984). Stress factors in the development of coronary artery disease. *Journal of Occupational Medicine* 26(10): 747–756.

Fawzy, Fawzy I.; Kemeny, Margaret E.; Fawzy, Nancy W.; Elashoff, Robert; Morton, Donald; Cousins, Norman; and Fahey, John L. (1990). A structured psychiatric intervention for cancer patients. *Arch. Gen. Psychiatry* 47:729–735.

Francis, Martha E., and Pennebaker, James W. (1992). Putting stress into words: The impact of writing on physiological, absentee, and self-reported emotional well-being measures. *American Journal of Health Promotion* 6(4): 280–287.

Gorman, Jack M., and Kertzner, Robert M. (1991). *Psychoimmunology update*. Washington, D.C.: American Psychiatric Press.

Gorman, James, and Locke, Steven (1989). Neural, endocrine, and immune interactions. In *Comprehensive Textbook of Psychiatry*. 5th ed. Baltimore: William and Wilkins.

Harris, Tirril (1991). Life stress and illness: The question of specificity. *An-*

nals of Behavioral Medicine 13(4): 211–219.

Heisel, J. Stephen; Locke, Steven E.; Kraus, Linda J.; and Williams, R. Michael (1986). Natural killer cell activity and MMPI scores of a cohort of college students. *Am. J. Psychiatry* 143(11): 1382–1386.

Helmer, Dianne C.; Ragland, D.; and Syme, S. Leonard (1991). *American Journal of Epidemiology* 133(2): 112–122.

Hiatt, J. F. (1986). Spirituality, medicine, and healing. *Southern Medical Journal* 79(6): 736–743.

Kabat-Zinn, J., and Chapman-Waldrop, Ann (1988). Compliance with an outpatient stress reduction program: rates and predictors of program completion. *Journal of Behavioral Medicine* 11(4): 333–351.

Kabat-Zinn, J.; Lipworth, L.; Burney, R.; and Sellers, W. (1987). Four-year follow-up of a meditation-based program for the self-regulation of chronic pain: Treatment outcomes and compliance. *Clinical Journal of Pain* 2:159–173.

Kaplan, G., and Camacho, T. (1983). Perceived health and mortality: A nine-year follow-up of the human population laboratory cohort. *American Journal of Epidemiology* 117:292–304.

Kaplan, Jay R.; Manuck, Stephen B.; Clarkson, Thomas B.; Lusso, Frances M.; Taub, David M.; and Miller, Eric W. (1983). Social stress and atherosclerosis in normocholesterolemic monkeys. *Science* 220:733–735.

Kiecolt-Glaser, Janice K., and Glaser, Ronald (1988). Psychological influences on immunity: Implications for AIDS. *American Psychologist* 43(11): 892–898.

Kiecolt-Glaser, Janice K.; Glaser, Ronald; Williger, Daniel; Stout, Julie; Messick, George; Sheppard, Sharon; Ricker, Denise; Romisher, Stephen C.; Briner, William; Bonnell, George; and Donnerberg, Roy (1990). Psychosocial enhancement of immunocompetence in a geriatric population. *Health Psychology* 4(1): 24–41.

Locke, S. E. (1983). *Mind and immunity: Behavioral immunology.* New York: Institute for the Advancement of Health. Annotated bibliography, 1976–1982.

Locke, S. E.; Ader, R.; Besedovsky, H.; Hall, N. R.; Solomon, G. F.; and Strom, T., eds. (1985). *Foundations of psychoneuroimmunology.* Hawthorne, N.Y.: Aldine.

Locke, S. E., and Gorman, J. R. (1989). Behavior and immunity. In *Comprehensive Textbook of Psychiatry,* 5th ed., edited by H. I. Kaplan and B. J. Sadock. Baltimore: William and Wilkins.

Locke, Steven E.; Kraus, Linda; Lesserman, Jane; Hurst, Michael W.; Heisel, J. Stephen; and Williams, R. Michael (1984). Life change stress psychiatric symptoms, and natural killer cell activity. *Psychosomatic Medicine* 46(5): 441–453.

Locke, Steven E.; Ransil, Bernard J.; Covine, Nicholas A.; Toczydlowski, Janice; Lohse, Christopher M.; Dvorak, Harold F.; Arndt, Kenneth A.; and Frankel, Fred H. (1987). Failure of hypnotic suggestion to alter immune response to delayed type hypersensitivity antigens. *Annals of the New York Academy of Sciences* 496:745–749.

Marx, Jean L. (1985). The immune system "belongs in the body." *Science* 227:1190–1192.

McCubbin, James A.; Kaufmann, Peter G.; and Nemeroff, Charles B., eds. (1991). *Stress, neuropeptides, and systemic disease.* San Diego: Academic Press.

Mechanic, D. (1977). Illness behavior, social adaptation, and the management of illness: A comparison of educational and medical models. *Journal of Nervous and Mental Disorders* 165:70–87.

Miller, Andrew H. (1989). *Depressive disorders and immunity.* Washington, D.C.: American Psychiatric Press.

Mossey, J., and Shapiro, E. (1982). Self-rated health: A predictor of mortality among the elderly. *American Journal of Public Health* 72:800–808.

Parkes, C.; Benjamin, B.; and Fitzgerald, R. (1969). Broken heart: A study of increased mortality among widowers. *British Medical Journal* 1:740–743.

Pelletier, K. (1979). *Holistic medicine: From stress to optimum health.* New York: Delta.

———(1984). Healthy people in healthy places: Health promotion programs in the workplace. In *Emotions in health and illness: Clinical applications,* edited by C. Van Dyke, L. Temoshok, and L. S. Zegans. New York: Grune and Stratton, 243–255.

———(1985). Holistic medicine. *World book encyclopedia.*

———(1986). Longevity: What can centenarians teach us? In *Wellness and health promotion for the elderly,* edited by E. Dychtwold, Rockville, Md.: Aspen.

———(1987). Behavioral medicine. In *Mind, body, and health: Toward an integral medicine,* edited by J. S. Gordon, D. T. Jaffe, and D. E. Bresler. New York: Human Sciences Press.

———(1992). *Mind as healer, mind as slayer: A holistic approach to preventing stress disorders.* New York: Delta.

Pelletier, K. R., & Herzing, D. L. (1988). Psychoneuroimmunology: Toward a mindbody model—A critical review. *Advances: Journal of the Institute for the Advancement of Health* 5(1):1–30.

Pilisuk, M., and Parks, K. (1985). Health and social support: Caring relationships and immunological protection. In *The healing web: Social networks and human survival,* edited by M. Pilisuk and S. Hiller. Boston: University of New England Press.

Raphael, B. (1977). Preventive intervention with the recently bereaved. *Archives of General Psychiatry* 34: 1450–1457.

Rosch, P., and Pelletier, K. R. (1987). Designing workplace stress management programs. In *Stress management in work settings,* edited by L. R. Murphy and T. F. Schoenborn. Washington, D.C.: Department of Health and Human Services, Publication No. 87–111.

Sieter, W. J.; Rodin, J.; Larson, L.; Ortega, S.; Cummings, N.; Levy, S.; Whiteside, T.; & Herlerman, R. (1992). Modulation of human natural killer cell activity by exposure to uncontrollable stress. *British Journal of Behavioral Immunity* 6:141–156.

Schnall, Peter L.; Pieper, Carl; Schwartz, Joseph E.; Karasek, Robert A.; Schlussel, Yvette; Devereux, Richard B.; Ganau, Antonello; Alderman, Michael; Warren, Katherine; and Pickering, Thomas G. (1990). The relationship between "job strain," workplace diastolic blood pressure, and left ventricular mass index. *JAMA* 263(14): 1929–1935.

Smith, G., and McDaniel, S. (1983). Psychologically mediated effort on the delayed hypersensitivity reaction to tuberculin in humans. *Psychosomatic Medicine* 45(1): 65–70.

Smith, G.; McKenzie, J.; Marmer, D.; and Steele, R. (1985). Psychologic modulation of the human immune response to varicella zoster. *Archives of Internal Medicine* 145:2110–2112.

Spiegel, D. (1991). Psychosocial aspects of cancer. *Current Opinion in Psychiatry* 4:889–897.

Spiegel, David (1991). A psychosocial intervention and survival time of patients with metastic breast cancer. *Advances, The Journal of Mind-Body Health,* 7(3): 10–19.

Spiegel, David; Bierre, Pierre; and Rootenberg, John (1989). Hypnotic alteration of somatosensory perception. *American Journal of Psychiatry* 146(6): 749–754.

Spiegel, David; Bloom, Joan R.; Kraemer, Helena C.; and Gottheil, Ellen (1989). Effect of psychosocial treatment on survival of patients with metastatic breast cancer. *The Lancet* 2 (October 14): 888–891.

Spratt, M. L., and Denney, D. R. (1991). Immune variables, depression, and plasma cortisol over time in suddenly bereaved parents. *J. Neuropsychiatry Clin. Neurosci.* 3:299–306.

Stein, M.; Miller, A. H.; and Trestmen, R. L. (1991). Depression, the immune system, and health and illness: Findings in search of meaning. *Archives of General Psychiatry* 48:171–177.

Tessler, R., and Mechanic, D. (1978). Psychological distress and perceived health status. *Journal of Health and Social Behavior* 19:254–262.

The mind, the body, and the immune system: Part I. (1992). *Harvard Mental Health Letter* 8(7): 1–3.

The mind, the body, and the immune system: Part II. (1992). *Harvard Mental Health Letter* 8(8): 1–3.

Vaillant, George E. (1977). *Adaptation to life.* Boston: Little Brown.

Volhardt, Lawrence T. (1991). Psychoneuroimmunology: A literature review. *American Journal of Orthopsychiatry* 61 (January): 35–47.

Yeung, Alan C.; Vekshtein, Vladimir I.; Krantz, David S.; Vita, Joseph A.; Ryan, Thomas J., Jr.; Ganz, Peter; and Selwyn, Andrew P. (1991). The effect of atherosclerosis on the vasomotor response of coronary arteries to mental stress. *New England Journal of Medicine* 325(22): 1551–1580.

CHAPTER FIVE

Barry, Joan; Selwyn, Andrew P.; Nabel, Elizabeth G.; Rocco, Michael B.; Mead, Kimberley; Campbell, Stephen; and Rebecca, George (1988). Frequency of ST-segment depression produced by mental stress in stable angina pectoris from coronary artery disease. *Am. J. Cardiol.* 61:989–993.

Bower, Bruce (1991). Stress goes to the dogs. *Science,* November 2, 285.

Browner, C. H. (1987). Job stress and health: The role of social support at work. *Research in Nursing and Health* 10(2): 93–100.

Case, Robert B.; Moss, Arthur J.; Case, Nan; McDermott, Michael; and Eberly, Shirley (1992). Living alone after myocardial infarction. *JAMA* 267(4): 515–520.

Crichton, Michael (1990). Greater expectations. *Newsweek,* September 24, 58.

Deanfield, John E.; Kensett, Malcolm; Wilson, Richard A.; Shea, Michael; Horlock, Peter; deLandsheere, Christian M.; and Selwyn, Andrew P. (1984). Silent myocardial ischaemia due to mental stress. *The Lancet,* November 3, 1991.

DeAngelis, Tori (1992). Cutting cholesterol—feeling feisty? *APA Monitor,* May, 8–9.

DeVreede, J. J. M.; Gorgels, A. P. M.; Verstraaten, G. M. P.; et al. (1991). Did prognosis after acute myocardial infarction change during the past 30 years? A meta-analysis. *J. Am. Coll. Cardiol.* 18 (September): 698–706.

Frankenhaeuser, Marianne (1991). Mini-series: Behavioral medicine: An international perspective. *Annals of Behavioral Medicine* 13(4): 197–204.

Hendrix, W. H. (1989). Job and personal factors related to job stress and risk of developing coronary artery disease. *Psychological Reports* 65 (December): 1136–1138.

House, James S.; Landis, Karl R; and Umberson, Debra (1988). Social relationships and health. *Science* 241 (July): 540–545.

Idler, Ellen L. and Kasl, Stanislav V. (1992). Religion, disability, depression, and the timing of death. *American Journal of Sociology* 97(4) January: 1052–1079.

James, G. D.; Cates, E. M.; Pickering, T. G.; and Laragh, J. H. (1989). Parity and perceived job stress elevate blood pressure in young normotensive working women. *American Journal of Hypertension* 2(8): 637–639.

Jemmot, John B., and Locke, Steven E. (1984). Psychosocial factors, immunologic mediation, and human susceptibility to infectious diseases: how much do we know? *Psychological Bulletin* 95(1): 78–106.

Johnson, Jeffrey V., and Hall, Ellen M. (1988). Job strain, work place social support, and cardiovascular disease: A cross-sectional study of a random sample of the Swedish working population. *AJPH* 78 (10): 1336–1342.

Kaplan, G. A., et al. (1988). Outcomes of the North Karetic, Sweden, project. *American Journal of Epidemiology* 128(2): 370–380

Kaplan, J. R., et al. (1983). Coronary blockages in monkeys with disrupted social networks. *Science* 220(4598): 733–735.

Karasek, R. (1989). The political implications of psychosocial work redesign: A model of the psychosocial class structure. *International Journal of Health Services* 19(3): 481–508.

Karasek, R. A.; Theorell, T.; Schwartz, J. E.; Schnall, P. L.; Pieper, C. F.; and Michela, J. L. (1988). Job characteristics in relation to the prevalence of myocardial infarction in the US Health Examination Survey (HES) and the Health and Nutrition Examination Survey (HANES). *American Journal of Public Health* 78(8): 910–918.

Karasek, Robert; Baker, Dean; Marxer, Frank; Ahlbom, Anders; and Theorell, Tores (1981). Job decision latitude, job demands, and cardiovascular disease: A prospective study of Swedish men. *AJPH* 71(7): 694–705.

Kawakami, N.; Araki, S.; Haratani, T.; Kaneko, T.; Masumoto, T.; and Hayashi, T. (1990). Job-stress and medical consultation rates for physical illness among blue collar workers of an electrical factory in Japan: A four-year prospective follow-up study. *Industrial Health* 28(1): 1–7.

Kawakami, N.; Araki, S.; Hayashi, T.; and Masumoto, T. (1989). Relationship between perceived job-stress and glycosylated hemoglobin in white-collar workers. *Industrial Health* 27(4): 149–154.

Kawakami, N.; Haratani, T.; Kaneko, T.; and Araki, S. (1989). Perceived job-stress and blood pressure increase among Japanese blue collar workers: One-year follow-up study. *Industrial Health* 27(2): 71–81.

Kiecolt-Glaser, J. K.; Dura, J. R.; Speicher, C. E.; Trask, O. J.; and Glaser, R. (1991). Spousal caregivers of dementia victims: Longitudinal changes in immunity and health. *Psychosom. Med.* 53:345–362

Kiecolt-Glaser, J., and Glaser, R. (1988). Lowered immune function among patients above average in loneliness measures. *Adv. Biochem. Psychopharmacol.* 44:217–224.

Kiritz, Stewart, and Moos, Rudolf H. (1974). Physiological effects of social environments. *Psychosomatic Medicine* 36(2): 96–114.

Kritz-Silverstein, Donna; Wingard, Deborah L.; and Barrett-Connor, Elizabeth (1992). Employment status and heart disease risk factors in middle-aged women: The Rancho Bernardo study. *American Journal of Public Health* 82(2): 215–219.

Kryder, Suzanne, and Wilde, Judith Busch (1991). Stressors, strain, health outcomes, and social support in bank employees. *Wellness Perspectives: Research, Theory and Practice* 8(2): 32–45.

Levi, L. (1989). Occupational stressors, biological stress reactions, and worker's health. *Sangyo Ika Daigaku Zasshi*, March 20, 11 Suppl, 480–481.

Marcelissen, F. H.; Winnubst, J. A.; Buunk, B.; and de Wolff, C. J. (1988). Social support and occupational stress: A casual analysis. *Social Science and Medicine* 26(3): 365–373.

Minkler, Meredith (1986). The social component of health. *American Journal of Health Promotion* 1(2): 33–38.

Nerem, R. M., et al. (1980). *Science* 208(4451): 1475–1476.

Niaura, R.; Herbert, P. N.; Saritelli, A. L.; Goldstein, M. G.; Flynn, M. M.; Follick, M. J.; Gorkin, L.; and Adhern, D. K. (1991). Lipid and lipoprotein responses to episodic occupational and academic stress. *Archives of Internal Medicine* 151(11): 2172–2179.

Orth-Gomer, K., et al. (1988). *Acta Med. Scand.* 224(3): 205–215.

Pelletier, K. R. (1985). The hidden hazards of the modern office. *New York Times,* September 8.

———(1986). Healthy people in healthy places: Health promotion programs in the workplace. In *Health and industry—A behavioral medicine perspective.* New York: John Wiley.

———(1988). Cost-effective data: Searching for the unicorn continues. *American Journal of Health Promotion* 3(1): 57–66.

———(1988). Psychoneuroimmunology: A new model of health. In *Eastern and western approaches to healing.* New York: John Wiley.

Pelletier, K. R.; Doellefeld, Howard C.; and Standley, M. (1988). Firms gain competitive advantage by targeting employee health. *Business and Health,* October, 44–45.

Pelletier, K. R., and Klehr, N. L. (1988). Town and gown: A lesson in collaboration. *Business and Health,* February, 34–39.

Pelletier, K. R.; Klehr, N. L.; and McPhee, S. J. (1988). Developing workplace health promotion programs through university and corporate collaboration. *American Journal of Health Promotion* 2(4): 75–81.

Pelletier, K. R., and Lutz, R. (1988). Healthy people—Healthy business: A critical review of stress management programs in the workplace. *American Journal of Health Promotion* 2(3): 5–12, 19.

Pelletier, K. R.; McPhee, S. J.; and Klehr, N. L. (1988). Corporate management and academic medicine. *Perspectives on Prevention: Journal of the Association of Teachers of Preventive Medicine* 3(3): 64–66.

Pennebaker, J. W., et al. (1988). *J. Consult. Clin. Psychol.* 56(2): 239–245.

Pieper, C.; LaCroix, A. Z.; and Karasek, R. A. (1989). The relation of psychosocial dimensions of work with coronary heart disease risk factors: A meta-analysis of five United States data bases. *American Journal of Epidemiology* 129(3): 483–494.

Razanski, Alan; Bairey, C. Noel; Drantz, David S.; Friedman, John; Resser, Kenneth J.; Morell, Marie; Hilton-Chalfen, Sally; Hestrin, Lisa; Bietendorf, James; and Berman, Daniel S. (1988). Mental stress and the induction of silent myocardial ischemia in patients with coronary artery disease. *New England Journal of Medicine* 318(16): 1005–1017.

Reed, D., et al. (1983). Protective effects on coronary heart disease among men of Japanese ancestry living in Hawaii. *American Journal of Epidemiolgy,* 117(4): 384–396.

Reed, D. M.; LaCroix, A. Z.; Karasek, R. A.; Miller, D.; and MacLean, C. A. (1989). Occupational strain and the incidence of coronary heart disease. *American Journal of Epidemiology* 129(3): 495–502.

Roberman, William (1992). Psychosocial influences on mortality of patients with coronary heart disease. *JAMA* 267(4): 559–560.

Rosch, P. J., and Pelletier, K. R. (1986). *Occupational Stress.* Monograph 14. New York: AMS Press.

Rothberg, Joseph M.; Bartone, Paul T.; Holloway, Harry C.; and Marlowe, David H. (1990). Life and death in the US army. *JAMA* 264(17): 2241–2244.

Ruberman, W., et al. (1984). Increased risk of cardiac death and all-cause mortality among socially isolated men. *New England Journal of Medicine* 311(9): 552–559.

Schnall, P. L.; Peiper, C.; Schwartz, J. E.; Karasek, R. A.; Schlusel, Y.; Devereux, R. B.; Ganau, A.; Alderman, M.; Warren, K.; and Pickering, T. G. (1990). The relationship between "job strain," workplace diastolic blood pressure, and left ventricular mass index. Results of a case-control study. *JAMA* 263(14): 1929–1935.

Schwartz, J. E.; Pieper, C. F.; and Karasek, R. A. (1988). A procedure for linking psychosocial job characteristics data to health surveys. *American Journal of Public Health* 78(8): 904–909.

Seeman, T. E. and Syme, S. L. (1987). Reduced coronary angiograph blockages among men and women with and without social support. *Psychosom. Med.* 49(4): 341–354.

Siegrist J.; Matchinger, H.; Cremer, P.; and Seidel, D. (1988). Atherogenic risk in men suffering from occupational stress. *Atherosclerosis* 69(2–3): 211–218.

Singh, R. G. (1990). Relationship between occupational stress and social support in flight nurses. *Aviation Space and Environmental Medicine* 61(4): 349–352.

Specchia, Giuseppe; de Servi, Stefano; Falcone, Colomba; Gavazzi, Antonello; Angoli, Luigi; Bramucci, Ezio; Ardissino, Diego; and Mussini, Antonio (1984). Mental arithmetic stress testing in patients with coronary artery disease. *American Heart Journal* 108:56.

Spiegel, D., et al. (1989). The beneficial effect of psychosocial treatment on survival of metastatic breast cancer patients: A randomized prospective outcome study. *The Lancet* 2(8677): 1447.

Syme, S. Leonard (1982). People need people. *American Health,* July/August, 49–51.

Theorell, T., and Karasek, R. (1989). Can the number of myocardial infarctions be reduced by improving the psychosocial work environment? (in Swedish). *Lakartidningen* 86(16): 1455–1456.

Theorell, T.; Karasek, R. A.; & Eneroth, P. (1990). Job strain variations in relation to plasma testosterone fluctuations in working men—A longitudinal study. *Journal of Internal Medicine* 227(1): 31–36.

Unden, Anna-Lena; Orth-Gomer, Kristina; and Elofsson, Stig (1991). Cardiovascular effects of social support in the work place: Twenty-four-hour ECG monitoring of men and women. *Psychosomatic Medicine* 53(1): 50–60.

Vaillant, George E. (1977). *Adaptation to life*. Boston: Little Brown.

Williams, Redford B.; Barefoot, John C.; Califf, Robert M.; Haney, Thomas L.; Saunders, William B.; Pryor, David B.; Hlatky, Mark A.; Siegler, Ilene C.; and Mark, Daniel B. (1992). Prognostic importance of social and economic resources among medically treated patients with angiographically documented coronary artery disease. *JAMA* 267(4): 520–524.

Wing, Steven; Barnett, Elizabeth; Casper, Michele; and Tyroler, H. A. (1992). Geographic and socioeconomic variation in the onset and decline of coronary heart disease mortality in white women. *American Journal of Public Health* 82(2): 204–209.

CHAPTER SIX

Anda, R. F.; Williamson, D. F.; Escobedo, L. G.; et al. (1992). Self-perceived stress and the risk of peptic ulcer disease. *Archives of Internal Medicine* 152 (April): 829–833.

Bennett, William I.; Goldfinger, Stephen E.; and Johnson, Timothy, eds. (1987). *Your good health: How to stay well, and what to do when you're not*. Cambridge: Harvard University Press.

Browner, Warren S.; Westenhouse, Janice; and Tice, Jeffrey A. (1991). What if Americans ate less fat? A quantitative estimate of the effect on mortality. *JAMA* 265:3285–3291.

Buchholz, William M. (1990). Hope (generic). *JAMA* 263(17): 2357–2358.

Chopra, Deepak (1989). *Quantum healing: Exploring the frontiers of mind/body medicine*. New York: Bantam Books.

Cousins, Norman (1988). Intangibles in medicine: An attempt at a balancing perspective. *JAMA* 260(11): 1610–1612.

Cowen, Emory L. (1991). In pursuit of wellness. *American Psychologist* 46(4): 404–408.

Cummings, Carol A.; and Nutter, June (1991). The relationship of stress management adaptive coping techniques to cardiovascular disease risk. *Wellness Perspectives: Research, Theory and Practice* 7(4): 38–50.

DeAngelis, Tori (1991). When going gets tough, "the hopeful keep going." *APA Monitor*, July 18–19.

Dienstbier, Richard A. (1989). Arousal and physiological toughness: Implications for mental and physical health. *Psychological Review* 96(1): 84–100.

Eisenberg, David M. (1993). Unconventional medicine in the United States: Prevalence, costs, and patterns of use. *New England Journal of Medicine* 328(4): 246–283.

Engel, George L., M.D. (1960). A unified concept of health and disease. *Perspectives in Biology and Medicine* 3:459–485.

Gardner, John W. (1970). *The recovery of confidence.* New York: W. W. Norton.

Harvard Health Letter (1992). The seven best tests. Special supplement, July, 9–12.

Haskell, William L. (1992). Role of water-soluble dietary fiber in the management of elevated plasma cholesterol in healthy subjects. *American Journal of Cardiology* 69:433–439.

Herzlinger, Regina E., and Schwartz, Jeffrey (1985). How companies tackle health care costs: Part 1. *Harvard Business Review,* July-August, 69–81.

———(1985). How companies tackle health care costs: Part 2. *Harvard Business Review,* September-October, 108–120.

Herzlinger, Regina E., and Calkins, David (1985). How companies tackle health care costs: Part 3. *Harvard Business Review,* November-December, 70–80.

Holman, Halsted (1991). Psychosocial support and the management of chronic illness. *Advances* 7(3): 8–9.

Kent, J.; Coates, T. J.; Pelletier, K. R.; and O'Regan, B. (1989). Unexpected recoveries: Spontaneous remission and immune functioning. *Advances: Journal of the Institute for the Advancement of Health* 6(2): 66–73.

Landi, Ann (1989). When having everything isn't enough. *Psychology Today* 23(4): 27–30.

LaRosa, Judith H. (1990). Executive women and health: Perceptions and practices. *American Journal of Public Health* 80(12): 1450–1454.

Locke, S. E., ed. (1986). *Psychological and behavioral treatments for medical disorders.* Vol. 2, *Disorders associated with immune function.* New York: Institute for the Advancement of Health. Includes annotated bibliography.

Murphy, Michael (1992). *The future of the body: Explorations into the further evolution of human nature.* Los Angeles: J. P. Tarcher.

Ornstein, Robert, and Sobel, David (1987). The healing brain. *Psychology Today,* March, 48–52.

Patrick, Cynthia (1992). Thoresen: Getting ahead vs. getting along may hold key to heart disease survival rates. *Campus Report* (Stanford University), Summer, 5.

Pelletier, K. R. (1990). The longevity game. *East West Journal,* January, 52–53.

———(1991). A review and analysis of the health and cost-effective outcome study of comprehensive health promotion and disease prevention programs. *American Journal of Health Promotion* 5(4): 311–315.

Pelletier, K. R.,; Joss, J.; and Locke, S. E. (1992). Personal efficacy: A research database for the clinical application of self-efficacy in mental health. White paper prepared for the Office of Prevention, California Department of Mental Health, Sacramento.

Popkin, B. M., and Patterson, R. E. (1987). Older Americans are uncertain about diet guidelines. *American Journal of Clinical Nutrition.* 55 (April): 823–830.

Quick, J. C.; Barab, J.; Hurrell, J. J.; Ivancevich, J. M.; Mangelsdorff, A. D.; Pelletier, K. R.; Raymond, J.; Smith, D. C.; Vaccaro, V.; and Weiss, S. (1990). Health promotion: Education and treatment. In *Work and well being: An agenda for the 90's.* American Psychological Association and National Institute of Occupational Health and Safety position paper. Washington, D.C.

Rivlin, Richard S., M.D. (1992). Nutrition. *JAMA* 268(3): 382–383.

Rosenblum, Gail (1990). Orient excess. *Longevity,* July, 86.

Rothberg, Joseph M.; Bartone, Paul T.; Holloway, Harry C.; and Marlowe, David H. (1990). Life and death in the US army. *JAMA* 264(17): 2241–2244.

Schafer, Walt, and Gard, Barbara (1988). Stress: How low-stress city managers differ from the rest. *Western City,* August, 15–17.

Thoresen, Carl E., and Low, Kathryn Graff (1991). Psychosocial interventions in females with CVD. Women, Behavior and CVD Conference, September 25–27. Standford University; Meyer Friedman Institute and Bates College.

Ullmann, Daniel; Phillips, Roland L.; Beeson, Lawrence; Dewey, Houston G.; Brin, Burton N.; Kuzma, Jan W.; Chacko, P. Mathews; and Hirst, Albert E. (1991). Cause-specific mortality among physicians with differing life-styles. *JAMA* 265(18): 2352–2357.

Walsh, Diana Chapman (1990). The private side of public health. *Journal of Public Health,* Winter, 405–411.

Wannamethee, G., and Shaper, A. G. (1992). Physical activity and stroke in British middle-aged men. *BMJ* 304 (March 7): 597–601.

Williams, Redford (1989). The trusting heart. *Psychology Today* 23(5): 36–42.

———(1990). The role of the brain in physical disease. *JAMA* 263(14): 1971–1972.

Winkleby, Marilyn A.; Jatulis, Darius E.; Frank, Erica; and Fortmann, Stephen P. (1992). Socioeconomic status and health: How education, income, and occupation contribute to risk factors for cardiovascular disease. *American Journal of Public Health* 82(6): 816–820.

Winslow, Ron (1991). New study shows inpatient treatment may be best course for problem drinkers. *Wall Street Journal,* September 12, B1–2.

CHAPTER SEVEN

Adler, Tina (1991). Optimists' coping skills may help beat illnesses. *APA Monitor,* February, 12–13.

———(1991). In terms of evolution, altruism makes sense. *APA Monitor,* April, 11–12.

Berney, K. (1987). Finding the ethical edge. *Nation's Business* 75 (August): 18–19.

Bishop, Morris (1974). *Saint Francis of Assisi*. Boston: Little, Brown.

Brody, Jane (1988). Those who volunteer to help others can discover a bounty of surprising benefits for themselves. *New York Times,* Deember 1.

Byrne, J. A. (1988). Businesses are signing up for Ethics 101. *Business Week,* February 15, 56–57.

Callahan, D. (1980). Contemporary biomedical ethics. *New England Journal of Medicine* 302:1228–1233.

Campbell, Donald T. (1972). On the genetics of altruism and the counter-hedonic components of human culture. *Journal of Social Issues* 28(3): 21–37.

Chapman, Larry S. (1986). Spiritual health: A component missing from health promotion. *American Journal of Health Promotion,* Summer, 38–42.

Cohen, Ronald (1972). Altruism: Human, cultural, or what? *Journal of Social Issues* 28(3): 39–57.

Colby, Anne, and Damon, William (1991). The uniting of self and mortality in the development of extraordinary moral commitment. Unpublished report.

Collipp, P. J. (1969). The efficacy of prayer: A triple-blind study. *Medical Times* 97:201–204.

Cousins, Norman (1982). *Healing and belief.* Cincinnati: Mosaic Press.

Curle, Adam (1972). *Mystics and militants.* London: Tavistock.

Dominian, J. (1983). Doctor as prophet: Medicine and religion. *British Medical Journal* 287(6409): 1925–1927.

Dossey, Larry (1989). *Recovering the soul: A scientific and spiritual search.* New York: Bantam.

Downing, Frederick L. (1986). *To see the promised land: The faith pilgrimage of Martin Luther King, Jr.* Macon, Ga.: Mercer University Press.

Dubovsky, S. L., and Schrier, R. W. (1983). The mystique of medical training: Is teaching perfection in medical house-staff training a reasonable goal or a precursor of low self-esteem? *JAMA* 250:3057–3058.

Eastwood, B. S. (1982). The place of medicine in a heirarchy of knowledge. *Sudhoffs Archives,* Band 66, Heft 1.

Edwards, K. S. (1981). In search of medicine's morals. *Ohio State Medical Journal,* December, 693–695.

Erikson, Erik H. (1963). *Childhood and society.* New York: Norton.

——(1969). *Gandhi's truth.* New York: Norton.

Fordyce, M. W. (1983). A program to increase happiness: Further studies. *Journal of Counseling Psychology* 130:483–498.

Francis, D. (1987). Morals of the money makers. *Macleans,* May 4, 7.

Freud, Anna (1937). *The ego and the mechanisms of defense.* London: Hogarth.

Fromm, Erich (1947). *Man for himself.* New York: Reinhart.

Galton, F. (1972). Statistical inquiries into the efficacy of prayer. *Fortnightly*

Review 12:125–135.

Gartner, Dave Larson, and George Allen (1991). *Journal of Psychology and Theology* 19:6–25.

Gilligan, Carol (1982). *In a different voice: Psychological theory and women's development*. Cambridge: Harvard University Press.

Glaser, Barney G., and Strauss, Anselm L. (1967). *The discovery of grounded theory: Strategies for qualitative research*. Chicago: Aldine.

Goldberg, A. D. (1986). The sabbath as dialectic: Implications for mental health. *Journal of Religion and Health* 25(3): 237–244.

Goleman, Daniel (1991). Therapists see religion as aid, not illusion. *New York Times,* September 10, 140.

Gordon, E. (1980). *Me, myself, and who? Humanism: Society's false premise*. Plainfield, N.J.: Logos International.

Gratzer, W. B. (1983). Science has lost its virtue, not its value. *Science,* January-February, 17.

Greer, K. (1988). Are American families finding new strength in spirituality? *Better Homes and Gardens* 66:15–16.

Guy, J. R. (1982). The episcopal licensing of physicians, surgeons and midwives. *Bulletin of History of Medicine* 56:528–542.

Halberstam, David (1992). *The best and the brightest*. New York: Random House.

Hall, C. M. (1986). Crisis as opportunity for spiritual growth. *Journal of Religion and Health* 25(1): 8–17.

Harsham, P. (1982). Physicians treat, God heals. *Medical Economics,* May 24, 2.

Hettler, G. (1983). High levels wellness: A quality of life. *Health Values* (11–12): 31–35.

Hoffman, Martin L. (1975). Developmental synthesis of affect and cognition and its implications for altruistic motivation. *Developmental Psychology* 11:607–622.

Idler, Ellen L., and Kasl, Stanislav V. (1992). Religion, disability, depression, and the timing of death. *American Journal of Sociology* 97(4): 1052–1079.

James, William (1958). *The varieties of religious experience*. Reprint, New York: New American Library.

Joyce, C. R. B., and Welldon, R. M. C. (1965). The objective efficacy of prayer: A double-blind clinical trial. *Journal of Chronic Disease* 18:367–377.

Klein, M. (1970). On observing the behavior of infants: On the theory of anxiety and guilt. In *Developments in psychoanalysis,* edited by J. Riviere. London: Hogarth.

Knaster, Mirka (1991). The good that comes from doing good. *East West Journal,* November/December, 65–70.

Kohlberg, Lawrence (1973). Continuities in childhood and adult moral development revisited. In *Lifespan developmental psychology: Personali-*

ty and socialization, edited by P. Baltes and W. Shaie. New York: Academic Press.

Kohn, Alfie (1988). Beyond selfishness. *Psychology Today,* January, 34–38.

Kuhn, Clifford C., M.D. (1988). A spiritual inventory of the medically ill patient. *Psychiatric Medicine* 6(2): 87–100.

Lacocque, P.E. (1986). An existential interpretation of success neurosis. *Journal of Religion and Health* 25(2): 96–106.

Lang, Sarah (1989). Extend your hand, extend your life. *Longevity,* October, 18–19.

Lowenthal, Marjorie Fiske, Thurner, M.; Chiriboga, D.; and associates (1975). *Four stages of life.* San Francisco: Jossey-Bass.

Maeir, D. M. (1983). The physician as a man . . . the man as a physician. *New York State Journal of Medicine* 133(813): 124–125.

Magnet, M. (1986). The decline and fall of business ethics. *Fortune,* December 8, 65–66.

Maslow, Abraham H. (1951). *Motivation and personality.* New York: Harper and Row.

Meyers, David (1993). *The pursuit of happiness: Who is happy and why.* New York: Morrow.

Muck, T. (1987). The Boesky couch. *Christ Today,* March 6, 14–15.

Noah, T. (1987). The business ethics debate. *Newsweek,* May 25, 36.

Novak, P. (1986). The Buddha and the computer: Meditation in an age of information. *Journal of Religion and Health* 25(3): 188–192.

———(1992). *Religion and altruism.* Research Report Series ASP-1. Sausalito, Calif: Institute of Noetic Sciences.

Osmond, H. (1982). God and the doctor. *New England Journal of Medicine* 302:555–558.

Ouellette Kobasa, S.; Maddi, S.; Puccetti, M.; and Zola, M. (1985). Effectiveness of hardiness: Exercise and social support as resources against illness. *Journal of Psychosomatic Research* 29:252–253.

Papper, S. (1983). *Doing right: Everyday medical ethics.* Boston: Little, Brown.

Pelletier, K. R. (1985). *Toward a science of consciousness.* New York: Delacorte and Delta/Seymour Lawrence, 1978. Revised ed. Celestial Arts: Berkeley, Calif.

———(1992). Mind-body health: Research, clinical, and policy applications. *American Journal of Health Promotion* 6(5): 345–357.

———(1993). Between mind and body: Stress, emotions, and health. In *Mind/body medicine.* New York: Consumer's Union Press.

Pelletier, K. R., and Garfield, C. (1976). *Consciousness: East and west.* New York: Harper and Row.

Pfeiffer, C. C., and Braverman, E. R. (1982). Zinc, the brain and behavior. *Biological Psychiatry* 17:513–532.

Pietroni, Patrick C. (1986). "Spiritual" interventions in a general practice setting. *Holistic Medicine* 1:253–262.

Pressman, Peter; Lyons, John S.; Larson, David B.; and Strain, James J. (1990). Religious belief, depression, and ambulation status in elderly women with broken hips. *American Journal of Psychiatry* 147(6): 758–760.

Preuss, J. (1978). *Biblical and talmudic medicine.* Translated by F. Rosner. New York: Hebrew Publishing Co.

Remen, Rachel Naomi (1988). Spirit: Resource for healing. *Noetic Science Review,* Autumn, 5–9.

Rockefeller, David (1988). *Remarks by David Rockefeller on the health benefits of altruism.* New York, N.Y.: Institute for the Advancement of Health.

Rohrlick, J. (1980). *Work and love.* New York: Summit.

Roof, Wade Clark (1993). *A generation of seekers.* San Francisco: Harper-Collins.

Rosenhan, David (1972). Learning theory and prosocial behavior. *Journal of Social Issues* 23(3): 151–163.

Rosner, F. (1984). *Medicine in the Mishnah Torah of Maimonides.* New York: KTAV.

Schachter, Z. and Hoffman, E. (1983). *Sparks of light: Counseling in the hasidic tradition.* Boulder, Colo.: Shambhala.

Seaward, Brian Luke; Meholick, Betsy; and Campanelli, Linda (1992). A spiritual well-being program at the United States postal service headquarters. *Wellness Perspectives: Research, Theory and Practice* 8(4): 16–30.

Sharabany, Ruth, and Bar-Tal, Daniel (1982). Theories of the development of altruism: Review, comparison, and integration. *International Journal of Behavioral Development* 5:49–80.

Sinetar, M. (1987). *Do what you love, the money will follow: Discovering your right livelihood.* Mahwah, N.J.: Paulist.

Steiner, C. (1975). *Scripts people live.* New York: Random House.

Stewart, J.; Harrison, W.; Quitkin, F.; and Baker, H. (1984). Low B-6 levels in depressed outpatients. *Biological Psychiatry* 19:613–630.

Zahn, Waxler, C.; Cummings, E. M.; and Iannotti, R. (1986). *Altruism and aggression: Biological and social origins.* Cambridge: Cambridge University Press.

Zautra, A., and Hempel, A. (1984). Subjective well-being and physical health: A narrative literature review with suggestions for future research. *International Journal of Aging and Human Development* 19:95–110.

Zborowski, Mark, and Herzog, Elizabeth (1962). *Life is with people.* New York: International Universities Press.

CHAPTER EIGHT

Abramson, Leonard (1990). Better quality through accountability. *Business and Health,* November, 64.

Aggressive treatment cuts heart risks. (1991). *Stanford University Campus Report,* November, 13, 9–10.

Becker, Edmund R.; Dunn, Daniel; Braun, Peter; and Hsiao, William C. (1990). Refinement and expansion of the Harvard resource-based relative value scale: The second phase. *AJPH* 80(7): 799–803.

Blair, Steven N.; Kohl, Harold W., III; Paffenbarger, Ralph S.; Clark, Debra G.; Cooper, Kenneth H.; and Gibbons, Larry W. (1989). Physical fitness and all-cause mortality. *JAMA* 262(17): 2395–2401.

Bodenheimer, Thomas (1992). Underinsurance in America. *New England Journal of Medicine,* July 23, 274–278.

Braveman, Paula A.; Egerter, Susan; Bennett, Trude; and Showstack, Jonathan (1991). Differences in hospital resource allocation among sick newborns according to insurance coverage. *JAMA* 266(23): 3300–3308.

Brennan, Troyen A.; Leape, Lucian L.; Laird, Nan M.; Liesi, Herbert; Localio, A. Russell; Lawthers, Ann G.; Newhouse, Joseph P.; Weiler, Paul C.; and Hiatt, Howard H. (1991). Incidence of adverse events and negligence in hospitalized patients. *New England Journal of Medicine,* February 7, 370–384.

Breo, Dennis L. (1992). Uwe Reinhardt, PhD—The economist as health evangelist. *JAMA* 268(10): 1332–1336.

Brody, Sam (1992). We have lost our humanity. *Newsweek,* September 7, 8.

Catalano, Ralph (1991). The health effects of economic insecurity. *AJPH* 81(9): 1148–1152.

Cella, D. F., et al. (1991). Socioeconomic status and cancer survival. *Journal of Clin. Oncol.* 9:1500–1509.

Consumer Reports (1992). Pushing drugs to doctors. February, 87–94.

Crichton, Michael (1990). Greater expectations. *Newsweek,* September 24, 58.

Egolf, Brenda; Lasker, Judith; Wolf, Stewart; and Potvin, Louise (1992). The Roseto effect: A 50-year comparison of mortality rates. *American Journal of Public Health* 82(8): 1089–1094.

Farquhar, John W.; Fortmann, Stephen P.; Flora, June A.; Taylor, Barr; Haskell, William L.; Williams, Paul T.; Maccoby, Nathan; and Wood, Peter D. (1990). Effects of communitywide education on cardiovascular disease risk factors. *JAMA* 264(3): 359–365.

Fielding, Jonathan (1989). Corporate health cost management. *Occupational Medicine* 4(1): 121–144.

Foege, William H. (1990). The growing brown plague. *JAMA* 264(12): 1580.

Goetzel, R. Z.; Thorpe, K. E.; Fielding, J. E.; and Pelletier, K. R. (1992). Behind the scenes of a POS program. *Journal of Health Care Benefits,* March/April, 33–37.

Goldman, L., et al (1992). Cost and health implications of cholesterol lowering. *Circulation* 85 (May): 1960–1968.

Hadley, Jack; Steinberg, Earl P.; and Feder, Judith (1991). Comparison of uninsured and privately insured hospital patients. *JAMA* 265(3): 374–380.

Hahn, Robert A.; Teutsch, Steven M.; Rothenberg, Richard B.; and Marks, James S. (1990). Excess deaths from nine chronic diseases in the United States, 1986. *JAMA* 264(20): 2654–2659.

Harkin, Tom (1991). Another pound of cure. *JAMA* 266(12): 1692–1693.

Herzlinger, Regina E. (1991). Healthy competition. *Atlantic Monthly,* August, 69–81.

Iglehart, John K. (1992). The American health care system. *New England Journal of Medicine,* September 3, 742–747.

Krause, Richard M. (1992). The origin of plagues: Old and new. *Science* 257:1073–1078.

Leaf, Alexander (1989). Potential health effects of global climatic and environmental changes. *New England Journal of Medicine* 321(23): 1577–1583.

Leaf, Alexander, and Ryan, Thomas J. (1990). Prevention of coronary artery disease. *New England Journal of Medicine,* November 15, 1416–1419.

Locke, Steven E.; Kowaloff, Hollis B.; Hoff, Robert G.; Safran, Charles; Popovsky, Mark A.; Cotton, Deborah J.; Finkelstein, Dianne M.; Page, Peter L.; and Slack, Warner V. (1992). Computer-based interview for screening blood donors for risk of HIV transmission. *JAMA* 268(10): 1301–1305.

Lundberg, George D. (1992). National health care reform. *JAMA* 267(18): 2521–2524.

Manson, JoAnn E.; Tosteson, Heather; Ridker, Paul M.; Satterfield, Suzanne; Hebert, Patricia; O'Connor, Gerald T.; Buring, Julie E.; and Hennekens, Charles H. (1992). The primary prevention of myocardial infarction. *New England Journal of Medicine,* May 21, 1406–1416.

Marshall, Eliot (1990). OTA peers into cancer therapy fog. *Science* 249(4975): 1369.

——(1991). Breast cancer: Stalemate in the war on cancer. *Science,* December 20, 1719–1720.

McBride, P. E., and Davis, J. E. (1992). Cholesterol and cost-effectiveness: Implications for practice, policy, and research. *Circulation* 85 (May): 1939–1941.

Moore, Thomas J. (1989). *Heart failure: A critical inquiry into american medicine and the revolution in heart care.* New York: Random House.

Morell, Virginia (1992). Oregon becomes a test case for health care reform. *Science* 257:1202–1203.

National Leadership Commission of Health Care (1989). *For the health of a nation: A shared responsibility.* Ann Arbor: Health Administration Press Perspectives.

Neu, Harold C. (1992). The crisis in antibiotic resistance. *Science* 257:1064–1072.

Palca, Joseph (1992). NIH unveils plan for women's health project. *Science* 254:792.

Paradis, Norman (1992). Making a living off the dying. *New York Times,*

April 25, 23.

Payer, Lynn (1988). *Medicine and culture: Varieties of treatment in the United States, England, West Germany and France.* Los Angeles: Henry Holt.

Pelletier, K. R.; Coates, T. J.; Fisher, E.; and Heins, J. M. (1993). Healthy people—Healthy business: Disease prevention and health promotion programs in business and industry. In *Introduction to occupational health and safety.* Chicago: National Safety Council.

Relman, Arnold S. (1992). The trouble with rationing. *New England Journal of Medicine* 323(13): 911–913.

Schroeder, Steven A. (1992). On squeezing balloons. *New England Journal of Medicine* 325(15): 1099–1100.

Specter, Michael (1990). Health care woes apparent; cure isn't. *Washington Post,* June 15, 2.

Sullivan, Louis W. (1991). Partners in prevention: A mobilization plan for implementing Healthy People 2000. *American Journal of Health Promotion* 5(4): 291–297.

Sultz, Harry (1991). Health policy: If you don't know where you're going, any road will take you. *American Journal of Public Health* 81(4): 418–420.

Sutherland, Ralph W., and Fulton, M. Jane (1988). *Health care in Canada: A description and analysis of Canadian health services.* Ottawa: The Health Group.

U.S. Senate Democratic Policy Committee (1992). How many is 37 million? *Business and Health,* January, 15.

Wasson, John; Gaudette, Catherine; Whaley, Fredrick; Savigne, Arthur; Baribeu, Priscilla; and Welch, H. Gilbert (1992). Telephone care as a substitute for routine clinic follow-up. *JAMA* 267(13): 1788–1793.

Weidner, Gerdi; Connor, Sonja L.; Hollis, Jack F.; and Connor, William E. (1992). Improvements in hostility and depression in relation to dietary changes and cholesterol lowering: The family heart study. *Annals of Internal Medicine* 117(10): 820–823.

Wenneker, Mark B.; Weissman, Joel S.; and Epstein, Arnold M. (1990). The association of payer with utilization of cardiac procedures in Massachusetts. *JAMA* 264(10): 1255–1260.

INDEX

Dr. Kenneth R. Pelletier is a clinical associate professor of medicine, Department of Medicine and the Stanford Center for Research in Disease Prevention, Stanford University School of Medicine, and is a vice president with Healthtrac Incorporated. At Stanford, Dr. Pelletier is director of the Stanford Corporate Health Program, a collaborative effort between the school and twenty major corporations including American Airlines, Aetna, AT&T, ARCO, Chevron, Bank of America, IBM, Kaiser Permanente, Lockheed, Levi-Strauss, Syntex, and Xerox.

Dr. Pelletier has served as president of the American Health Association since 1980, and in 1992 was appointed a founding board member of the California Wellness Foundation and served as Chairman of the Board. He is the author of more than 225 professional journal articles and seven books which have been translated into fifteen languages, including the classic bestseller *Mind as Healer, Mind as Slayer,* first published in 1977 and revised in an updated edition in 1992. At sea, Dr. Pelletier is an avid open ocean sailor; on land, he is an equestrian and lives on a farm in Danville, California, with his wife, Elizabeth, and their thoroughbred horses, Shaughnessy and Sullivan.